Research Recipes for Midwives

Research Recipes
for Midwives

FIRST
EDITION

Caroline J. Hollins Martin

Edinburgh Napier University

Edinburgh

UK

WILEY Blackwell

This edition first published 2024

Registered Offices
John Wiley & Sons, Inc., 111 River Street, Hoboken, NJ 07030, USA
John Wiley & Sons Ltd, The Atrium, Southern Gate, Chichester, West Sussex, PO19 8SQ, UK

For details of our global editorial offices, customer services, and more information about Wiley products visit us at www.wiley.com.

Wiley also publishes its books in a variety of electronic formats and by print-on-demand. Some content that appears in standard print versions of this book may not be available in other formats.

Library of Congress Cataloging-in-Publication Data applied for
[Paperback ISBN: 9781394180080]

Cover Design: Wiley
Cover Images: © FatCamera/Getty Images; MartinPrescott/E+/Getty Images; mith_67/E+/Getty Images; svetikd/E+/Getty Images

Set in 9.5/12pt STIXTwoText by Straive, Pondicherry, India
Printed and bound by CPI Group (UK) Ltd, Croydon, CR0 4YY

C9781394180080_090124

With great pride, I would like to dedicate this book to my niece Anna Hollins, who is studying at Robert Gordon University in Scotland (UK) to become a midwife. Anna and her cohort of peers at all universities worldwide are the future of midwifery clinical practice. Welcome aboard.

Contents

6   Accessing Populations of Participants and Sampling Them   122

7   Data Collection Methods   135

8 Analyzing Qualitative Data   152

10 The Role and Procedures Involved in Gaining Ethical Approval 191

11 An Empty Template for Designing a 16-STEP Research Proposal 207

About the Author

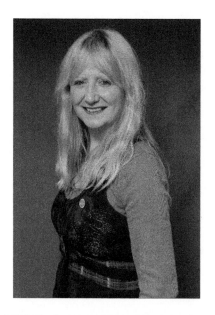

Prof Caroline J. Hollins Martin PhD MPhil BSc RM RGN MBPsS Senior Fellow HEA is a Professor in Midwifery within the School of Health and Social Care (SHSC) at Edinburgh Napier University (ENU) in Scotland (UK). Caroline's professional experience covers a career in women's reproductive health that spans 38 years. The first 11 years were spent as a clinical midwife working in Ayrshire (Scotland), and the remaining 27 have been spent teaching and researching women's reproductive health in a variety of settings. Caroline is a Nursing and Midwifery Council (NMC) registered midwife and lecturer/practice educator. She is also a graduate and postgraduate in psychology and a Member of the British Psychological Society (MBPsS). Caroline's research interests principally lie in psychology that speaks to childbearing women's reproductive health, with her earlier work relating to midwives' autonomy, evidence-based practice, and providing choice and control to women over the childbirth continuum. Of late, her interests have transferred to research that produces functional tools for midwives to use in clinical practice. For instance, the *Birth Satisfaction Scale-Revised* (*BSS-R©*), which measures women's experiences of labour and childbirth (https://www.bss-r.co.uk/). More current research interests lie in the midwife's role in providing perinatal bereavement care to women, partners, and families. To date, Caroline has published 135 papers and has a lot of experience of writing research proposals.

Prof Caroline J. Hollins Martin PhD MPhil BSc RM RGN MBPsS Senior Fellow HEA
Professor in Midwifery, School of Health and Social Care, Edinburgh Napier University
Worktribe: https://www.napier.ac.uk/people/caroline-hollinsmartin
Research Gate: https://www.researchgate.net/profile/Caroline_Hollins_Martin
Scopus Author ID: 8665735000
Orcid ID: https://orcid.org/0000-0002-3185-8611/print

Foreword

Nothing has such power to broaden the mind as the ability to investigate systematically and truly all that comes under thy observation of life (Marcus Aurelius, 120–180 AD).

Professor Hollins Martin had a wealth of clinical midwifery experience before moving into the field of teaching and research. To many midwives (and many others), research can seem a taunting task, with a confusing method and an uncertain end. Caroline's book shows a clear path to help that uneasy traveler along the research process road. It is important for those involved in clinical practice to understand that the collection of data is vital towards providing the best and safest of care.

It is a capital mistake to theorise before one has data (Arthur Conan Doyle).

T.V. Nivison Russell (FRCOG)
Ayrshire, Scotland (UK) (2023)

A Memorandum from the Author

The information provided in this book is designed to guide the reader gently through the processes involved in writing a research proposal. As such, the 16-step model will equip the student midwife with sufficient knowledge to prepare each section of a 'research proposal', and once complete, they will have a recipe to answer their pre-decided research question. As part of the modern midwifery curriculum in the West, student midwives are required to complete a research methods module as a component of their degree program. Two main objectives of undertaking a research methods module are to first teach the student midwife how to read published papers from which they can evidence-base their clinical practice, and second, how to write a research proposal. To direct this endeavour, a 16-step model has been developed, which is in essence a written recipe that the student can follow while designing their study. Examples of where a completed 'research proposal' will be required includes:

- As modular assessment at the end of a research methods module.

- As part of, or whole of, a dissertation.

- To outline a proposed doctorate study (e.g. PhD, Prof Doc, Doc Ed, etc.).

- To apply for a research grant.

- To design an audit or evaluation of maternity care.

Writing of a research proposal is entirely achievable but requires input of time, effort, practice, and patience. Anticipating this commitment, I am certain that any engaged student midwife can write a research proposal. Nonetheless, during its writing, they are likely to find the steps involved both challenging and rewarding. To meet the challenges, this book will gently guide the student midwife through the 16-step model to produce a written research proposal. To view a summary of the 16 steps involved (see Table 1) and a blank template (see Table 2).

Table 1   The 16 steps involved in writing a research proposal.

STEP (1):	Give the research proposal a title.
STEP (2):	Provide relevant personal and professional details.
STEP (3):	Provide a short abstract or summary of around 300 words.
STEP (4):	Supply six keywords to describe the research proposal.
STEP (5):	Construct an introduction that contains a relevant literature review and rationale.
STEP (6):	State the objectives, aim(s), research question(s), sub-question(s), hypotheses & null hypotheses, of the proposed research study.
STEP (7):	Outline the research method.
STEP (8):	Select setting, participants, sampling method, inclusion & exclusion criteria and method of recruitment.
STEP (9):	Describe data collection instruments.
STEP (10):	Detail intended data processing and analysis.
STEP (11):	Declare any ethical considerations and outline data protection procedures.
STEP (12):	Produce a timetable and consider potential problems that may occur.
STEP (13):	Estimate resources that may be required.
STEP (14):	Detail a public engagement plan.
STEP (15):	Append a reference list.
STEP (16):	Appendix relevant additional material.

Table 2   BLANK TEMPLATE: The 16 steps involved in writing a research proposal.

STEP (1): Give the research proposal a title.

STEP (2): Provide relevant personal and professional details.

Name & title of Principle Investigator (PI):

Professional qualifications:

Telephone number:

Email number:

Role(s) in study:

(CV Appendix 1)

Name of Co-applicant (C1):

Professional qualifications:

Telephone number:

Email number:

Role(s) in study:

(CV Appendix 2)

Table 2   (Continued)

Name of Co-applicant (C2):

Professional qualifications:

Telephone number:

Email number:

Role(s) in study:

(CV Appendix 3)

STEP (3): Provide a short abstract or summary of around 300 words.

Background:

Aim:

Method:

Participants:

Setting:

Proposed data collection:

Proposed data analysis:

Proposed reporting of results:

Potential relevance of conclusions:

Potential recommendations for practice:

STEP (4): Supply six keywords to describe the research proposal.

1

2

3

4

5

6

STEP (5): Construct an introduction that contains a relevant literature review and rationale.

Introduction:

Literature review:

Rationale:

STEP (6): State the objectives, aim(s), research question(s), sub-question(s), hypotheses & null hypotheses, of the proposed research study.

Objectives:

Aim(s):

Research question(s):

Sub-question(s):

Hypotheses:

Null hypotheses:

(Continued)

Table 2   (Continued)

Step (7): Outline the research method.

Method:

Rationale for choice of method:

STEP (8): Select setting, participants, sampling method, inclusion & exclusioncriteria and method of recruitment.

Setting:

Participants:

Sampling method:

Inclusion criteria:

Exclusion criteria:

Method of recruitment:

STEP (9): Describe data collection instruments.

STEP (10): Detail intended data processing and analysis.

STEP (11): Declare any ethical considerations and outline data protection procedures.

Ethics committee(s):

Ethical considerations:

Informed consent:

Confidentiality:

Data protection:

Conflicts of interest:

Proposed publications:

STEP (12): Produce a timetable and consider potential problems that may occur.

The duration of the proposed project will be (e.g. 36 months) and in accordance with the following timetable. Tweak this timetable to match your own research proposal, and place X's in the boxes for the months each activity will take place in (see Step 12, *Chapter 1*).

Table 2   (Continued)

*Q = quarter of a year (3-month period) Place the marker at the time point of expected delivery, e.g. ☐

Gantt Chart Project PAL	Project Year 1 1/1/24–31/12/25 1–12 months				Project Year 2 1/1/25–31/12/26 13–24 months				Project Year 3 1/1/26–33/12/27 25–36 months			
Preparation (P) for Named Project	Q1	Q2	Q3	Q4	Q5	Q6	Q7	Q8	Q9	Q10	Q11	Q12
P.1: Research fellow – advertising & recruitment												
P2: Ethics submission/approval												
P3: Meet with partner institutions												
P4: Set up Steering Group (SG)												
P6: Develop optimal recruitment strategy												
Study (S) process	Q1	Q2	Q3	Q4	Q5	Q6	Q7	Q8	Q9	Q10	Q11	Q12
S.1: Full research team meeting (incl co-applicants, collaborators, & research fellow)												
S.2: Steering Group (SG) meetings												
S.3: Literature review-update												
S.4: Develop study protocol												
S.5: Data collection – qualitative												
S.6: Data entry and transcription												
S.7: Data analyses												
S.8: Write up report/paper(s)												
S.9: Annual report to funder												
Final acts	Q1	Q2	Q3	Q4	Q5	Q6	Q7	Q8	Q9	Q10	Q11	Q12
F.1: Dissemination to stakeholders – Conferences												
F.2: Finished report to funders												

STEP (13): Estimate resources that may be required.

	Year 1	Year 2	Year 3	*TOTAL*
Personal Support of Applicants Named person (e.g. 1 day a week)	State amount (330 hours)	State amount (330 hours)	State amount (330hours)	State amount (990 hours)
Named person (e.g. 1 hour a week)	State amount (52 hours)	State amount (52 hours)	State amount (52 hours)	State amount (156 hours)
Named person (e.g. 1 hour a week)	State amount (52 hours)	State amount (52 hours)	State amount (52 hours)	State amount (52 hours)
NB: Add increments on salaries per year				
Research Assistance Grade: 7 (e.g. Full Time (FT)	State amount (FT)	State amount (FT)	State amount (FT)	State amount (FT)
NB: add increments on salaries per year				

(Continued)

Table 2 (Continued)

Consumables				
• Print costs x e.g. 800 etc.	State amount	0	0	Stated amount
Patient Public Involvement (PPI)				
e.g. (n=?) service users	State amount(s)	State amount(s)	State amount(s)	State amount(s)
e.g. 2 steering groups a year				
• Venue				
• Refreshments & lunch				
• Thank you voucher.				
• Travel costs				
• Stationary				
Travel and subsistence home				
University–maternity unit–participants home	State amount	State amount	State amount	State amount
Travel and subsistence				
To international conferences			State amount	State amount
Payment to partner university				
e.g. named statistician	State amount	State amount	State amount	State amount
Contribution to Maternity Unit				
• Lighting	State amount(s)	State amount(s)	State amount(s)	State amount(s)
• Toilets				
• Water				
• Heat				
Equipment				
e.g. Monitors X 6	State amount	0	0	State amount
Estates charge	State amount	State amount	State amount	State amount
Indirect costs	State amount	State amount	State amount	State amount
TOTAL COSTS				State amount
ESIMATED RECOVERY (80%)				State amount

STEP (14): Detail a public engagement plan.

(1) Public perceptions of the importance of the proposed study:

(2) Public acceptance of activities involved in taking part in the study:

(3) Personal motivation to participate in study and what would prevent interest:

Table 2   (Continued)

(4) Members of the public will be involved in:

  • Design of the study.   YES/NO

  • Management of the research (e.g. Steering Group (SG).   YES/NO

  • Developing Participant Information Sheets (PIS).   YES/NO

  • Undertaking the project and/or analysing the data.   YES/NO

  • Contributing to reporting or writing of the study report.   YES/NO

  • Dissemination of research findings.   YES/NO

(5) Details of user group(s):

  (Group 1) User group (e.g. will consist of 3 women from. . .. . .etc.):

  (1) Name, place of work, & email

  (2) Name, place of work, & email

  (3) Name, place of work, & email

  (Group 2) Expert group (e.g. will *consist* of 2 midwives, 1 physiotherapist from. . ..etc.):

  (1) Name, place of work, & email

  (2) Name, place of work, & email

  (3) Name, place of work, & email

  The above, e.g. 6 people have agreed to be part of the *Steering Group* (SG).

STEP (15): Append a reference list.

References:

Author(s) Surname, Initials. (Publication Year). Article title, Journal name. Volume (issue), Pages. Doi or Available at and date accessed.

STEP (16): Appendix relevant additional material.

Appendix 1:

Appendix 2:

Appendix 3:

Appendix 4:

Appendix 5:

Appendix 6:

Appendix 7:

Appendix 8:

Signature ....

Name ....

Date ....

Acknowledgements

I dedicate this book to all the student midwives I have taught over the years, along with colleagues past and present who have worked with me on research projects that have delivered papers to evidence-base midwifery practice. I also dedicate this manuscript to all the booklovers I have known, which includes my father, mother, teachers, and university lecturers, who, akin to me, love the smell of a freshly published book. I blame you all for injecting me with an addiction to writing, acknowledging that without your input, my path as a researcher, educator, and writer would not have been possible. I would also like to thank my beloved companion, Arnie Burgoyne, who has always kept the kettle on and looked up at the stars with me. I would like to thank you Arnie for all the coffee, coffee, coffee, prosecco, and more coffee. Furthermore, I dedicate this book to those also awed by the incredible voyage of the research process, which includes my lifelong research mentor Prof. Colin Martin and the many great research students, doctors, and professors I have worked with and published with across my lifetime. Thank you all for your company, humour, teaching, patience, support, and nurturing.

Introduction to Research Methods

1.1 WHAT IS RESEARCH?

The word *research* is used in everyday speech to cover a broad spectrum of meaning. This makes it a confusing term for learners. Much of what student midwives are taught, they may sometime later down the line be told to unlearn. Merchandisers use the word research to suggest the discovery of a revolutionary product, with the term used as an attention-grabbing sales pitch. When in truth, there may be only a minor alteration to the existing product. Other activities have been called research, but more appropriately should be called information gathering, library skills, documentation, or self-enlightenment. Real research follows a systematic set of steps, which are prescribed like a recipe. The process involves a systematic way of collecting and analyzing information (data), for the purpose of increasing understanding of a particular phenomenon.

The word research has a certain amount of mystique about it. Researchers may be considered to be mystical people who hide in laboratories, in scholarly libraries, or within the academic institutions. Generally, the public is unaware of what activities are undertaken by a researcher or of the important contributions their work may make to people's comfort or general welfare. The intention of this book is to dispel any misconceptions the student midwife may have about research and present an accurate outline of its function and purpose. The first concept to grasp is that research is not:

1. Simply information gathering.

2. Mere transportation of facts from one place to another.

3. Purely delving for information.

4. A slogan to simply sell a product.

Instead, research is a formal process which follows a set of concrete repeatable steps. To define the term research:

1.1.1 DEFINITION

Research is a systematic process which produces data to answer a specific question. Several processes (recipes) may be followed, each of which has distinct characteristics. The generic term given to each possible recipe that could be used is *research methods*. As such, the variety of _research methods_ that a researcher chose from have distinct and shared characteristics. That is, every *research method* (recipe):

Research Recipes for Midwives, First Edition. Caroline J. Hollins Martin.
© 2024 John Wiley & Sons Ltd. Published 2024 by John Wiley & Sons Ltd.

1. Originates from an identified problem.

2. Is guided by a research question, and if quantitative in approach a hypothesis.

3. Follows a specific set of systemic steps and procedures.

4. Requires data to be collected and interpreted in attempts to resolve the problem that initiated commencement of the study.

A large amount of knowledge about certain subjects is incomplete, along with many unsolved problems. Hence, to address a recognized void in knowledge, researchers ask questions and formulate plans to answer them. There are many ways to answer a research question, with the choice made dependent upon the specifics of the question asked. In other words, the suitable 'research method' or recipe selected, involves a prescribed sequence of steps specific for the situation. At present, you may not understand what each of the different 'research methods' are, e.g. grounded theory (Birks and Mills, 2023), ethnography (O'Reilly, 2012), phenomenology (Smith et al. 2009), discourse analysis (Paltridge, 2021), randomized controlled trial (RCT) (Shih and Aisner, 2021), or survey (Groves et al. 2009), with the specifics of each different 'research method' (recipe) explained further on. In essence, 'research methods' involves a whole new glossary of terms, which the student midwife requires to learn for the purpose of passing a university research module, to evidence-based clinical midwifery practice, and take part in recruitment and data collection for the organization they work for.

1.2 GLOSSARY OF RESEARCH TERMS

A dictionary of research terms is helpful towards educating student midwives to understand the meaning of words used in 'research methods'. It is impossible to cover all research terms used; however, a few have been selected to help you get on your feet (see Activity 1.1). Outside of the selected list, it could be useful to purchase a dictionary of terms used in research methodology (Sharmer and Navar, 2020).

Activity 1.1

Look up the internet and write down definitions of the following terms.

Control _____

Control group _____

Correlational studies _____

Deduction _____

Epidemiology _____

Ethics _____

Experiment _____

Hypothesis _____

Induction _____

Informed consent _____

Likert scale _____

Literature review _____

Null hypothesis _____

Objective measures _____

Qualitative methods _____

Quantitative methods _____

Quasi-experimental designs _____

Questionnaire _____

Range _____
Relationships _____
Repeated measures _____
Phenomenology _____
Sample _____
Sampling error _____
Sampling method _____
Subjective measures _____
Validity _____
Variable _____

1.3 ONTOLOGY

Ontology is the study of the nature of reality. Traditionally listed as part of philosophy, ontology deals with questions concerning what entities exist or can be said to exist and how they can be grouped within a hierarchy and subdivided according to similarities and differences. One common approach is to divide the existent entities into groups called categories. Such lists of categories differ widely from one another, and it is through the co-ordination of different categorical schemes that ontology relates to fields of information. For example:

1.3.1 SUBJECTIVISM

Subjectivity holds that the nature and existence of everything depend solely on a person's individual personal awareness of it. For example, one person may perceive that cricket is exciting, whilst another finds it boring. The tenet of qualitative research is to study individuality, which involves the assumption that all is not the same. In other words, the way each person views the world is different, with each of us having (like glasses) different prescriptions.

1.3.2 RELATIVISM

Relativism is the idea that aspects of experience are dependent upon incidents that we encounter. For example, what is true to one person may differ from another. That is, in relation to internal forces, such as religious beliefs, people hold different ideas about what does and does not matter.

1.3.3 OBJECTIVISM

Objectivism is the belief that reality is independent of thinking. An objective account is one that captures the nature of an object, which is studied in a way that it is not influenced by features of the person who studies it. In other words, it stands outside individuality (subjectivism). An objective account is an impartial interpretation, which is not influenced by a person's perceptions of the object under discussion. Objectivism does not draw on assumptions, prejudices, beliefs, or values of the participant. Objectivism is the tenet of quantitative research and deals in numbers from which a conclusion is derived.

Scientific research (objectivism) involves clearly defined actions, which are carried out in a laboratory or distinctly defined environment. Objectivism is the general approach taken by the theoretical sciences, e.g. ecology, chemistry, biology, and psychology. Objectivism is deductive in nature and is called the quantitative approach. Deductive means that the answers are reduced to one single outcome.

In contrast, social researchers find the objective approach concerning, since the idea of individuality is impossible to define as one thing. What people mean in each situation is influenced by their beliefs, e.g. religious convictions (see Figure 1.1).

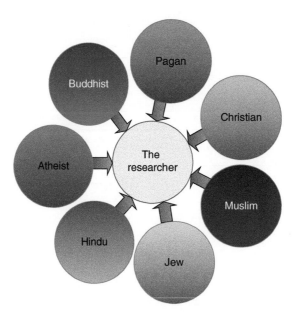

FIGURE 1.1   A model of religious value systems that persuade an individual's perceptions.

Heidegger suggests that our way of being human and the way the world is perceived by us is underpinned by ontological assumptions that are part of our language (Heidegger, 2010). This assumption provides the context for communication, which is influenced by a horizon of unspoken background of meaning. Each person's individual assumptions are embedded and recycled within everyday interactions, with the locus of being rooted in the language used to communicate events. This appreciation is the premise of the qualitative (inductive) research approach, which includes many points of view.

1.4 EPISTEMOLOGY

Epistemology is a branch of philosophy that addresses philosophical problems surrounding the theory of knowledge. What is knowledge? How is knowledge obtained? What makes knowledge fact? Rene Descartes provided strong evidence against empiricism, scientific objectivism, or the quantitative approach (Descartes and Moriarty, 2008).

1.4.1 THE THEORY OF KNOWLEDGE

The theory of knowledge is tied up with the history of its evolution, with new ideas developed on top of foundations created by earlier philosophers (Nagael, 2014). For example, Socrates (Ahbel-Rappe, 2011) and Plato (Allen, 2012) were amongst the first group of philosophers to study knowledge and its social influence. In essence, epistemology tackles the deeper philosophical issues surrounding knowledge, such as the question about what it is possible to know, which is underpinned by the following influential elements.

- *Sources*: Sources of knowledge can be either perception or reason.

- *Reason*: Some people believe that reason or abstract knowledge is superior to sensory perception.

- *Basic beliefs*: Knowledge provides a basis for reason, and it is argued that some beliefs can be taken as true and certain.

- *Perception*: Some believe that perception is not a valid source, whilst others argue that without perception there is nothing to reason about.

- *Representation*: The holder of the knowledge must represent knowledge formed from perception or reason. This representation is about the thing that is knowledge but is used by the holder of the knowledge.

- *Knowledge*: For something to be classified as knowledge, it must be traceable to true and justified beliefs, which are based upon basic beliefs and/or valid perceptions.

- *Not knowledge*: Evaluation may result in rejection of a belief.

- *Justification: If beliefs* can be justified and held as true, then they can be classed as knowledge.

- *Justified true belief*: Knowledge is justified true belief.

Epistemology is concerned with knowledge and how we know what we know (Nagael, 2014). A range of epistemologies exist. At one extreme, the epistemology of objectivism asserts that there exists a singular, concrete reality that can be understood by logical means. This is the epistemology that underpins science and the quantitative paradigm. At another extreme, constructionism rejects this view of knowledge. Constructionists assert that individuals generate meaning as they engage with the world they are interpreting. This is the epistemology that underpins the qualitative paradigm. Accordingly, multiple realities exist and there is no objective reality to be discovered. The lines between epistemologies have become blurred and so most researchers do not operate at these extreme poles of objectivism and constructionism. They may work somewhere between.

1.5 GENERIC STAGES OF THE RESEARCH PROCESS

This section reports the contents of a short paper published by the author in 2010 (Hollins Martin and Fleming, 2010), which discusses the 16 steps involved in writing a research proposal. This initial paper has been elaborated upon quite considerably. Initially, the 15-step model was designed by the author to guide student midwives through the process of writing a research proposal, either for assessment, for dissertation, to apply for a grant, to or present a potential future research supervisor. The contents reported in *Section 1.5* underpin the substantial evolution of this book, which comprises 25 years of knowledge accumulated by the author during teaching university-based research methods modules. What follows is a template of the generic 16 steps involved in writing any research proposal (Table 1.1).

Table 1.1   The 16-step model to writing a research proposal.

STEP (1): Give the research proposal a title.
STEP (2): Provide relevant personal and professional details.
STEP (3): Provide a short abstract or summary of around 300 words.
STEP (4): Supply six keywords to describe the research proposal.
STEP (5): Construct an introduction that contains a relevant literature review and rationale.
STEP (6) State the objectives, aim(s), research question(s), sub-question(s), hypotheses, and null hypotheses of the proposed research study.
STEP (7): Outline the research method.
STEP (8): Select setting, participants, sampling method, inclusion and exclusion criteria, and method of recruitment.
STEP (9): Describe data collection instruments.
STEP (10): Detail intended data processing and analysis.
STEP (11): Declare any ethical considerations and outline data protection procedures.
STEP (12): Produce a timetable and consider potential problems that may occur.
STEP (13): Estimate resources that may be required.
STEP (14): Detail a public engagement plan.
STEP (15): Append a reference list.
STEP (16): Appendix relevant additional material.

Source: Hollins Martin and Fleming, 2010 / MA Healthcare Ltd.

1.5.1 THE HOLLINS MARTIN 16-STEP MODEL TO WRITING A RESEARCH PROPOSAL

STEP (1): Give the Research Proposal a Title

The title should accurately reflect the content and scope of the proposed study. It is important to present a consistent title throughout all of the regulatory documents; this includes the proposal itself, the ethics and grant application, and all associated appendices, forms, and questionnaires. An example of a project title is provided below to facilitate understanding of the first step in developing a research proposal.

STEP 1: Example project title (Acronym: Physical Activity Labour (PAL)
Describing and quantifying maternal physical activity and postures during first stage of labour and determining relationships with length of first stage, pain experience, infant condition immediately post birth, and birth satisfaction.

STEP (2): Provide Relevant Personal and Professional Details

On the first page of the research proposal, it is imperative to state the names and titles of the principal researcher(s), supervisor(s), their professional qualifications, the intended study site(s), and contact information. In addition, the principal researcher should appendix a curriculum vitae (CV), which cites their publishing record. The writer of the research proposal will need to justify why members of the research team are suitable people to deliver the project, which will be evidenced in their qualifications, CV, publications, and experience. Amongst the myriad of appendices attached to the final proposal, an up-to-date version of each team members CVs will need to be attached.

STEP 2: Example of relevant and professional details.
STAFF DETAILS 1 (see *Appendix 1*)
Name: Caroline J. Hollins Martin (Proposed Principal Investigator [PI])
Grade: Professor
Professional certifications and academic qualifications, date obtained, and who awarded
Employing organization: Named university
Education
Work experience, skills, and awards
Contact information
Prior projects delivered to completion
Personal statement of why suitable to deliver the research project
Publications
Conference presentations.
STAFF DETAILS 2 (see Appendix 2) etc.

STEP (3): Provide a Short Abstract or Summary of Around 300 Words

The purpose of the abstract is to present a clear summary of the intended project. It is normal to write this concise synopsis at the end of the proposal development, once the project has been methodically assembled and written. Since the writer is limited to 300 words, they must be brief in abridging the relevant sections.

A good abstract should present:

a. A brief background to the proposed study.

b. The aim(s) of the proposed study.

c. The research methodology (recipe) that will be used.

d. The study design (i.e. declare measuring tools, variables (if quantitative), and describe data to be collected).

e. The setting of the research (i.e. where the research will be conducted).

f. Who the intended participants are (i.e. population, sampling method, groups, and numbers).

g. Proposed data processing and analysis (i.e. proposed descriptive and inferential statistics if numeric quantitative data are to be collected. Thematic analysis and coding processes if qualitative data are to be collected).

h. The potential use of outcomes for developing professional practice.

STEP 3: Example abstract (283 words)

Background: A Cochrane collaboration review of 21 studies (Lawrence et al. 2009) concluded that the first stage of labour was around an hour shorter for women who labour upright instead of semi-recumbent. None of the 21 studies used physical activity monitors to record maternal activity or measured birth satisfaction and outcomes for babies.

Aim: To measure the effects of activity in the first stage of labour upon specified maternal and neonatal outcomes.

Method: An observational analytical experimental research methodology will be used.

Design: At commencement of labour, an activity monitor (ActivPAL) will be taped to the consenting woman's right thigh. Quantitative scales will be used to measure:

(i) length of first stage (partogram), (ii) perinatal condition (Apgar scores), (iii) pain (Wong–Baker scale), and (iv) maternal birth satisfaction (Hollins Martin Birth Satisfaction Scale [BSS).

Setting: Maternity unit (specify).

Participants: A convenience sample of healthy childbearing women:

(i) Primigravidas ($n = 40$) and (ii) Multiparous ($n = 40$).

Data processing and analysis: Participants will be sorted into 1 of 4 groups according to ActivPAL results: (i) No activity (control), (ii) Mild activity, (iii) Moderate activity, and (iv) High activity. Means and standard deviations will be presented in tables and graphs. ANOVA' will produce 'p' values for mean differences between groups.

Triangulation component: A phenomenological study will be conducted six weeks postpartum to explore women's experiences of being active in labour and their reports of birth satisfaction and pain ($n = 10$). This qualitative component that will consist of women's opinions will enrich quantitative findings. Interview scripts will be analyzed using inductive thematic analysis.

Use of outcomes: Results should facilitate midwives with providing evidence-based information to childbearing women about the advantages/disadvantages of being active during first stage of labour whilst birth planning.

STEP (4): Supply Six Keywords to Describe the Research Proposal

Keywords are intended to facilitate the reader who wants to search databases and electronic journals for pertinent research studies cited in the literature review.

STEP 4: Example keywords

(1) Physical
(2) Activity
(3) Labour
(4) Childbearing
(5) Midwife/midwives
(6) Experiment

STEP (5): Construct an Introduction that Contains a Relevant Literature Review and Rationale

Present a literature review that summarizes and critically appraises previous research in the field, draws attention to gaps in current knowledge, and cites key references. Relevant research papers are accessed from appropriate databases (e.g. MEDLINE, CINAHL, APA PsycInfo, and Cochrane Library) and electronic journals (e.g. *Midwifery, Women and Birth, and Journal of Reproductive and Infant Psychology*). These research studies are analysed, and the findings are summarized and discussed in relation to the aim of the proposed research study. Where appropriate the research methodology used in previous studies should be reviewed, making comment on relative strengths and weaknesses. An example summary of a literature review follows.

STEP 5: Example summary of a literature review

In a Cochrane systematic review of studies on first stage of labour, 21 controlled studies from a number of countries randomly assigned a total of 3706 women to

(i) upright or (ii) recumbent positions during the first stage of labour (Lawrence et al. 2009). Results found length of second stage and use of opioid analgesia to be similar between groups, although women randomized to upright positions were less likely to have epidural analgesia (Lawrence et al. 2009). Five studies in the review that examined position and mobility of women receiving epidural analgesia ($n = 1176$ women), upright or recumbent position in first stage, did not change length or rates of spontaneous vaginal, assisted, or caesarean delivery. No research on maternal satisfaction or outcomes for babies has yet been conducted. Overall from the studies reviewed, first stage of labour was assessed to be around an hour shorter for women who are upright or walking.

None of the studies reviewed used ActivPAL physical activity monitors to measure maternal activity during labour and its effects on maternal and neonatal outcomes. Use of activity recorders should allow for more precise quantification of maternal movement in relation to length of first stage and measured pain experience. Since no research on maternal satisfaction or outcomes for babies has been conducted, this merits some research attention.

Give the background and justification for the research study. This rationale provides information to the reader that will promote their understanding of the purpose of undertaking the study. This justification communicates the link between the research question and its relationship to advancing the literature and improving professional practice.

STEP 5: Example rationale for study

Women in western countries generally lie in the semi-recumbent position during the first stage of labour, when perhaps it is more natural for women to labour standing, sitting, kneeling, or walking around (Hollins Martin et al. 2015). Woman semi-reclining during first stage of labour has evolved because it is more convenient for midwives to monitor progress and assess foetal condition whilst the woman is lying down (Gizzo et al. 2014). In addition, current obstetric interventions, e.g. cardiotocography, epidurals, and intravenous infusions, limit maternal movement during labour (Akyıldız et al. 2021).

The literature that relates to activity in first stage of labour and its effects upon maternal and neonatal outcomes is insufficient at providing evidence to underpin midwifery practice. That is, there is a dearth of literature (research studies) to support or reject the idea that midwives should or should not encourage women to be physically active or otherwise during the first stage of labour.

STEP (6): State the Objectives, Aim(s), Research Question(s), Sub-question(s), Hypotheses, Null Hypotheses of the Proposed Research Study

Research forms a circle. In other words, it starts with a problem and ends with a solution to the problem and/or a roadmap for further research. The researcher should think about what stimulated them to research the problem. Are there questions about the stated problem to which answers have not been found? The research aims and questions should be stated in a way that leads to analytical thinking and potential concluding solutions to the stated problem.

Stating the objectives, aim, research questions, hypotheses, and null hypotheses makes explicit the purpose of the proposed research study. That is, what the researcher hopes to achieve (hypotheses are only relevant in quantitative studies).

The introduction should provide some background that stands in support of the aim. The objectives, aim, research questions, and hypotheses should be grammatically correct and avoid meaningless words. Demarcating the research study into manageable parts by dividing the main problem into sub-problems is of utmost importance. The following serves as an example:

Objectives Research objectives describe the processes involved in carrying out the research proposal.

STEP 6: Example objectives

(1) Publish a systematic literature review that reports on what research already states about maternal physical activity and postures adopted during labour, and their effects upon length of first stage, pain experience, infant condition, and birth satisfaction.

(2) Develop an evidence-based guideline for midwives, which evidences the effects maternal physical activity and postures have upon length of first stage of labour, pain experience, infant condition, and birth satisfaction.

(3) Build an education program for pregnant couples to practice and learn about the value of walking, moving, and postures and their effects upon length of labour, their pain experience, baby's condition, and birth satisfaction.

The aim A clear statement of the aim of the research study is crucial. This statement cannot be vague and should sum up the goal of the research study. In summary, it encapsulates what precisely the researcher intends to do?

STEP 6: Example aim(s)

To measure the effects of women's activity in the first stage of labour and its effects upon specified maternal and neonatal outcomes. Based on our current understanding, the postures and activities adopted by women during labour will influence key physiological processes which in turn may influence maternal and infant outcomes. We also know that these postures and activities can have profound psychological impact on women's experiences of labour. However, previous studies have limitations in terms of adequately detailing time spent and what in fact constituted particular positions and activity, and hence failed to clearly establish relationships with specified labour outcomes. An improved understanding of these relationships would be of great value (benefit) to childbearing women's (patients') obstetricians and midwives. In this study, guided by our PPI input, we plan to address this clear gap in the current literature in an interdisciplinary project involving midwifery academics, practicing midwives, an obstetrician, and biomedical engineers. Specifically, we will ask women and service providers for their views of physical activity in labour. We will also use an unobtrusive activity monitoring system to record and describe the amount of time women in the first stage of labour elect to adopt different postures and activities and look at relationships to four clinical outcomes (length of first stage, pain experience, infant condition immediately post birth, and birth satisfaction).

AIMS:

(1) To explore women's and service providers' views of physical activity during labour.

(2) To adapt and find out if the system we have designed to measure maternal activity in labour is accurate and acceptable in an NHS context and by maternity care providers.

(3) To provide immediate patient benefit through enabling midwives and obstetricians to answer part of the unanswered question about benefits/drawbacks of having an 'active or passive' birth.

The research question(s) The research study is underpinned by a question. Why? What is the cause of that? What does it mean? The research question is the first step the investigator takes when designing the project. It precedes selection of an appropriate research method (recipe) to answer the question. The question must be clearly articulated since it underpins the entire project.

STEP 6: Example research question(s)

(1) What are women's and service providers' views of physical activity during labour?

(2) Is the activity monitoring system designed by the research team, acceptable to women in labour and staff working in NHS maternity services, and is it able to measure maternal physical activity during real labour?

(3) What are the effects of time spent in different postures (measured using a novel activity monitoring system) during labour upon length of fist stage (measured on a partograph), pain experience (measured using the Wong–Baker Pain Scale), infant condition immediately post birth (measured using Apgar scores at 1, 5, and 10 minutes postdelivery), and maternal perceptions of birth satisfaction (using the Birth Satisfaction Scale-Revised [BSS-R])?

The sub-questions The research question may be divided into further manageable sub-questions. A simple primary question may require answering before the overarching principal research question can be attended to.

<u>STEP 6: Example of sub-questions</u>
What are the effects of women's physical activity during labour upon:

(1) Length of first stage?
(2) Perinatal outcomes?
(3) Pain experience?
(4) Maternal birth satisfaction?

Hypotheses/null hypotheses If a quantitative numerical approach has been adopted, the attendant sub-questions are further encapsulated in objective hypotheses. A hypothesis is a logical statement which the statistical results of the study either support or reject. Each hypothesis provides information that is pertinent to answering the sub-questions and ultimately the overarching research question. A hypothesis is stated in an explanatory form, because it indicates the expected reference of the difference between two variables. The research hypothesis may be stated in a directional or non-directional form. A directional hypothesis statement indicates the expected direction of results, while a nondirectional one indicates no difference or no relationship. A hypothesis should be:

1. Testable.

2. A tentative answer to the stated problem.

3. Specific, logical, and simplistic (not vague).

4. Supported or rejected post statistical analysis.

<u>STEP 6: Example hypotheses and null hypotheses</u>

Hypothesis 1:
Maternal activity shortens length of first stage of labour.

Null Hypothesis 1:
Maternal activity makes no difference to length of first stage of labour.

Hypothesis 2:
Maternal activity in first stage of labour raises perinatal Apgar scores.

Null Hypothesis 2:
Maternal activity in first stage of labour makes no difference to perinatal Apgar scores.

Hypothesis 3:
Maternal activity in first stage of labour reduces women's reports of pain experience.

Null Hypothesis 3:
Maternal activity in first stage of labour makes no difference to women's reports of pain experience.

Hypothesis 4:
Maternal activity in first stage of labour improves women's reports of birth satisfaction.

Null Hypothesis 4:
Maternal activity in first stage of labour makes no difference to women's reports of birth satisfaction.

STEP (7): Outline the Research Method

The research method (recipe) provides practical details of the sequential processes involved in answering the research question(s). A well-designed research proposal should be written in such a way that an unfamiliar person could pick up the proposal and repeat the study. Each research method (recipe) follows a recognizable template, e.g. randomized controlled trial (RCT), grounded theory, phenomenology, ethnography, or survey, to name but a few. The selected research method is declared and referenced. It is also underpinned by a written rationale for why the indicated method (recipe) is the most appropriate choice to answer the research question(s).

Selecting an appropriate research method Research follows a carefully planned formula or recipe. That is, it follows a specific plan, with several methods available to select from. The method (recipe) chosen should be a suitable formula to answer the research question(s). The researcher then outlines the steps of the selected research method. It is not enough to follow the research procedures without an intimate understanding that the research method directs the whole endeavour. The research method clearly outlines the steps involved from beginning to the end of the study. For example, it dictates how data will be acquired and arranges it into logical relationships. The entire process is a unified effort, as well as an appreciation of its component parts.

An analogy to selecting an appropriate research method is as follows. When a person organizes a dinner party, they typically select an appropriate recipe for the occasion. Choices that a person makes are influenced by characteristics of the occasion, such as resources, applicability (e.g. Christmas or a Burn's supper), and specifics of the guests' requirements. In an analogous fashion, the researcher may elect to follow the recipe for a grounded theory study or alternatively use an experimental design, such as an RCT. There is a vast array of research methods to select from, with each following a universally prescribed process. An important factor to grasp is that the research method of choice is selected from one of two camps. That is, either from the 'quantitative' (deductive) or 'qualitative' (inductive) camp. What are the differences between the two?

Quantitative research In quantitative research, the information collected takes the form of measurements or numbers that can be analysed statistically to determine whether or not a treatment has made a real difference. This type of research requires standardized procedures, which involve specific research methods (e.g. RCT, quantitative survey, and experimental design), all of which involve statistical analysis of numerical data designed to maximize objectivity.

A deductive approach is taken by quantitative researchers. Deductive reasoning works from the more general to the more specific. This is sometimes informally called a 'top-down' approach. The researcher begins by thinking up a *theory* about a topic of interest. This is again narrowed down into more specific *hypotheses* that can be tested. This is narrowed down even further, with *observations* collected to address the hypotheses. Ultimately processes involved equip the researcher to test the hypotheses using specific data that provides *confirmation* (or not) of the original theory.

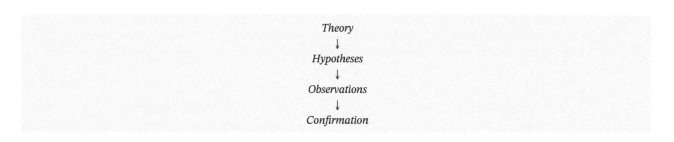

Quantitative research is:

1. Experimental
2. Manipulative
3. Controlled

4. Hypotheses are stated

5. Empirically based

6. Data collection precedes analysis

In stark contrast:

Qualitative research Qualitative research aims to understand the processes that lie behind patterns of behaviour, people's emotions, or their responses to certain situations. Qualitative methods (recipes) (e.g. grounded theory, phenomenology, and ethnography) use different ways of collecting data (e.g. interviews, qualitative surveys, and notes), with words and phrases gathered and analysed in nonmathematical ways.

Quantitative research takes an inductive approach. Inductive reasoning works the other way round from the quantitative approach, through moving from specific observations to broader generalizations and theories. This is sometimes informally called the 'bottom-up' approach, with the researcher attempting to detect patterns and regularities in the data that can be explored, with qualitative approaches usually ending in the development of conclusions and/or theories.

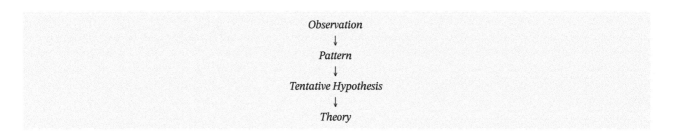

Observation
↓
Pattern
↓
Tentative Hypothesis
↓
Theory

Inductive reasoning, by its very nature, is more open-ended and exploratory. In comparison, deductive reasoning is narrower in nature and is concerned with testing or confirming hypotheses.

Qualitative research is:

1. Interpretive

2. Reflective

3. Inductive

4. Data collection and analysis are often concurrent

Examples of qualitative research methodologies include grounded theory, ethnography, phenomenology, and discourse analysis. The main differences between quantitative and qualitative research methodologies are summarized below:

Quantitative (Deductive)	Qualitative (Inductive)
Reductionalist – one answer	Holistic – many answers
Deals with absolutes – same for all	Individual context important
Objective – researcher is detached from participants. Exerts no influence on participant responses	Subjective – researcher interacts with participants. Inevitably influences their responses
Many participants	Few participants
Interested in findings that apply to many	Interested in personal meaning
Produces accurate replicable findings	Produces diversity in answers
Numerical data that supports/rejects hypothesis	Produces many themes
Predicts findings	No prediction of findings made

When choosing the most appropriate method to answer the research question(s), the method selected will depend upon:

a. The type of question(s) the researcher wants to answer.

b. Whether the best approach to answer the research question(s) is qualitative or quantitative in approach.

At this point, it is time to decide which research method (recipe) to use to answer the selected research question(s). It may be helpful to retrieve a published research paper that has used the particular method of choice. From this paper, the generic pathway (ingredients of the recipe) may be identified. What follows are some examples of both quantitative and qualitative research methods.

Quantitative methods (recipes)

(1) Descriptive
(2) Randomized Controlled Trial (RCT)
(3) Quasi experimental
(4) Quantitative survey
(5) Action research
(6) Clinical audit

Qualitative methods (recipes)

(7) Content analysis
(8) Grounded theory
(9) Phenomenology
(10) Ethnography
(11) Qualitative surveys
(12) Case study
(13) Historical

STEP 7: Example of a research method:
An experimental method will be used to answer the proposed research question(s). At commencement of labour, an activity monitor (ActivPAL) will be taped to the consenting woman's right thigh. The ActivPAL is intended to measure physical activity undertaken during first stage of labour. Post data collection, participants will be allocated to an appropriate group based on level of activity achieved during first stage of labour. The design will involve allocation of participants to 1 of 4 groups.

The information from the ActivPAL will be downloaded onto a computer and a graph of physical activity produced in terms of upright, walking, sitting, etc. Scores are attached to no, mild, moderate, and extensive activity undertaken during first stage of labour.

Groups:
(1) No physical activity during first stage of labour (control).
(2) Mild activity during first stage of labour.
(3) Moderate activity during first stage of labour.
(4) High activity during first stage of labour.

Quantitative scales will be used to measure:
(a) Length of first stage.
(b) Perinatal Apgar scores.
(c) Pain experience.
(d) Birth satisfaction.

A quantitative method has been selected since numeric scores attached to the measuring tools will allow for statistical analysis. The results will provide absolute answers about the relationship between maternal physical activity during first stage of labour and the assessed maternal and neonatal outcomes. Significant/insignificant differences between groups will provide concrete 'yes' or 'no' answers to support or reject the hypotheses and answer the research question(s).

STEP (8): Select Setting, Participants, Sampling Method, Inclusion/Exclusion Criteria, and Method of Recruitment

Consider the setting, participants, and numbers to be included. Alternatively, details of the data are to be collected if no participants are being included. Choice of population, sampling method, and inclusion/exclusion criteria should be considered (e.g. age, absence of disease, and native English speaker). Method of recruitment should be declared and justified. In quantitative studies, data collected is submitted to a significance test to assess the viability of the null hypothesis, with the p-value produced used to reject the null hypothesis. A power analysis conducted during the planning stage will estimate the number of participants necessary to yield an acceptable significant difference between groups. Generally, the larger the effect size wanted, the larger the sample size should be. The goal of a power analysis is to find an appropriate balance by taking into account the substantive goals of the study and the resources available to the researcher.

STEP 8: Example setting
Maternity Unit (specify).

Example participants
Childbearing women, both primigravidas and parous will be invited to participate:

(i) Group 1 – 1st baby ($n = 40$)
(ii) Group 2 – 2nd baby ($n = 40$)

Example sampling method
A convenience sampling method of women who meet the prescribed criteria.

Example inclusion criteria
Healthy
Uncomplicated pregnancy
Term (37–42 weeks)
Spontaneous onset of labour
Age range = 18–35
Caucasian

Example exclusion criteria
Presence of a medical diagnosis
Poor obstetric history
Premature (<37 weeks) /postmature (>42 weeks)
Prescribed induction
<18 years or >35 years of age
Non-Caucasian

Example method of recruitment
Consenting participants will be recruited from the antenatal clinic at the cited maternity unit.

STEP (9): Describe Data Collection Instruments

Provide details of the data collection instruments intended for use in the study, e.g. medical records review, questionnaire, interviews, observation, or apparatus to be employed. Describe how they will be used and the items of data that will be collected, e.g. demographic data and medical conditions. Justification for choices should be provided. If existing validated data collection instruments are being used, these should be referenced as such. If new measuring tools are being specifically developed for the intended research study, information should be provided on how validity and reliability will be established. The design and methods should be described in sufficient detail to allow external people to cost the workload and estimate an achievable timetable.

<u>STEP 9: Example measuring tools</u>

(a) Length of first stage will be recorded on a partograph in numerical values of time (measured in minutes) and cervical dilatation (measured in centimetres (1–10)) (see Figure 1.2).

(b) Neonatal condition immediately post birth will be measured using Apgar scores (0–10) at five minutes immediately post birth (see Figure 1.3).

(c) Pain will be measured using the Wong–Baker pain scale (scores 1–5) (see Figure 1.4).

(d) Birth satisfaction will be measured using the Birth Satisfaction Scale-Revised (BSS-R) (see Figure 1.5).

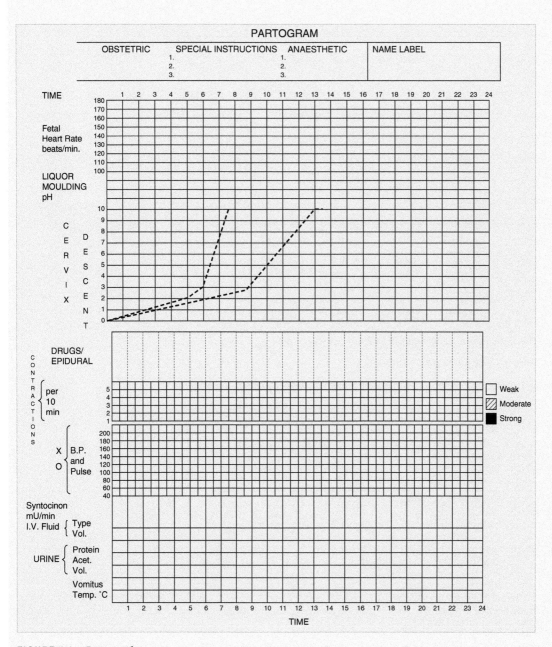

FIGURE 1.2   Partograph.

	Score of 0	Score of 1	Score of 2	Component of acronym
Skin colour	Blue all over	Blue at extremities body pink (acrocyanosis)	No cyanosis body and extremities pink	Appearance
Pulse rate	Absent	<100	>100	Pulse
Reflex irritability	No response to stimulation	Grimace/feeble cry when stimulated	Sneeze/cough/pulls away when stimulated	Grimace
Muscle tone	None	Some flexion	Active movement	Activity
Breathing	Absent	Weak or irregular	Strong	Respiration

FIGURE 1.3   Apgar scoring system.

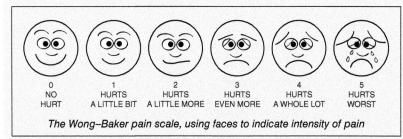

The Wong–Baker pain scale, using faces to indicate intensity of pain

(Adapted from Wong–Baker FACES Foundation, 2021).

FIGURE 1.4   Wong–Baker pain scale. (*Source:* Adapted from Wong–Baker FACES Foundation, 2021).

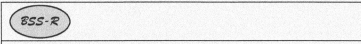

- Quality of care provision (4-items)
- Women's personal attributes (2-items)
- Stress experienced during labour (4-items)

(1) I came through childbirth virtually unscathed.
(2) I thought my labour was excessively long.
(3) The delivery room staff encouraged me to make decisions about how I wanted my birth to progress.
(4) I felt very anxious during my labour and birth.
(5) I felt well supported by staff during my labour and birth.
(6) The staff communicated well with me during labour.
(7) I found giving birth a distressing experience.
(8) I felt out of control during my birth experience.
(9) I was not distressed at all during labour.
(10) The delivery room was clean and hygienic.

FIGURE 1.5   Birth Satisfaction Scale-Revised (BSS-R). *Source:* Adapted from Hollins-Martin, C.J. and Martin, C. (2014).

The partograph is a graphical representation of the changes that occur in labour, including cervical dilatation, foetal heart rate, maternal pulse, blood pressure, and temperature; it also shows a numerical record of features such as urine output and volume and type of intravenous infusions (including oxytocin drips). It is therefore possible at a glance to identify deviations from normal in any of these variables and progress of labour (adapted from WHO, 1994; Bedwell et al. 2017).

<u>Interpretation of Apgar scores</u>
The test is generally done at one and five minutes after birth and may be repeated later if the score is and remains low. Scores 3 and below are generally regarded as critically low, 4–6 fairly low, and 7–10 generally normal (adapted from Apgar, 1953; ACOG, 2021).

The Birth Satisfaction Scale-Revised (BSS-R) is available at: https://www.bss-r.co.uk

The BSS-R is recommended as the key global clinical measure of birth satisfaction by the ICHOM Standard Set for Pregnancy and Childbirth: www.ichom.org/medical-conditions/pregnancy-and-childbirth/

To obtain a copy of the *BBS-R* and marking grid contact Prof. Caroline J. Hollins Martin.

Email: c.hollinsmartin@napier.ac.uk

STEP (10): Detail Intended Data Processing and Analysis

The next step is to consider the intended data processing and analysis. Specifically, what descriptive and inferential statistics are going to be produced? What comparisons might be made 'if any' with the data, e.g. by age, sex, and socioeconomic status? The projected analyses should relate to the aim and the research questions cited. For qualitative research, describe the processes involved in analysis of the interview transcripts.

Once data has been collected, it will be organized into meaningful patterns that can be interpreted. The significance of findings depends on the way the human brain extracts meaning. No rules or formula leads the researcher to correct interpretation. Analysis is subjective and depends entirely on the logical mind, inductive reasoning skills, and objectivity of the researcher. For advice on appropriate statistical analysis, it may be helpful to seek the advice of a statistician.

<u>STEP 10: Example of proposed data processing and analysis</u>
Data will be entered into a software package (SPSS) and appropriate statistical analysis carried out.

<u>Descriptive statistics</u>
Means and standard deviations will be calculated from numerical scores collected using the 4 data collection instruments.

(1) Length of first stage on partogram in minutes.
(2) Apgar scores at five minutes postpartum.
(3) Pain scale scores.
(4) Birth Satisfaction Scale scores.

Participants will be sorted into 1 of 4 groups according to ActivPAL results quantified in mean group numeric scores.

(a) No activity (control)
(b) Mild activity
(c) Moderate activity
(d) High activity

The data collected will be submitted to a significance test to assess the viability of each null hypothesis, with the p-value produced used to reject or accept. Tables and graphs of results will be produced.

Inferential statistics

(1) Length of first stage on partogram:
2 (groups 1 and 2)×4(a, b, c, d) ANOVA will produce 'p' values between groups.

(2) Apgar allocation at five minutes:
2 (groups 1 and 2)×4(a, b, c, d) ANOVA will produce 'p' values between groups.

(3) Pain scale:
2 (groups 1 and 2)×4(a, b, c, d) ANOVA will produce 'p' values between groups.

(4) Birth Satisfaction Scale:
2 (groups 1 and 2)×4(a, b, c, d) ANOVA will produce 'p' values between groups.

Reliability and validity of BSS will be analysed using:

(a) Correlation coefficients
(b) Cronbach alpha
(c) Factor analysis

Please note that not all quantitative studies are subjected to significance testing. In descriptive studies, the aim is to summarize the data set quantitatively without employing probabilistic formulation, e.g. to produce measures of central tendency, dispersion, or association.

1.6 TRIANGULATION

Triangulation is the application and combination of several research methods in the same study. By combining multiple observers, theories, methods, and/or empirical materials, researchers can hope to overcome the weakness or intrinsic biases and problems that arise from using one single research method. Triangulation combines research strategies for the purpose of achieving a multidimensional view of the phenomenon of interest.

Content analysis may be qualitative or quantitative in nature. First, in most basic terms, qualitative content analysis (Schreier, 2012) induces elements of text into labelled categories. In addition to this, during quantitative content analysis, the researcher further proceeds to allocate numeric codes to these labelled bundles of meaning.

Example triangulation method

A qualitative study will be conducted simultaneously to explore women's experiences of being active in labour and their reports of birth satisfaction and pain. Data will be collected six weeks postdelivery. A phenomenological method like Interpretative Phenomenological Analysis (IPA) (Smith et al. 2009) is appropriate since the 'lived-in' experiences of labour as reported by the childbearing women are being explored. The qualitative component, consisting of women's opinions discussed during interview, will enrich the quantitative findings. The questions asked in a semi-structured interview will include:

(1) What was it like being physically active during labour?
(2) What sort of physical activities did you undertake during the first stage of labour?
(3) How do you believe activity/inactivity altered your pain experience during labour?
(4) What impact did activity/inactivity have upon how satisfied you are with your birth experience?

The intention is to interview randomly selected consenting participants ($n = 10$). The interviews will be carried out in a clinic side room at the maternity unit after the six-week postnatal check. Interviews will be transcribed verbatim and imported into a NVivo (2020) software program. The scripts will be analysed using inductive thematic analysis. Coding will be derived from the comments using an iterative process.

1.6.1 A SCIENTIFIC SUMMARY OF MIXED METHODS RESEARCH FOLLOWS

The researcher will be asked to provide a structured summary of the entire mixed methods research study, which in the case of *Project PAL* would look akin to the following.

Further example triangulation method

TITLE: Physical activity in the first stage of labour and its effects upon specified maternal and neonatal outcomes: an observational analytical experimental study (Project PAL).

SUMMARY: Childbearing women often ask midwives what the benefits are of being active in different ways during first stage of labour. At present this question remains unclearly answered. In a Cochrane review of 21 controlled studies from a number of countries ($n = 3706$ women) (Lawrence et al. 2009), findings were contradictory and a recommendation for more sophisticated research was advised. This mixed methods study will gather patient perspectives and describe and observe current activity habits of labouring women using sophisticated equipment never used before in this context. It will allow us to accurately quantify what positions and activities childbearing women actually adopt during labour and determine relationships with four defined variables. It is proposed that understanding more about maternal activity and movement during labour will benefit women through providing information to educate and engage them in their maternity care rather than simply following ritualized practise. This mixed methods study has three overlapping phases.

STUDY DESIGN: The study will use mixed methods:

In PHASE 1, the aim is to explore women and service providers' views of maternal physical activity during labour using a qualitative ethnographic methodology. A comparison of data from women, midwives, and obstetricians will enable us to consider how the meaning and experience of maternal activity during labour may differ according to the perspective of the informant.

In PHASE 2, an internal pilot/acceptability study will determine if the system designed to measure maternal postures and movement during labour actually works in an NHS context with both service users and providers. The aim is to test the designed system to measure activity of women in a real labour ward setting and determine its acceptability to childbearing women, midwives, and obstetricians. The final protocol will be informed by the work undertaken by the research team, childbearing women, and the steering group.

In PHASE 3, an observational study will aim to observe the natural behaviour of labouring women and measure the effects of time spent in different specific postures and movements upon length of first stage, pain experience, infant condition, and birth satisfaction. We will observe what activity women actually undertake and in what percentages, which has never been quantified before using validated objective monitoring with body-worn sensors.

ETHICS: Approval will be sought from NHS IRIS and R&D at NAMED maternity unit.

SHORT- AND LONG-TERM PUBLIC BENEFIT: Quantifying benefits/deficits of maternal physical activity will improve understanding of health outcomes for mothers and neonates. Improving birth satisfaction may have mental health impacts and facilitate information giving to inform joint decision-making between women and midwives whilst birth planning.

IMPACT BEYOND FUNDING PERIOD: Results will immediately impact upon national intranatal guidelines and provide an evidence base to underpin decision-making about suitable maternal activity and epidural option. Information produced will both in the short and long-term develop how midwives manage intranatal care.

The summary of the triangulated research method for Project PAL will be further outlined in a more developed research plan.

RESEARCH PLAN

PHASE 1: QUALITATIVE STUDY (1–24 months).

TITLE: An exploration of women's and service providers' views of physical activity during labour.

AIM: To explore women's and service providers' views of physical activity during labour.

DESIGN: The study will use qualitative methodology and draw on the principles and practices of ethnographic research methodology.

SAMPLE: The sample of 70 participants in total: 40 (20 prenatal/20 postnatal) women, 10 midwives, and 10 obstetricians will be drawn from Bolton Maternity Unit (partners). Current records show that there is ethnic diversity in Bolton, with an appropriate cross section sampled to represent this. We also intend to recruit older and younger women from different socioeconomic groups. Consecutive sampling will be used, with attention to age, socioeconomic background, and ethnicity. We have estimated the sample size, but flexibility will be maintained as the aim is to reach data saturation, with increases or decreases in sample size as appropriate. This approach will support us in developing theoretically informed contrasts that reflect the complexity of the phenomenon and valid comparisons across subgroups. Robust conclusions can be developed using this approach.

INCLUSION CRITERIA: Inclusion criteria are women who are pregnant ($n = 20$) and postnatal women ($n = 20$) around six to eight weeks. There will be no exclusion criteria except for those with severe cognitive impairment and those who do not speak English. Ten obstetricians and a cross section of ten midwives working at different grades at named Maternity Unit will be invited to participate.

PROCEDURE: We will recruit childbearing women, midwives, and obstetricians in the following way. The researcher will attend antenatal and postnatal clinics to recruit participants. This will enable the researcher to give potential participants information about the study and researcher contact details. Participants will be afforded an informed consent process and then a venue agreed to conduct a face-to-face interview. We will recruit obstetricians and midwives through letters of invitation and a direct contact point of the researcher. Key areas for discussion will include participant experiences of activity during labour, their understanding of benefits/ drawbacks, their interpretation of what is or is not sanctioned, and beliefs about the detail and context of accommodation/provision by midwives and obstetricians. In this way, we will be able to understand users, midwives, and obstetricians' priorities and concerns and whether they match.

DATA ANALYSIS: Interviews will be taped and transcribed. NVivo version 9 will be used to support the management, retrieval, and analysis of data. Framework analysis will be the analytical technique. After initial reading and rereading of transcripts, a process of indexing and mapping will be conducted to enable researchers to explore the complexity of experiences across participants. This will support the identification of typologies across the sample.

RIGOUR: We will ensure methodological rigour and enhance quality by using referenced approaches. We will adopt a systematic approach with a clear audit trail and provide a comprehensive description of the methods we have used. As part of the analytical process, we will engage in a reflexive process in which we will consider our prior assumptions and experiences and how these may influence our interpretations. We will pay particular attention to participants' accounts that deviate from preliminary interpretations and consider how these might be explained. Our research partners who are service users and NHS staff on the steering group will contribute to the interpretative process through scrutinizing the interpretation.

OUTPUTS: An in-depth account of views of physical activity during labour from the perspectives of women and service providers will be reported. A comparison of data from women, midwives, and obstetricians will enable us to consider how the meaning and experience of maternal activity during labour may differ from the perspective of the informant.

RESEARCH PLAN

PHASE 2: INTERNAL PILOT/ACCEPTABILITY STUDY (1–12 months)

TITLE: Measuring activity in real labour and user acceptability of study.

AIM: To adapt and find out if the system we have designed to measure maternal activity in labour is viable and acceptable in an NHS context and by maternity care providers.

DESIGN: In a previously conducted preliminary study we have shown that the appropriately processed output of 2 ActivPAL™ monitors, one on the shank and one on the thigh, can be used to accurately classify the posture adopted by the wearer at any instant in time into one of six different classes: lying, sitting, standing, all fours, stepping, and transition (research paper pending). As stated earlier in the proposal, we have also carried out PPI work suggesting participants will accept wearing the monitoring system during labour. The work in Phase 2 is to demonstrate that we can collect high-quality data with women in an actual labour ward setting. Pilot labouring women will wear 2 ActivPAL™ activity monitors adhered to their right thigh and shank and will complete the other outcome measures. We will use the results to refine our recruitment and data collection methods until we have shown that the care providers and participants can use the system and that our data collection methods are appropriate for the next stage. The midwives in the labour room will be fully trained to work with the research team.

OUTCOMES: Those working on the project will receive continued support. The midwives' information sheet will be amended in accordance with findings from this pilot. Topics that emerge will be discussed with local service users to identify if they understand and any new dimensions they may like added. The final protocol will be a refinement of collaborative work undertaken by the research team, childbearing women, and the steering group. During this period of time, ethical approval will be sought.

RESEARCH PLAN

PHASE 3: OBSERVATIONAL ANALYTICAL EXPERIMENT (13–36 months)

TITLE: Describing and quantifying maternal physical activity and postures during first stage of labour and determining relationships with length of first stage, pain experience, infant condition immediately post birth, and birth satisfaction.

AIM: To measure and describe the amount of time women in first stage of labour elect to adopt six pre-identified postures (lying, sitting, standing, all fours, stepping, and transition) and conduct a regression analysis to identify the relationships of time spent in these postures with four clinical outcomes (length of first stage, pain experience, infant condition immediately post birth, and birth satisfaction).

DESIGN: An observational analytical experimental design will be used.

SAMPLE: A convenience sample of informed and consenting nulliparous childbearing women will be recruited from the antenatal clinic at named maternity unit ($n = 110$). Initially, 150 participants will be recruited to allow for a withdrawal rate due to complications. The rationale for only recruiting nulliparous women is that the labouring process differs considerably between nulliparous and multiparous women, with this limitation an attempt to reduce variables that influence outcome.

INCLUSION CRITERIA:
  Nulliparous
  Occipito anterior position at commencement of data collection
  <2 cm dilated and uneffaced at commencement of data collection
  Healthy
  Uncomplicated pregnancy
  Term (3–42 weeks)
  Spontaneous onset of labour
  Age range = 16–40 years
  Have arrived in the labour ward still in latent phase of labour
  Singleton pregnancy
EXCLUSION CRITERIA:
  Multiparous
  Foetal position other than occipito anterior at commencement of data collection
  >2 cm dilated
  Presence of a medical diagnosis
  Premature (<37 weeks)/postmature (>42 weeks)
  <16 years or >40 years of age
  Waterbirth (as monitors not waterproof)
  Stillbirth, perinatal/neonatal death
  Have arrived in the labour ward in active phase of labour
  Physical disability

METHOD OF RECRUITMENT: At the first clinic booking, a leaflet will be given to interested participants providing an overview of the study and a contact point for interested parties. Substantive explanations will be provided, with time for questions and answers afforded. Potential participants will be given the opportunity to opt out at any point with assurance of continuation of quality care provision. To view participant information sheet and consent form see supporting documentation. If the woman's interest in participating is secured, she will be given a two-week window to consider and after a question-and-answer session asked to sign a consent form. A research midwife will be employed to undertake these activities, providing continuity of care.

PHYSICAL ACTIVITY MONITORING SYSTEM: The system consists of two synchronized ActivPAL™ monitors, with one worn midline on the anterior aspect of the thigh and another worn on the anterior aspect of the lower leg (Figure 1.6).

Each ActivPAL contains an accelerometer that produces a signal related to inclination and movement. Based on the inclination and movement of each of the monitors at each instance in time, the system classifies posture into one of six classes (lying, sitting, standing, all fours, stepping, and transition). The ActivPAL device has previously been used to measure posture[13], has been validated for step count and cadence[14], step count in adults at a variety of treadmill and outdoor speeds[15], and step state function in a group of females[16].

At commencement of active labour (2 cm dilatation + 2–3 contractions in 10 minutes), two activity monitors ($1 \times 3 \times 0.5$ cm) (ActivPAL™) will be adhered to the consenting woman's right thigh and right shank. The participant will be in latent stage of labour at time of admission. She will be asked to phone the research midwife as soon as contractions commence. Monitors will be adhered and the time of commencement of 'active phase' of first stage recorded (<2 cm dilatation + 2–3 contractions in 10 minutes). Data used in the study will commence from point of diagnosis of 'active phase' (as opposed to 'latent phase' of first stage of labour). The ActivPAL™-based system will record maternal posture and movement from that point onwards, against which outcome measures will be compared.

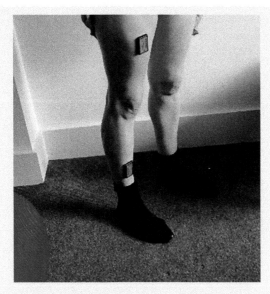

FIGURE 1.6 Photograph to illustrate ActivPAL activity monitors in situation.

MEASURING TOOLS AND ASSESSMENTS: Measuring tools will record:

(a) Length of first stage
(b) Pain experience
(c) Infant condition immediately post birth
(d) Birth satisfaction

(a) *Length of first stage will be measured using a partograph*
   The partograph is a graphical representation of changes that occur during labour. These include cervical dilatation, descent of presenting part, foetal heart rate, number of contractions in 10 minutes, and their strength. From records, it is possible to identify deviations from normal and progress made during labour. On the partograph, length of labour is routinely mapped in relation to cervical dilatation, with total duration recorded postpartum.

(b) *Pain experience will be measured using the Wong–Baker Pain Scale (WBPS)*
   Scores of 1–10 will be used to measure pain experience in labouring women at three points during labour at 3, 6, and 9 cm cervical dilatation, based on graphical representation on a partograph. The WBPS is represented by faces with expressions that indicate intensity of pain and it follows the same guideline as a numerical scale. Zero is represented by a smiley face, whilst 10 corresponds to a distraught crying face. The numbers are appended on the card and the woman will be facilitated by the attendant midwife with process of completion. Visual analogue scales have been extensively used and validated in pain research and are considered to produce consistent measurements of pain, with the WBPS useful for rating pain in children and adults who are compromised.

(c) *Neonatal condition will be measured using Apgar scores*
   Perinatal condition immediately post birth will also be measured using Apgar scores at 1, 5, and 10 minutes postdelivery (Scores of 3 and below are regarded as critically low, 4–6 fairly low, and 7–10 normal) (to view Apgar system, see supporting documentation).

(d) *Birth satisfaction measured using the Birth Satisfaction Scale-Revised (BSS)*
   At 4 postnatal weeks, participants will respond to a posted BSS consisting of 10 statements on a 5-point Likert scale based on level of agreement or disagreement with the statement placed. The possible range of scores is 10–50, where a score of 10 represents least satisfied and 50 most.
   DATA ANALYSIS: We will describe the sample in terms of important patient characteristics. A descriptive analysis will be used to explore the nature and extent of maternal activity and/or positioning assumed by childbearing women in the first stage of

labour. We will document the time spent and pattern of the following activities and summarize using descriptive statistics (lying, sitting, standing, all fours, stepping, and transition).

We will report descriptive statistics for the four primary outcome measures for the sample: duration of first stage of labour, maternal pain experience, neonatal condition, and birth satisfaction. Inferential statistics will be used to relate the type and duration of maternal activity on the maternal and neonatal outcomes. Multilevel modelling will be used where repeated observations are recorded. Regression models will be employed, appropriate to the type of outcome variable (nominal, ordinal, or continuous). The primary analysis will explore the relationship between nature and duration of activity on each outcome. Ancillary analysis will explore the effects of maternal activity, taking into account important environmental and clinical characteristics. This is a novel study of the use of this technique in a maternity setting, and as such the sample size will be influenced by pragmatic considerations. These include the number of primigravidas accessed through the midwife-led unit, which the research unit midwife is able to recruit during the recruitment period. To give an indication of the power of the study, a sample size of 110 patients assuming a medium effect size and 10 predictors for a linear multiple regression would result in a power of 0.76; a sample size of 110 patients assuming a medium effect size and five predictors for a linear multiple regression would result in a power of 0.88.

STEP (11): Declare Any Ethical Considerations and Outline Data Protection Procedures

Detail any ethical considerations and how these will be dealt with. Provide practical particulars of the measures taken to ensure confidentiality for participants and in relation to the data collected. All research studies require approval from the appropriate Ethics Committees. Particularize these in the research proposal and complete the associated committee's application forms.

It is requisite to declare any 'conflicts of interest'. For example, a researcher affiliated to a company closely related to the proposed area of research may stand to profit from steering the study in a specific direction. The general principle to consider is whether or not the circumstances could reasonably be perceived to affect the judgement or decision-making processes of the researcher during process. In attempts to remove potential 'conflicts of interest', transparency in procedures is required. This involves the researcher declaring any 'conflicts of interest' in the research proposal for scrutiny by the relevant ethics committees. The researcher should report the offer and take advice over whether or not to accept the funding, gift, or hospitality.

STEP 11: Example of ethical considerations

Collecting data from women who are in pain and stressed at a key life event could be considered an invasion of privacy. Nevertheless, collection of the data may ultimately improve the labour experience of subsequent childbearing women, especially if it were found that activity in labour shortened first stage and improved Apgar scores, pain experience, and birth satisfaction. A means of circumventing the problem of invasion would be to ask women during their pregnancy for cooperation with wearing an ActivPAL (www.palt.com) and rating pain experience on a scale during labour. In the prenatal period, prospective participants would be able to effectively process the information that is given to them. Asking for cooperation at a time when the woman is able to think about and ask questions before agreement would provide due consideration to the ethical principle of **voluntary participation** and **informed consent.** **Confidentiality** will be respected, with information restricted from anyone not directly involved in the study. **Anonymity** will be provided with questionnaires tagged with numbers and stored in a locked filing cabinet. There are no _conflicts of interest_ that relate to this study.

Does the proposed research raise ethical issues? YES

Collecting data from women who are in pain and stressed at a key life event could be considered an invasion of privacy. A means of circumventing some of the ethical issues would be to ask women earlier in their pregnancy for cooperation with wearing ActivPAL™ (www.palt.com) monitors and rating pain experience on a scale during labour. In the antenatal period, prospective participants will be able to view and handle an ActivPAL™ monitor and process what procedures will be involved in data collection during this study. The aim is to seek informed consent when the woman is not stressed by labour. This may be achieved during the prenatal period at the antenatal clinic when prospective participants would be able to effectively process information, ask questions, and provide informed consent.

Please detail how and when you intend to get ethical review completed

The PI and RM will register on the NHS NRES and complete the online application as indicated on the timeline (STEP 12). Research and Development (R&D) for the maternity unit will also be applied for in this application. As this is a single-site project, no multisite forms are required. This ethics application will cover the time span of four years. The university ethics committee will be kept fully informed of process and results. Due consideration to the ethical principle of _voluntary participation_ and _informed consent will be afforded._

In addition, ethical judgements require to be stated for why the study is worth undertaking, which is captured in a statement of beneficial expected outputs and potential research impact.

STEP 11: Expected outputs and research impact

(1) Childbearing women will benefit in the short and long term from the knowledge produced from this study. Pending further investigation, information generated may provide information from which women can make informed choices when 'birth planning'.

(2) The study will provide understanding of women's natural behaviours during labour, with activity monitors never before used in this context. Post study we will understand more about the time women choose to spend in different positions during labour and how this effects length of first stage, pain experience, infant condition, and birth satisfaction.

(3) If the length of labour is shortened by particular types of maternal activity and positioning, this may save money in terms of time spent providing care, equipment, and skill provision.

(4) If foetal outcomes are improved because of shortened labours, this may save money in terms of risk reduction and need to perform Caesarean Section (CS).

(5) Birth satisfaction may be improved because women are active during labour.

(6) If maternal pain experience is reduced, women are less likely to request expensive methods of pain relief, e.g. epidural.

Data protection   It is also important for the researcher to address their data protection plans, which are outlined in a Data Management Plan (DMP). In this DMP, the researcher outlines what will happen to: (i) existing data, (ii) information about data collected, (iii) quality assurance, (iv) backup and security, (v) ethical issues, (vi) expected difficulties with data sharing, (vii) copyright and intellectual property right, (viii) responsibilities, and (ix) preparation for data sharing and archiving.

STEP 11: Data protection plan for Project PAL

(a) *Existing data*
The research objectives require that qualitative data be gathered which is not available from other sources. No data to date is known to have addressed the aims of Project PAL.

(b) *Information about data collected*
This research project involves primary data collection. The qualitative approach involves semi-structured interviews which will be conducted face-to-face with women, with the use of appropriate personal protection equipment. When face-to-face interviews are not possible, the university's approved secure virtual tool will be utilized (e.g. Teams). Qualitative data will be collected and stored using digital audio recording (e.g. MP3), with soundtracks typed according to agreed formats and standards. All transcripts will be written in Microsoft Word, with methods of note-taking, recording, transcribing, and anonymizing interview data developed and agreed with the supervisory team in advance of commencing data collection. Interview transcripts will be coded within a suitable qualitative software package. With similarity, the quantitative data collected will be stored in SPSS or a similar system that allows analysis.

(c) *Quality assurance*
Detailed protocols for extracting data will be developed, piloted, refined, and agreed with the supervisory team. Quality will be assured through routine monitoring and periodic cross-checks against the protocols written and agreed with the supervisory team. Whilst the interview schedules are being developed, standards and systems for note taking, recording (if consented), transcribing, and storing of data will be clearly outlined. Quality control for data collection will be assured, with members of the research team checking through transcripts for consistency in accordance with agreed standards. With similarity, collection, analysis, and storage of quantitative data will be outlined in the protocol.

(d) *Backup and security*
Data will be backed up regularly, which will include regular email sharing with the supervisory team. In addition, up-to-date versions will be coded and stored on the appropriate university server (e.g. allocated X drive). This X drive is a managed data storage service, which is secure and backed up regularly as per the University Research Data Management (RDM) policy and the RDM requirements. Data collected will be backed up and secured on a regular basis, which will involve clear labelling of versions and dates. The team will establish a system for protecting data, which will include the use of passwords and safe backup hardware.

(e) *Ethical issues*

A letter explaining purpose, approach, and the dissemination strategy will be prepared. A clear verbal explanation will also be provided to each participant prior to interview. Commitments to ensure confidentiality will be maintained by ensuring recordings are not shared, those transcripts are anonymized, and details that identify participants are removed from transcripts or concealed in write-ups. The highly focused nature of the research project means that several participants may be easily identifiable, despite efforts to ensure anonymity or confidentiality. Where there is such a risk, participants will be shown sections of transcript to ensure they are satisfied that no unnecessary risks are being taken with their interview data. In addition, interviewees may be more comfortable if some sections of their interview are not recorded or made public, and when stated such requests will be respected. In such circumstances, recordings will be paused or sections of text removed from shared transcripts, with an indication made that this is the case.

(f) *Expected difficulties with data sharing*

Transcripts will be recorded and transcribed in English, which will limit accessibility of the data to alternative-speaking cultures.

(g) *Copyright and intellectual property right*

The institutional partners (Health Board (HB) and named university) will jointly own the data generated. Online and archival sources will be cited and clearly acknowledged in the database and research outputs. Permission will be sought from other sources to share the findings of the research, e.g. on public websites.

(h) *Responsibilities*

The Principal Investigator (PI) and supervisory team will direct the data management process, with the Research Midwife (RM) responsible for ensuring data production, day-to-day cross-checks, backup, and other quality control activities are maintained. Data extraction, processing, and inputting for the data set will be undertaken by the RM, with guidance from the PI and supervisory team. The RM will take responsibility for collecting all data and transcribing interview data, with the PI and supervisory team supporting process as necessary. The RM will be responsible for dealing with quality, sharing, and archiving of data.

(i) *Preparation for data sharing and archiving*

The most appropriate method of sharing the data generated will be through publications, online (e.g. Worktribe), and institutional websites. The project will have a dedicated space on the university website, for purpose of sharing and archiving, with the HB also encouraged to host data on their websites.

STEP (12): Produce a Timetable and Consider Potential Problems that May Occur

Provide a summary of the planned programme of work using a bar, Gantt chart, or table which highlights significant phases of the project. A Gantt chart is a type of bar chart that illustrates the schedule for the research proposed. Gantt charts illustrate the beginning and completion dates of the procedures involved in the proposed research study. For example, timescales for expected ethics approval, literature review completion, recruitment of participants, completion of data collection, and write-up of study. Outline any potential organizational, practical, or methodological problems that might occur and how you intend to overcome these. For example, when determining the projected length of the study, it is important to incorporate interview and employment plans and the total time required to train relevant people. If new staff members are also to be employed and trained, the procedures involved may add an additional four months to the projected timetable.

STEP 12: Example of a research timetable

The duration of the proposed project will be 36 months and in accordance with the following timetable:

◆Q = quarter of a year (three-month period)

Gantt chart project PAL		Project year 1 1/1/24–31/12/25 1–12 months				Project year 2 1/1/25–31/12/26 13–24 months				Project year 3 1/1/26–33/12/27 25–36 months		
Preparation for Project PAL		Q1	Q2	Q3	Q4	Q5	Q6	Q7	Q8	Q9	Q10	Q11	Q12
P.1: Research fellow-advertising and recruitment	◆											
P2: Ethics submission/approval	◆ ◆ ◆											
P3: Meet with SIMBA partnerships	◆											

Gantt chart project PAL	Project year 1 1/1/24–31/12/25 1–12 months				Project year 2 1/1/25–31/12/26 13–24 months				Project year 3 1/1/26–33/12/27 25–36 months			
Preparation for Project PAL	Q1	Q2	Q3	Q4	Q5	Q6	Q7	Q8	Q9	Q10	Q11	Q12
P4: Set up steering group (SG)	◆											
P6: Develop optimal recruitment strategy	◆	◆										
Project PAL	Q1	Q2	Q3	Q4	Q5	Q6	Q7	Q8	Q9	Q10	Q11	Q12
2.1: Full research team meeting (including co-applicants, collaborators, and research fellow)	◆				◆				◆			
2.2: Steering group (SG) Meetings	◆		◆		◆		◆		◆		◆	
2.3: Literature review-update	◆					◆					◆	
2.4: Develop study protocol	◆											
2.5: Data collection – qualitative	◆	◆	◆	◆	◆	◆	◆	◆				
2.6: Data entry and transcription	◆	◆	◆	◆	◆	◆	◆	◆	◆			
2.7: Data analyses	◆	◆	◆	◆	◆	◆	◆	◆	◆	◆		
2.8: Write-up report/paper(s)										◆	◆	◆
2.9: Annual report to funder				◆				◆				◆
Final project PAL												
F.1: Dissemination to stakeholders – conferences											◆	◆
F.2: Final report to funders											◆	◆

STEP (13): Estimate Resources that May Be Required

Provide a summary of the estimated costs and requirements for the project pending, e.g. time, travel, consumables such as researchers' time, stationery, postage, and equipment. The researcher may be asked to explain why the project is value for money. For example, this research project provides value for money because never before have biophysical engineers worked with midwives in a childbearing capacity, which makes the proposed project novel and exciting. Results of the proposed study will benefit childbearing women (patients) in the short and long term. Evidence produced will quantify the specifics of type, level, and extent of maternal physical activity actually undertaken by women during the first stage of labour. Advancing knowledge about childbirth has practical relevance for maternity staff, since women in the United Kingdom more often lie in the semi-recumbent position during first stage of labour, when perhaps it is more natural for them to labour standing, sitting, kneeling, or walking around. In addition, many obstetric interventions hamper opportunity for maternal movement during first stage, with epidural by its very nature restricting mobilization. At present there is confusion over type, level, and extent of maternal physical activity that maternity staff should offer/support during labour, with conflicts of interests between protocols and movement-limiting technology. This makes providing choice and control to childbearing women an arduous task and leaves maternity care staff unclear about how to counsel women. Providing information about environmental influences is important for service users since interventions and behaviours that increase or diminish the likelihood of having the type of birth desired increase women's chances of having such. The researcher will be asked to explain how the research costs have been calculated and justify how they have been allocated, with the following example explaining this.

STEP 13: PAL costing sheet	Year 1	Year 2	Year 3	TOTAL
Personal support of applicants				
Prof. Caroline Joy Hollins Martin (1 d a wk)	£15343	£15489	£15636	£46468
	(330h)	(330h)	(330h)	(990h)
Dr Graham Smith (1 h a wk)	£2134	£2164	£2184	£6482
	(52h)	(52h)	(52h)	(156h)
Dr Mary McDonald (1 h a wk)	£2814	£2841	£2868	£8523
	(52h)	(52h)	(52h)	(156h)
Research Assistance				
Grade: 0730	£41381	£43684	£45892	£130957
Consumables				
Birth satisfaction scales (print costs × 400)	£1000	0	0	£1000
Pain scales (print costs × 400)	£1440			£1440
Patient Public Involvement (PPI)				
4 members of the public who are users	£1000	£1000	£1000	£3000
2 steering groups a year				
• Venue • Refreshments and lunch at • Thank you voucher • Travel costs • Stationery				
Travel and subsistence home				
University-maternity unit-participants home	£4000	£5000	£5000	£14000
Travel and subsistence			£6000	£6000
To international conferences				
Payment to partner university				
Tanya Sinclair (statistician)	£5293	£5293	£5293	£15879
Contribution to maternity unit	£2850	£4000	£3000	£9850
• Lighting • Toilets • Water • Heat				
Equipment				
ActivPAL™ monitors × 8	£8000	0	0	£8000
Estates charge	£9574	£9574	£9574	£28722
Indirect costs	£47306	£47306	£47306	£141918
Total costs				£434239
Estimated recovery (80%)				£347391

Clarification of team responsibilities Clarifying each member of the research team's individual responsibilities will help avoid duplication and identify gaps that have not been covered in the project. This delineation should enhance teamwork and will allow more effective planning, implementation, and evaluation of project delivery. In relation to Project PAL, this has been explained as follows.

STEP 13: Clarification of team responsibilities in Project PAL

<u>Prof. Caroline Hollins Martin</u> has been calculated at one day a week of her university salary. In her role as PI, she will spend part of this time in the named maternity unit setting up the project and supporting the RM in her role of managing data collection and actual data collection. The rest of her allotted time will be spent:

- Recruiting and training the RM.
- Organizing ethics applications.
- Preparing participant and staff information sheets and consent forms.
- Helping with participant recruitment and preparation.
- Preparing maternity care staff for the study.
- Organizing the SG and writing of minutes.
- Managing public involvement components of the study.
- Formulating a system of data storage.
- Working with the team on data analysis components of the study.
- Writing budget expenditure reports.
- Writing research papers with the team.
- Day-to-day running of the project and supervision of the RM.

Dr Graham Smith and Dr Mary McDonald have both been calculated one hour a week of their university salary (together two hours a week). Their responsibilities will be to teach the RM about storage and analysis of activity monitor data. They will liaise with the statistician about appropriate data analysis and writing of reports. They will present these reports at SG meetings and aid the research team to understand the findings. They will support supervision of the RM and help resolve issues that relate to activity monitor data, its analysis, and writing of relevant sections of the reports.

Research Midwife has been calculated as five days a week and is yet to be employed. The RM will spend part of her time as necessary in the named maternity unit setting up the project with the PI and once operational managing data collection and being involved in actual data collection. The rest of the allotted time will be spent undertaking the following activities:

- Liaising and working in conjunction with the PI.
- Organizing ethics applications.
- Preparing participant and staff information sheets and consent forms.
- Recruiting and preparing participants.
- Preparing and providing continual support to maternity care staff at Bolton maternity unit.
- Reporting processes to the steering group.
- Working on public involvement components of the study.
- Appropriately entering and storing data.
- Working with team on data analysis components of the study.
- Writing in conjunction with the whole team the research reports and papers.
- Day-to-day running of the project.

<u>Contribution to named Maternity Unit</u>: The named maternity unit has asked for £10 000 across the three years to cover general costs. For example, lighting, toilets, water, and heat.

<u>Equipment costs</u>: Will cover only the essential instruments for appropriately conducting the study.

<u>Materials and consumables</u>:

Travel and subsistence

Members of the research team require to:

- Travel from the university to the maternity unit (£6 a return trip).
- SG travel expenses and liaising with partners.

- Present conference papers in year three to disseminate methods and findings. If the outcomes are successful, then this component is really important. Caroline J Hollins Martin (CJHM) and the Research Midwife (RM) will disseminate findings to midwives, obstetricians, and allied health care professionals through national and international conferences, such as the Royal College of Midwives (RCM), Nursing Midwifery Council (NMC), and education forums.
- Purchase of measuring tools.
- Ad hoc purchases.

What is listed is essential for progressing the study:

- Providing refreshments for participants and members of the SG.
- Paper, envelopes, and stamps for communications.
- Print room to produce measuring tools with face validity.
- Photocopying and printing of documents.
- Open access conference paper.

Estates cost and indirect costs have been calculated into the budget. Any money not spent will be returned to the funder at the end of the project.

Research management arrangements Processes about how the project will be managed may need to be outlined. For example, a *Core Project Management Group* may be established, which comprises of named individuals. This *Core Project Management Group* will meet on a bimonthly basis to review overall management of the project. A *Steering Group* (SG) will be established, which consists of an independent chair, maternity unit representation, a participant (once study established), the *Research Team,* and members of the public from two advisory groups. For example.

(*Group 1*) *A user group* may consist of three to four service users from the named maternity unit, with names and contact numbers listed.

(*Group 2*) *An educators' group* may consist of three to four midwives, with names and contact numbers listed.

The SG may meet twice a year to advise on design and management of the project. Costs of meetings and travel should be built into the budget. Appropriate reports will require to be written by the PI and submitted to the funder at the required points. The financial aspects of the project will be managed by the university finance team.

Success criteria and barriers to proposed work To justify the costs, you may be asked to outline the success criteria and barriers that may obstruct project completion. For example, there are minimal risks to the completion of your project. In the case of Project PAL, the biggest risk is failure to recruit participants or the study overrunning its allocated timescale. One contingency that may be afforded is an assurance that were the timescale to be breached then there will be a no cost extension until the project is finished. For example:

Actions taken to assure delivery of Project PAL

In relation to the potential recruitment problem, the following actions have been agreed:

Commitment has been obtained from Dr. Named Obstetrician and Named Midwifery Manager at the Maternity Unit, who have agreed to support the study. To view letters of support, see supporting documentation in numbered Appendix. These people have also agreed to be part of the SG. They will help by preparing delivery suite staff for the project and will facilitate recruitment of participants. The named maternity unit averages 4500 deliveries a year and therefore the population of childbearing women is infinite. The research team will continue until full recruitment of participants has been achieved.

Rationale for length of project To justify the costs, a rationale for your chosen length of project may be requested. For example, three years length may be allocated, because data collection may be lengthy (approximately two to three a week), with 150 participants recruited to accommodate drop-out due to exclusion criteria, emergency situations, or withdrawal out of personal choice.

Projected outputs and dissemination To justify the costs, you may be asked to outline papers that will be written and how you will disseminate the project results. For example, appropriate audiences will be targeted through writing user-friendly reports that are uploaded onto University/NHS trust websites and sent to those involved in the project. Dissemination will take place via presentations at local, national, and international conferences relevant to interprofessional and interagency working. Reports will be sent to peer-reviewed journals, service users, and voluntary organizations' newsletters, magazines, websites and will be used to inform curriculum. The service user group will be involved in writing material and drafting or voicing podcasts. Opportunities for dissemination through the media may be explored. For example, presenting results on 'Woman's Hour' or other television programs that address women's issues. You may also be asked to outline potential publishable research papers that will be delivered from your proposed research project. For example:

Projected papers from Project PAL

Hollins Martin et al. Describing and quantifying maternal physical activity and postures during first stage of labour.

Hollins Martin et al. Measuring maternal physical activity in labour and its effect upon length of first stage, neonatal condition, pain experience, and birth satisfaction using ActivPAL™ professional monitors: an observational analytical experimental study.

Other anticipated outputs
Benefits for childbearing women are that the evidence produced from this feasibility study may underpin a future multisite trial, which includes women in their first, second, third, and fourth baby, with differing foetal positions at commencement of labour. The knowledge produced would benefit women through producing concrete information that can be used to inform decision-making about whether to opt for an 'active' or 'passive' labour or immobilizing epidural.

STEP (14): Detail a Public Engagement Plan

As part of process, you will be asked how patient and public involvement has informed and/or influenced development of your research proposal. For research midwives, this means that women, partners, and families must be actively involved in writing your proposal and delivering it (Bee et al. 2018). Public inclusion helps the researcher gain greater understanding and improves ability to respond to women's needs. The process should include families from all types of social backgrounds and ethnic representation. Public involvement in your study will improve women's access to services and help the researcher see the story through the eyes of those who actually use related facilities (NIHR, 2022). We need women to share their insight and experience, which ultimately hands them power to live healthier lives and have improved childbearing experiences. Hence, from initiation to completion of your research study, the public should play a part in prioritizing, designing, delivering, and disseminating the research study. In relation to Project PAL, the public was involved during writing of the research proposal, with an example report provided.

Public involvement report for Project PAL

The research team successfully applied for a public involvement bursary of £400. Using this grant, a group of six named service users were given a short presentation about the proposed study. They were then shown two activity monitors and the pain scale and asked if they considered them acceptable for use during labour. They were also asked if they thought whether knowing about maternal activity during labour is important in relation to:

(a) Women's pain experience
(b) Birth satisfaction
(c) Infant condition at birth
(d) Length of first stage of labour

(1) *Perceptions of the importance of maternal activity during the first stage of labour*
Service users reported wanting to have choice during their labour. They voiced the importance of understanding benefits/detriments of adopting different positions and activities in relation to length of labour, the baby's condition at birth, pain experience, and their satisfaction with the experience, which are the four outcome measures of this study.

(2) *Acceptance of wearing two activity monitors and completing pain charts during labour*

Having handled the monitors and tested wearing, all agreed that they were noninvasive and that they would be happy to participate in the study. They also expressed that responding to the pain face questionnaire at three points during labour may facilitate the midwife to understand what they were experiencing.

The main concern articulated was being free to move around during labour. This study permits the women to freely adopt whatever position suits them personally, with no activity events prescribed. All of those interviewed perceived that the information gained would benefit women in terms of birth planning and that this knowledge would empower them to make informed choices, particularly in relation to electing to have an epidural.

You may also be asked to indicate ways in which the public will be actively involved in delivering your proposed research study.

Members of the public will be involved in:

Design of the study.	YES/NO
Management of the research (e.g. Steering Group).	YES/NO
Developing participant information sheets.	YES/NO
Undertaking the project and/or analyzing the data.	YES/NO
Contributing to reporting or writing of the study report.	YES/NO
Dissemination of research findings.	YES/NO

Public involvement in design of Project ActivPAL

We plan to involve two groups to advise on design and delivery: (1) a user group and (2) an expert educators' service group:

(Group 1) User group consisting of three women from named maternity unit recruited during preparation of the study via the community midwives' office:

(1)   Name, place of work, and email
(2)   Name, place of work, and email
(3)   Name, place of work, and email

(Group 2) Expert educators' service group consisting of three midwives:

(4)   Name, place of work, and email
(5)   Name, place of work, and email
(6)   Name, place of work, and email

The above six people will be invited to be part of the Project PAL Steering Group (SG).

Management of the research:
Group 1 (user group), *Group 2* (expert educators' service group), and the *Research Team* will comprise the SG. An independent chair will be appointed to steer these meetings, which will take place twice a year over three years (six in total). The SG will inform the development, progress, and dissemination of the study and will meet twice a year (or more often if problems arise) to advise on the design and management of the project. The purpose is to ensure that issues raised are contextualized into the lived experience of childbearing women and to maintain the validity of the research. Participant information sheets will also be piloted on service users for comprehension. In addition, information resources will be viewed by members of the SG for comments. Costs of meetings and travel to the venue have been built into the budget.

Undertaking/analyzing the research
Study results produced will be viewed by members of the public and the SG for comments about interpretation and meaning. Service users will input into the type of analysis they would like to see pertaining to dissemination to the public.

Contributing to the reporting of the study

Service users from the user group will be asked to read the study reports and contribute towards writing a user-friendly synopsis of the study. These reports will also be viewed by the SG.

Dissemination of research findings

Members of the user group will be provided with opportunities to participate in writing reports and presenting at conferences. As such, these members of the public can present jointly decided components of the study in collaboration with the PI and other relevant members of the research team.

STEP (16): Append a Reference List

Appendix questionnaires, interview schedules, diagrams of equipment, and any relevant information that will aid understanding of the intended project. Remember to reference these in text.

STEP 14: Example of relevant appendices in Project PAL

Appendix 1 = Principal researcher(s) curriculum vitae
Appendix 2 = Partograph
Appendix 3 = Apgar system
Appendix 4 = Wong–Baker pain scale
Appendix 5 = Birth Satisfaction Scale
Appendix 6 = Interview schedule

STEP (15): Append a Reference List

The university recommended referencing format should be used throughout your research proposal.

STEP 15: Example references list for Project PAL

Hollins Martin, C.J., Fleming, V. (2010). A 15-step model for writing a research proposal. _British Journal of Midwifery_. 18(12): 791–798. 10.12968/bjom.2010.18.12.791.

Hollins-Martin, C.J., Martin, C. (2014). Development and psychometric properties of the Birth Satisfaction Scale-Revised (BSS-R). _Midwifery_. 30: 610–619. 10.1016/j.midw.2013.10.006.

Hollins Martin, C.J., Kenney, L., Pratt, T., Granat, M.H. (2015). The development and validation of an activity monitoring system for use in measurement of posture of childbearing women during first stage of labour. _Journal of Midwifery_ and _Women's Health_. 10.1111/jmwh.12230.

Lawrence, A., Lewis, L., Hofmeyr, G.J., Dowswell, T., Styles, C. (2009). Maternal positions and mobility during first stage labour. _Cochrane Database of Systematic Reviews_. (2). CD003934. 10.1002/14651858.CD003934.pub2.

STEP (16): Appendix Relevant Additional Material

Appendix questionnaires, interview schedules, diagrams of equipment, and any relevant information that will aid understanding of the intended project. Remember to reference these in text.

STEP 14: Example of relevant appendices in Project PAL

Appendix 1 = Principal researcher(s) curriculum vitae
Appendix 2 = Partograph
Appendix 3 = Apgar system
Appendix 4 = Wong–Baker pain scale
Appendix 5 = Birth Satisfaction Scale
Appendix 6 = Interview schedule

Post data analysis, a discussion, conclusions, and implications for practice are written in light of the study findings. Suggestions for future research may also be projected. Well-designed research proposals include a method of evaluating the success of the project post implementation, e.g. development of an audit tool. Most sponsors request that a process of evaluation and outcome statement be part of the submitted research proposal.

Conclusion

The written template in this chapter outlines STEPS 1–16 involved in writing a research proposal. This outline of the intended research project requires to be sent to the appropriate ethics committee(s) for approval prior to commencing the study. If the researcher is seeking funding, the proposal will be scrutinized for value before money is awarded from the specified grant body or being accepted by a doctorate research supervisor. The final completed research proposal will be the common understanding from which the researchers, clinical staff, and participants will operate. It is the template from which tasks are allocated, divided, and discussed. Remember to be realistic when designing your study. Overly optimistic ideas of what the project can accomplish may detract from the chances of being approved. To summarize, basically the research process follows a set of logical developmental steps and is cyclical (Figure 1.7):

(a) A questioning mind observes a particular situation and asks: Why? What caused that? How come? (the subjective origin of research).

↓

(b) A reason for carrying out the research is justified (the rationale).

↓

(c) A review of literature is carried out to find out what has already been discovered and published by researchers. The problems may already have been resolved.

↓

(d) The research question is written.

↓

(e) An appropriate research recipe (method) is selected.

↓

(f) Participants are justified in terms of numbers and appropriateness.

↓

(g) Specific data collection instruments are designed to take measurements.

↓

(h) Data are collected from participants using these purposeful measuring tools.

↓

(i) The body of data is processed, interpreted, and findings established. These results should answer the research question(s) and support/reject the hypotheses if a quantitative method.

↓

(j) A discussion takes place of the discovery made and a conclusion reached. The question and hypothesis are either supported by the data and the question partially or completely answered or not.

↓

(k) The cycle is complete.

FIGURE 1.7   The research cycle.

1.7 INTRODUCTION TO RESEARCH METHODS CHAPTER SUMMARY

The core concept underlying all research is its method (recipe). It is not enough to follow the research procedures without an intimate understanding that the research method directs the whole endeavour. The method controls the study, dictates the acquisition of data, and arranges them in logical relationships. The entire process is a unified effort as well as an appreciation of its component parts. To help you decide on an appropriate method (recipe) to answer a specific research question, please first formulate responses to the questions outlined in Activity 1.2. *Chapter Two* will now look at the differences between inductive and deductive approaches to research.

Activity 1.2

Formulate responses to the following questions:

(1)   Consider an area within maternity care that you perceive deserves more research attention.

(2)   In relation to your selected area of interest, construct an aim for your research proposal.

(3a) In relation to your selected area of interest, construct a research question for this research proposal.

(3b) Are there any sub-questions that this research proposal could answer?

(4)   If this is a quantitative research study, what are the hypotheses and null hypotheses?

(5)   What are the objectives for this research study?

1.7.1 CHAPTER CONCLUSION

Fundamentally each research method follows a generic pathway, which we have compared to the concept of following a recipe. To draw an analogy, if you make an apple pie, the generic steps in process are similar regardless of the recipe you follow. However, there may be small deviations in content between pies, which may involve whether you add ginger, syrup, type of apples, or otherwise. The point is, at the end of your makings, we can all identify that you have created an apple pie. In addition, *Chapter One* has introduced some basic concepts surrounding research methods. For example, we have familiarized you with a glossary of research terms and have presented a general outline of the generic steps involved in any research study. We have familiarized you with the terms ontology and epistemology, differences between quantitative and qualitative approaches, and the possibility of triangulating studies. We have also discussed the importance of including laypeople in development, management, and dissemination of research studies. Having laid these fundamental paving slabs, we will now move on to *Chapter Two* where we discuss the differences between qualitative (inductive) and quantitative (deductive) approaches in more detail. Also, to test and develop your understanding, we now list some *Self-Assessment Questions (SAQs)*.

1.8 SELF-ASSESSMENT QUESTIONS (SAQs)

Please circle the answer you think is most applicable.

1.1   The dependent variable is:

(a)   The measuring tool (i.e. scale) used by a quantitative researcher.

(b)   An ethical issue surrounding the research.

(c)   A schematic diagram of themes.

(d)   A clear-cut hypothesis.

1.2   A control group is a:

(a)   Researcher who keeps participants in order.

(b)   Placebo.

(c)   Matched group of participants who do not receive the intervention.

(d)   Manipulation strategy.

1.3 **Surveys involve data collection using questionnaires.**

(a) Only when a treatment reduces participants' symptoms.

(b) False

(c) True

(d) Only when an intervention is given.

1.4 **A researcher posts a questionnaire to 100 women asking whether they are happy with the professional care they have received. The research method used is:**

(a) Phenomenology.

(b) Grounded theory.

(c) An RCT.

(d) A survey.

1.5 **Phenomenology:**

(a) Is a research method that looks into an organizations' culture.

(b) Involves writing hypotheses.

(c) Is an attempt to capture experience in the process as lived.

(d) Is a research method that uses large number of participants.

1.6 **Ethnography:**

(a) Involves constant comparison.

(b) Is a quantitative methodology.

(c) Involves use of a control group.

(d) Has its roots in anthropology.

1.7 **Ethnography is a type of:**

(a) Qualitative study of women's lived birth experiences.

(b) Quantitative study comparing two treatments.

(c) Descriptive qualitative study of how culture affects childbearing women's behaviour.

(d) Quantitative study about non-English-speaking communities.

1.8 **Grounded theory involves:**

(a) The researcher conducting an extensive literature review in advance of data collection.

(b) Data collection stopping when saturation has been reached.

(c) Issue of drugs to matched groups.

(d) Issue of scored questionnaires.

1.9 **Historical research:**

(a) Attempts to look at trends in events over a period of years.

(b) Is an outdated research method.

(c) Involves the researcher living among the population.

(d) Looks at comparisons in behaviour between groups.

1.10 Triangulation:

    (a) Combines research strategies for the purpose of achieving a multidimensional view of the phenomenon of interest.

    (b) Is used to establish average efficacy of a treatment.

    (c) Is a quasi-experimental design.

    (d) Is a form of qualitative research.

ANSWERS TO CHAPTER 1 SAQs

1.1 **a**

1.2 **c**

1.3 **c**

1.4 **d**

1.5 **c**

1.6 **d**

1.7 **c**

1.8 **b**

1.9 **a**

1.10 **a**

Inductive Versus Deductive Approaches

'How do I begin to learn about research methods'?

2.1 INTRODUCTION TO INDUCTIVE VERSUS DEDUCTIVE APPROACHES

In response to this question, the first important factor to understand is that there are many recipes that could be followed by a researcher attempting to answer a research question. An analogy to selecting an appropriate method is when a person organizes a dinner party; they choose a suitable recipe for the occasion. Choices that a person makes are influenced by characteristics of the occasion, such as resources, applicability, and specifics of the guests' requirements. In an analogous fashion, the researcher may elect to follow the recipe for an ethnographic study or alternatively use an experimental design. There is a vast array of research methods to select from, with each following a universally prescribed process. An important factor to grasp is that the research method of choice is selected from one of two camps. That is either the 'quantitative' (deductive) or 'qualitative' (inductive) camp. The main differences between these two camps are *quantitative research (deductive)* and *qualitative research (inductive)*:

Quantitative Research (Deductive) is the systematic scientific investigation of properties and phenomena and their relationships. The objective of quantitative research is to develop and employ mathematical models, theories, and/or hypotheses pertaining to natural phenomena. The process of measurement is central to quantitative research because it provides the fundamental connection between empirical observation and mathematical expression of quantitative relationships.

Qualitative Research (Inductive) is a field of inquiry that crosscuts disciplines and subject matters. It involves an in-depth understanding of human behaviour and the reasons that govern human behaviour. Unlike quantitative research, qualitative research relies on reasons behind various aspects of behaviour. Simply put, it investigates the *why* and *how* of decision-making as compared to *what*, *where*, and *when* of quantitative research. Hence, the need is for smaller but focused samples rather than large random samples, which qualitative research categorizes data into patterns as the primary basis for organizing and reporting results. Qualitative researchers typically rely on four methods for gathering information: (i) participation in the setting, (ii) direct observation, (iii) in-depth interviews, and (iv) analysis of documents and materials.

Research Recipes for Midwives, First Edition. Caroline J. Hollins Martin.
© 2024 John Wiley & Sons Ltd. Published 2024 by John Wiley & Sons Ltd.

2.2 MORE ABOUT THE (QUANTITATIVE) DEDUCTIVE APPROACH

Quantitative Research
In quantitative research, the information collected takes the form of measurements or numbers that can be analyzed statistically to determine whether or not a treatment has made a real difference. This type of research requires standardized procedures, specific methods, and statistical analysis and so maximizes objectivity.

A deductive approach is taken by quantitative researchers. Deductive reasoning works from the more general to the more specific. This is sometimes informally called a 'top-down' approach. The researcher begins by thinking up a *theory* about a topic of interest. This is again narrowed down into more specific *hypotheses* that can be tested. This is narrowed down even further with *observations* collected to address the hypotheses. This ultimately equips the researcher to test the hypotheses using specific data that provides *confirmation* (or not) of the original theory (see Figure 2.1).

Quantitative research is:

1. Experimental.

2. Manipulative.

3. Controlled.

4. Hypothesis is stated.

5. Empirically based.

6. Data collection precedes analysis.

To view an example of a *quantitative* research study, which has used a *survey* research method (recipe) (see Activity 2.1a & 2.1b).

Activity 2.1a

An example of a *quantitative* research study, which follows the research method called a *survey* is:

Hollins Martin, C.J., Patterson, J., Paterson, C., et al. (2021). ICD-11 Complex Post Traumatic Stress Disorder (CPTSD) in parents with perinatal bereavement: Implications for treatment and care. *Midwifery* 96: 102947. https://doi.org/10.1016/j.midw.2021.102947.

Access the information services within your university or place of work and download the above-referenced research paper.

Activity 2.1b

Read the Hollins Martin et al. (2021) paper and attempt to answer the following questions:

(1) What is the focus of this research paper?
(2) Do the authors present a reason for undertaking this piece of research?
(3) What is the aim of the research? (usually immediately before methods section).
(4) How was the data collected?
(5) Who or what makes up the sample?
(6) Are there clear inclusion and exclusion criteria?
(7) How are the results presented, e.g. tables, bar graphs, pie charts, and percentages?
(8) What is the most important result?
(9) What is the conclusion of the study?
(10) What questions does this study raise for professional practice and further study?

Theory

↓

Hypotheses

↓

Observations

↓

Confirmation

FIGURE 2.1   Premise of quantitative research.

2.3 MORE ABOUT THE (QUALITATIVE) INDUCTIVE APPROACH

Qualitative Research
Qualitative research aims to understand the processes which lie behind patterns of behaviour, people's emotions, or their responses to certain situations. It uses different ways of collecting data, e.g. the words and phrases people use in interviews and focus groups and employs specialized nonmathematical analysis. Choosing the correct method to address a research question involves many considerations, such as medical ethics, patient acceptability, number of patients required, and whether it is likely to produce a clear answer.

In contrast to quantitative research, a qualitative inductive approach can be taken by researchers. Inductive reasoning works the other way around from the quantitative approach, moving from specific observations to broader generalizations and theories. This is sometimes informally called the 'bottom-up' approach. In inductive reasoning, specific observations are taken from the data, from which the researcher detects patterns and regularities, which are captured in themes (categories) and subthemes (subcategories). From the resulting themes (categories), the researcher can then formulate tentative hypotheses, draw general conclusions, and develop underpinning theories (see Figure 2.2).

These two methods of quantitative (deductive) and qualitative (inductive) reasoning have a very different 'feel' to them. Inductive reasoning, by its very nature, is open-ended and exploratory. Whilst, in contrast, deductive reasoning is narrow in nature and is concerned with testing or confirming hypotheses. Even though a particular study may look like it is straightforwardly deductive (e.g. an experiment designed to test the effects of a treatment upon a specified outcome), most research is triangulated to use both methods. As such, triangulation combines both qualitative inductive and quantitative deductive reasoning processes at the same time within one project. This is illustrated in the paper you read in *Activity 1*, which incorporates both a quantitative (survey) and qualitative thematic analysis. The difference is quantitative deductive data can demonstrate a relationship between two variables using numbers, which will not explain cause and effect, feelings, and thoughts underpinning relationships. In fact, it is not difficult to observe that the two illustrations (Figures 2.1 and 2.2) can be assembled into a single circular one, which continually cycles from theories down to observations and back up again to theories. Even in the most controlled experiment, the researcher may observe deductive patterns in the numerical quantitative data, which leads them to develop qualitatively informed new theories.

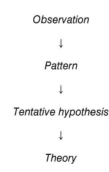

Observation

↓

Pattern

↓

Tentative hypothesis

↓

Theory

FIGURE 2.2   Premise of qualitative research.

Qualitative research is:

1. Interpretive.

2. Reflective.

3. Inductive.

4. Data collection and analysis are often concurrent.

Examples of qualitative research methods (recipes) include, e.g. grounded theory (Birks and Mills 2023), ethnography (O'Reilly 2012), phenomenology (Smith et al. 2009), and discourse analysis (Paltridge 2021), to name but a few.

Activity 2.2a

An example of a *qualitative* study, which follows the research method called interpretative phenomenological analysis (IPA) is:

Norris, G., Hollins Martin, C.J., Dickson, A. (2020). An exploratory interpretative phenomenological analysis (IPA) of childbearing women's perceptions of risk associated with having a high body mass index (BMI). *Midwifery* 89 (2020): 102789. https://doi.org/10.1016/j.midw.2020.102789

Access the information services within your university or place of work and download the above-referenced research paper.

Activity 2.2b

Read the Norris et al. (2020) paper and attempt to answer the following questions:

(1) What is the focus of this research paper?
(2) Do the authors present a reason for undertaking this piece of research?
(3) What is the aim of the research? (usually immediately before methods section).
(4) How was the data collected?
(5) Who or what makes up the sample?
(6) Are there clear inclusion and exclusion criteria?
(7) How are the results presented?
(8) What is the most important finding?
(9) What questions does this study raise for professional practice and further study?

Table 2.1 presents a summary of the main differences between quantitative (deductive) and qualitative (inductive) research methods.

Table 2.1 Summary of the main differences between quantitative and qualitative research methods.

Quantitative (deductive)	Qualitative (inductive)
Reductionist – one answer	Holistic – Many answers
Deals with absolutes – same for all	Individual context important
Objective – researcher is detached from participants Exerts no influence on participant responses	Subjective – researcher interacts with participants Inevitably influences participant responses
Many participants	Few participants
Interested in findings that apply to many	Interested in personal meaning
Produces accurate replicable findings	Produces diversity in answers
Numerical data that supports/rejects hypothesis	Produces many themes from the data
Predicts findings	No prediction of findings made

2.4 THE QUALITATIVE VERSUS QUANTITATIVE DEBATE

There has probably been more energy spent debating the differences between and relative advantages of whether to use qualitative (inductive) or quantitative (deductive) research methods (recipes), compared with almost any other topic in research. The 'qualitative versus quantitative debate' is a hot-button issue which almost invariably triggers intense debate. This contest is 'much ado about nothing'. To say that one or the other approach is 'superior', is simply trivializing a far more complicated issue than a dichotomous debate can settle. Both quantitative (deductive) and qualitative (inductive) approaches originate from a variety of traditions and disciplines. Both approaches can be employed to address almost any research topic. In fact, there is value in consciously combining both qualitative and quantitative approaches in mixed methods or triangulation projects, dependent upon what the researcher wants to find out and what the research question(s) are.

2.5 THE DIFFERENCE(S) BETWEEN QUALITATIVE AND QUANTITATIVE DATA

It is possible to argue that there is little difference between qualitative and quantitative data. This is because qualitative data typically consists of words, whilst quantitative data comprises of numbers. Both could be viewed to fundamentally not differ from one another for the following reason(s).

2.5.1 ALL QUALITATIVE DATA CAN BE CODED QUANTITATIVELY

Anything that is qualitative can be assigned meaningful numerical values. These values can then be manipulated to help achieve greater insight into the meaning of the data and to help examine specific hypotheses. Consider the following example. Many surveys have one or more short open-ended questions that ask the respondent to supply written responses. The simplest example is after a question on a scale that is responded to on a 1–10 Likert scale; there is often added a 'please add any additional comments' section. Any written responses are individual and personal and therefore categorized as qualitative. Such responses can be classified into categories and a short label that represents the theme allocated.

This simple act of categorizing similar responses placed by a number of participants can be viewed as quantitative as well as qualitative. For instance, a researcher develops five themes that respondents provided in the open-ended responses of a survey questionnaire. If there were 10 respondents, a simple coding table like the one in Table 2.2 may be set up to represent the coding of the participants' 10 responses into five themes. This is qualitative thematic coding of the data gathered.

Please note the same data may be analyzed quantitatively, as displayed in Table 2.3.

Table 2.3 illustrates the exact same data as Table 2.2. The first represents qualitative coding, whilst the second represents quantitative coding. The quantitative coding provides additional useful information, which makes it possible for the researcher to undertake statistical analyses that could not be done with just qualitative coding. For instance, from Tables 1.2 and 1.3, Theme 3 was the most frequently mentioned, with all respondents stating 2 or 3 of the themes. The point being made is that the line between qualitative and quantitative research methods (recipes) is less distinct than perhaps you previously thought. All qualitative data can be quantitatively coded in a variety of ways, which does not detract from the personal qualitative information provided. Researchers can carry out many types of analyses on both qualitative and quantitative data gathered, which opens new possibilities for interpretation of the data.

Table 2.2 Inducing themes from the data (qualitative approach).

Participant	Theme 1	Theme 2	Theme 3	Theme 4	Theme 5
1	✓		✓		
2		✓	✓	✓	
3			✓		✓
4	✓			✓	
5	✓				
6			✓		✓
7		✓		✓	
8	✓		✓		
9			✓	✓	
10	✓	✓	✓		

Table 2.3 Deducing numbers from the data (quantitative approach).

Participant	Theme 1	Theme 2	Theme 3	Theme 4	Theme 5	TOTAL
1	①		①			2
2		①	①	①		3
3			①		①	2
4	①			①		2
5	①					1
6			①		①	2
7		①		①		2
8	①		①			2
9			①	①		2
10	①	①	①			3
TOTAL	5	3	7	4	2	

2.5.2 ALL QUANTITATIVE DATA IS BASED ON QUALITATIVE JUDGEMENTS

Numbers cannot be interpreted without understanding the assumptions which underlie them. For example, take a simple 1–5 rating scale:

Question (1) Punishment is the best way to deal with adolescent smokers.

	Strongly Agree	Agree	Neither Agree or Disagree	Disagree	Strongly Disagree
Scores	5	4	3	2	1

In the example above, the participant responded to the Likert scale by underscoring the numeric of 2 (Disagree). What does this mean? In other words, how does the researcher interpret the value of 2 the participant underlined? To interpret this quantitative numerical value, the researcher requires to uncover the judgements and assumptions of the participant, which underpin their response:

1. Did the participant understand the term punishment?

2. Did the participant understand that a '2' means that they are disagreeing with the statement placed above?

3. Does the participant have any idea about alternatives to punishment (otherwise how can they judge what is best?

4. Did the participant read the question carefully enough to determine that the statement was limited only to 'addicted smokers' and how was this term defined?

5. Does the participant care or were they just circling anything arbitrarily?

6. How was this question presented in the context of the survey (i.e. did the questions immediately before bias the response in any way)?

7. Was the participant mentally alert (especially if this question was presented last in a long survey, or the respondent had other things to attend to simultaneously)?

8. What was the setting whilst the participant was completing the survey (e.g. lighting, noise, and other distractions)?

9. Was the survey anonymous and confidential?

10. In the participant's mind, is the difference between a 1 and a 2 the same as between a 2 and 3 (i.e. is this an interval scale)?

The point being made is all numerical information involves numerous judgements about what the number means. Quantitative and qualitative data are at some level virtually inseparable. Neither exists in a vacuum nor can be considered totally devoid of the other. To ask which is the better research approach, or more valid, ignores the intimate connection between the two camps. To undertake a quality research project, both qualitative and quantitative methods may be required.

2.6 QUALITATIVE AND QUANTITATIVE ASSUMPTIONS

What are the most common myths about the differences between qualitative and quantitative research? Many researchers believe the following:

- Quantitative research is *confirmatory* and *deductive* in nature.

- Qualitative research is *exploratory* and *inductive* in nature.

There is some truth in each of these statements. In general, a lot of quantitative research tends to be *confirmatory* and *deductive* (reduced to one answer). But there is lots of quantitative research that can be classified as *exploratory* as well. And while much qualitative research does tend to be *exploratory*, it can also be used to confirm very specific *deductive* hypotheses. The problem is that these statements do not acknowledge the richness of both traditions. They do not recognize that both qualitative and quantitative research can be used to address almost any kind of research question. So, if the difference between qualitative and quantitative is not along the *exploratory–confirmatory* or *inductive–deductive* dimensions, then where is it? The *quantitative* or *qualitative* debate is philosophical, not methodological.

For instance, many qualitative researchers believe that the best way to understand any phenomenon is to view it in its context. For some qualitative researchers, the best way to understand what is going on is to become immersed in the situation. Move into the culture or organization that is being studied and experience what it is like to be a part of it. It is important that the researcher is flexible in their inquiry of people in context. Rather than approaching measurement with the idea of constructing a fixed instrument or set of questions, allow the questions to emerge as the researcher becomes familiar with what they are studying. Many qualitative researchers also operate using different assumptions about the world. They do not assume that there is a single unitary reality apart from our perceptions. Each person experiences from their own point of view, a different reality. Conducting research without taking this into account violates the fundamental view of the individual. Consequently, the qualitative researcher may be opposed to methods that attempt to aggregate across individuals on the grounds that each person is unique. They also argue that the researcher is a unique individual and that all research is essentially biased by each researcher's individual perceptions. There is no point in trying to establish validity in any external or objective sense. All that the researcher can hope to do is interpret a view of the world as they perceive it.

Any researcher steeped in the qualitative tradition would certainly take issue with comments about the similarities between quantitative and qualitative data. They would argue that it is not possible to separate their research assumptions from the data. Some would claim that a person's perspective on data is based on assumptions common to the quantitative tradition. Others would argue that it does not matter if you can code data thematically or quantitatively because they would not do either. Both forms of analysis impose artificial structure on the phenomena and consequently introduce distortions and biases. In fact, it is better to see the point on both sides of the qualitative–quantitative debate.

In the end, people who consider themselves primarily qualitative or primarily quantitative researchers tend to be almost as diverse as those from the opposing camps. In either camp, there is intense and fundamental disagreement about both philosophical assumptions and the nature of data. Albeit, increasingly more researchers are interested in blending the two traditions in attempts to gain advantages of each. There is no resolution to this debate and social research is richer for the wider variety of views and methods that the debate generates.

Activity 2.3

(1) Consider the area within midwifery practice, which you are both interested in and consider to have been under researched. (*Chapter 1 Activity 1.1*)

(2) Justify why either a quantitative (deductive) or qualitative (inductive) approach would be the best way of answering your research question(s).

2.6.1 CHAPTER CONCLUSION

Chapter 2 intended to develop your understanding of the differences between qualitative (inductive) and quantitative (deductive) approaches to carrying out research. Now that you have developed greater appreciation of the 16 STEPS involved in developing a research proposal, *Chapter 3* will now elaborate on STEP 5, which addresses how to construct an introduction to your research proposal which contains a literature review and relevant rationale. As you progress through *Chapter 3*, you will learn about the different types of literature review and their individual purpose. You will also learn the importance of appraising research papers for inclusion or exclusion in your literature review. You will also be introduced to established tools for carrying out evaluation of individual primary research papers. Again to test and develop your understanding, we now list some more *self-assessment questions (SAQs)*.

2.7   SELF-ASSESSMENT QUESTIONS (SAQs)

Please circle the answer you think is most applicable.

2.1   Quantitative researchers:

  (a)   Focus on individuals behaving in their natural environments.

  (b)   Empathize with the participants' point of view.

  (c)   Take a holistic approach to persons.

  (d)   Test clear-cut hypotheses using purpose-built measuring tools.

2.2   Which of the following is not characteristic of qualitative methods?

  (a)   Few participants

  (b)   Inductive

  (c)   Prediction of findings

  (d)   Subjective

2.3   Which of the following professional disciplines are more likely to utilize qualitative research methods?

  (a)   Pharmacists

  (b)   Anthropologists

  (c)   Geneticists

  (d)   Neurologists

2.4   A midwife is interested in the effects of a drug on a Urinary Tract Infection (UTI). The research method they are likely to select is:

  (a)   A quantitative study, i.e. a randomized controlled trial (RCT).

  (b)   A qualitative study, i.e. phenomenology.

  (c)   Interviews.

  (d)   A holistic approach.

2.5   Which of the following is an example of quantitative research:

  (a)   A social worker forms a support group for school truants and writes about its success at improving school attendance.

  (b)   A radiographer spends a day in a wheelchair and writes-up a report of their experiences.

  (c)   A midwife compares two rival methods of treatment to reduce pain during labour.

  (d)   A podiatrist lives with an African tribe for the purpose of finding out about their approach to footwear and care.

ANSWERS TO CHAPTER 2 SAQs

2.1   **d**

2.2   **c**

2.3   **b**

2.4   **a**

2.5   **c**

Literature Searching and How to Critique a Research Paper

STEP (5): Construct an introduction that contains a relevant literature review and rationale.

3.1 DEFINE THE TERM LITERATURE REVIEW

The creation of a literature review is one of the most challenging and important tasks faced by a researcher. The process requires use of many skills, which include a systematic library search, logical arrangement of information, and quality academic writing. Before researchers commence a study, they are required to retrieve and read what previous related studies have discovered in relation to the topic of interest. The role of a good literature review is to present applicable findings from prior research studies and logically arrange their conclusions in a way that enlightens readers about what research has preceded the study you want to undertake. As a student, you may not be planning to carry out an actual research study, yet you are still required to learn the skills involved in undertaking a literature review that can be used to evidence-based your clinical practice as a midwife.

3.2 OUTLINE THE PURPOSE OF RESEARCH

The first step is to prepare an outline of the research study, alternatively known as the research proposal. As such, this process enables the researcher to clarify structure for the ethics committee, which assess appropriateness of fact conducting the study. The acceptance of the research proposal (recipe) by the ethics committee is a precondition to conducting the study. Post acceptance, this template is the document the research team and clinicians work from. The research proposal is a clear recipe outlining:

Research Recipes for Midwives, First Edition. Caroline J. Hollins Martin.
© 2024 John Wiley & Sons Ltd. Published 2024 by John Wiley & Sons Ltd.

(1) What the researcher intends to do.
(2) Why they intend to do it.
(3) How they intend to do it.
(4) When they intend to complete.

3.3 WHAT IS A LITERATURE REVIEW?

As part of a research proposal, the literature review is the synopsis of the total present state of knowledge on the chosen topic as found in reports from prior published research studies (the literature). There are several reasons why a literature review may be conducted:

a. As an assignment to assess a module whilst undertaking a degree at university.

b. As a dissertation in final year of a degree program of study.

c. To provide evidence that underpins a professional practice guideline or protocol.

d. As an introduction to a project.

e. As preparation for a subsequent research study.

f. As part of writing a research proposal.

3.4 WHAT IS THE PURPOSE OF A LITERATURE REVIEW?

1. To provide the reader with information about an identified topic. The researcher selects high-quality relevant published papers and summarizes their findings into one complete report.

2. To provide a starting point for researchers beginning to undertake an investigation into a specific area of interest.

3. To enlighten the reader of research that has already been conducted, which will prevent duplication and allow identification of areas where published papers are scarce.

4. To direct the researcher's focus.

5. To highlight key findings.

6. To emphasize inconsistencies, gaps, and contradictions in prior research evidence.

7. To accommodate constructive appraisal of processes involved in prior research studies.

One way to understand the format of a literature review is to retrieve one from the library, read it, and observe the steps in process it follows. There are different types of research methods (recipes) a literature review may follow (e.g. narrative literature review, systematic review, and metanalytic review). The literature review method (recipe) selected is dependent upon the purpose of the research proposal you are writing and what research method you intend to use. For example, a narrative review is more suited to undertaking a qualitative study, whilst a systematic review will precede carrying out a randomized controlled trial (RCT).

3.5 WHAT SHOULD A LITERATURE REVIEW CONSIST OF?

3.5.1 INTRODUCTION

The introduction explains the focus of the literature review and establishes its worth. A discussion is then presented of the kind of work that has been done before on the topic of interest. Any controversies in relation to research approaches used (e.g. qualitative versus quantitative) or research method selected, will be identified. Each study may be ranked for value using tools such as the critical appraisal skills programme checklists (CASP 2018).

Table 3.1 CASP checklist for qualitative studies.

(1)	Was there a clear statement of the aims of the research?
(2)	Is a qualitative methodology appropriate?
(3)	Was the research design appropriate to address the aims of the research?
(4)	Was the recruitment strategy appropriate to the aims of the research?
(5)	Was the research collected in a way that addressed the research issue?
(6)	Has the relationship between research and participants been adequately considered?
(7)	Have ethical issues been taken into consideration?
(8)	Was the data analysis sufficiently rigorous?
(9)	Is there a clear statement of findings?
(10)	How valuable is the research?

Table 3.2 CASP checklist for a Cohort Study.

(1)	Did the study address a clearly focussed issue?
(2)	Was the cohort recruited in an acceptable way?
(3)	Was the exposure accurately measured to minimize bias?
(4)	Was the outcome accurately measured to minimize bias?
(5a)	Have the authors identified all important confounding factors?
(5b)	Have they taken account of the confounding factors in the design and/or analysis?
(6a)	Was the follow-up of subjects complete enough?
(6b)	Was the follow-up of subjects long enough?
(7)	What are the results of the study?
(8)	How precise are the results?
(9)	Do you believe the results?
(10)	Can the results be applied to the local population?
(11)	Do the results of this study fit with other available evidence?
(12)	What are the implications of this study for practice?

(see Tables 3.1 and 3.2 for examples). Such checklist consists of questions for consideration when assessing quality of each primary study being scrutinized. Such checklists guide the researcher to consistently assess each published primary research paper identified in the literature review.

The purpose of the review should be clearly stated, along with where the findings took the researcher next.

3.5.2 BODY

The body of a literature review should contain headings and subheadings. A summary of an evaluation of the present state of knowledge in the research area under question is presented. Major themes or topics identified, along with trends and findings about what researchers agree or disagree upon. If the review is preliminary to a reader's own research project, the purpose is to make an argument that will justify the study they propose. In essence, a review should only discuss research that leads directly to a project.

3.5.3 CONCLUSION

The conclusion summarizes the evidence presented and should explain its significance. If the review is an introduction to a research study, it should highlight gaps in the literature and indicate how previous research led to the proposed project and selected research methodology. If the review is a stand-alone article, it should suggest some practical applications along with implications and possibilities for future research should be suggested.

Providing a Background to the Study (Literature Review)

Without a sound background, a study's worth in terms of contribution to the body of knowledge becomes shaky. The background is the review of related literature (literature review) in which prior studies support the main claim of the research study you wish to carry out. Through presenting a review of literature that relates to the research question, the researcher builds an argument for the relevance of conducting the study. This review of the literature provides a foundation to the research study, creating a root to the worth of the research question and its relationship to what is already known.

Justification for Carrying Out the Project and Expected Gains (Rationale)

The rationale is the reason for conducting the study. For example, a rationale for conducting a particular research study may be:

Example rationale for conducting a research study:
Midwives, researchers, and policymakers are concerned about the role of healthcare professionals in role modelling smoking to child-bearing women whom they are expected to support with smoking cessation. Research that focuses upon psychological evaluations of the effectiveness of role modelling behaviours of healthcare professionals in relation to influencing smoking behaviours is explained in the literature review, followed by evidence that smoking is harmful, and why in the context of interest. For example:

- Causing foetal growth retardation
- Causing artery damage in diabetics
- Causing cancer
- Placing the obese at risk

3.6 STEPS INVOLVED IN WRITING A LITERATURE REVIEW

1. Identify a topic of interest (select an area of research that is due for review).

2. Using relevant keywords search the databases and electronic journals. Reference lists at the back of articles can also lead to valuable papers.

3. Include studies that support and oppose your view (both qualitative and quantitative).

4. Keep a narrow focus and select papers accordingly (apply inclusion and exclusion criteria)

5. Read the selected articles thoroughly and evaluate them using tools (e.g. CASP tools [CASP 2018]).

6. Identify assumptions that researchers are making.

7. Critically discuss the research methods used.

8. Draw conclusions.

9. Identify conflicting theories, methods, and findings.

10. Observe how theories change over time.

11. Organize the papers into themes and subthemes, e.g. in terms of common findings, trends, and most convincing theories.

12. Write a statement that summarizes the conclusion reached about trends and developments identified.

13. Organize the paper into headings and subheadings. On a cleared table surface place post-it notes to organize findings into categories. Take a look at a published paper and see how the researcher organized it. For example:
    - Patterson et al. (2019) for a systematic review.
    - Hollins Martin et al. (2019) for a scoping review.

14. Write the body of the paper. Follow the plan developed ensuring each section links logically to the one before and after. Sections should be divided by themes (not by the work of individual researchers).

15. Focus on analysis and not description.

16. Thoroughly proofread the paper and ensure it is error free. Make sure all the references are present and follow the journal's house style.

The literature review should contain:

(1) *Introduction*
   (1a) An introduction explains the focus of the review and establishes its worth.
   (1b) A discussion of the kind of work previously published on the subject, which identifies any controversies in relation to approach, findings, or method.
   (1c) The purpose of the review should be clearly stated, along with how findings could possibly lead to a research question.

(2) *Body (The body should contain headings/subheadings)*
   (2a) A summary of the literature reviewing method used.
   (2b) An evaluation of the present state of knowledge in the research area under question.
   (2c) Major themes or topics identified, along with trends and findings about what researchers agree or disagree upon.

(3) *Conclusion*
   (3a) Summarizes the evidence presented and explain its significance.
   (3b) Highlight gaps in the literature and indicate potential for a research project.
   (3c) Suggest some practical applications along with implications and possibilities for future research.

To view a paper that has used a Scoping Review method (recipe) to explore prior published literature (see Activity 3.1).

Activity 3.1

Download the following scoping review and read it:

Hollins Martin, C.J., and Reid, K. (2022). A scoping review of therapies used to treat psychological trauma post perinatal bereavement. *Journal of Reproductive and Infant Psychology*. https://doi.org/10.1080/02646838.2021.2021477.

The following summary displays the steps involved in the process of writing the Hollins Martin and Reid (2022) *scoping review*:

Phases involved in writing the Hollins Martin and Reid (2022) *scoping review* (could not get a textbox around this)

(1) *Introduction*
   (1a) *An introduction explains the focus of the review and establishes its worth.*
     - This paper tells us that the focus is on perinatal death and examples of the proportion that occur each year.
     - An explanation of the relationship between perinatal death and the percentage of women who experience subsequent Post-traumatic stress disorder (PTSD) is provided.
     - The features of PTSD are clearly defined to emphasize the importance of suffering that women may experience post having a perinatal death.

(1b) *A discussion of the kind of work previously published on the subject, which identifies any controversies in relation to approach, findings, or method.*

- The fact that many women who have experienced perinatal death proceed to develop PTSD, emphasizes the value of providing psychological therapy/treatment.
- Many references are provided to demonstrate the effectiveness of using a variety of trauma treatments in other contexts. For example, the effectiveness of cognitive behavioural therapy (CBT) and eye movement desensitization and Reprocessing (EMDR) for treating PTSD post-rape, childhood abuse, post-combat, or car accident.

(1c) *The purpose of the review should be clearly stated, along with how findings could possibly lead to a research question.*

- *Purpose*: Delivering treatment for PTSD post perinatal bereavement is important because it impairs social interaction and capacity to work. Examples of symptoms experienced include reexperiencing the trauma event in the form of nightmares, flashbacks, continual replay, intrusive thoughts, and images.
- *Lead to research question*: Hence, the aim of advancing treatments for women who have developed PTSD post perinatal bereavement is important.
- *Aim leading to research question stated later*: To determine potential content of a treatment package, the aim of this scoping review was to identify what therapies have already been used to treat psychological trauma post perinatal bereavement.

(2) *Body (The body should contain headings/subheadings.)*

(2a) *A summary of the literature reviewing method used.*

- A *scoping review* was selected because the aim was to map the variety of treatments that have been used in the past to treat psychological trauma post perinatal bereavement. The intention was not to describe findings in detail but instead map treatments that have previously addressed this area of interest. In addition, a *scoping review* was selected as it allows the author to include research studies that have used a wide range of research methods (recipes). The stages of Arksey and O'Malley (2005) were followed:

  (1) *Identifying the research question*
  What research has evaluated effectiveness of therapies used to treat psychological trauma post perinatal bereavement?

  (2) *Identifying relevant studies*
  Studies were identified via electronic databases (MEDLINE, CINAHL, APA PsycInfo, and Cochrane Library), reference lists, and hand searching of key journals. A combined free text and thesaurus approach identified relevant papers for inclusion. In addition, the search terms used are declared.

  (3) *Study selection*
  The inclusion and exclusion criteria for studies to be included in the scoping review are stated.

  (4) *Charting the data*
  Papers reviewed were sifted, recorded, and organized into themes according to trauma treatments used to treat traumatized postnatal women. Two researchers validated and agreed the choice of papers, which was finalized at 23. A PRISMA diagram is included (see https://prisma-statement.org/prismastatement/flowdiagram.aspx).

  (5) *Collating, summarizing, and reporting results*
  As this was a *scoping review*, no 'weighting' of evidence was carried out using critical appraisal tools. Both validators (authors) agreed the 10 categories of trauma treatments identified.

(2b) *An evaluation of the present state of knowledge in the research area under question.*

- Due to the dearth of research that has been carried out in the area of PTSD post perinatal bereavement, the net has been widened to understand the 'lay of the land' of prior therapies used to treat psychological trauma post perinatal bereavement.

(2c) *Major themes or topics identified, along with trends and findings about what researchers agree or disagree upon*
Ten treatments for psychological trauma were identified in this paper, and their success evaluated.
Treatment 1: CBT
Treatment 2: EMDR
Treatment 3: Debriefing
Treatment 4: Counselling

        Treatment 5: Expressive writing
        Treatment 6: Self-help materials
        Treatment 7: Family support programme
        Treatment 8: Tetris
        Treatment 9: Yoga
        Treatment 10: Compassion focused therapy (CFT)

(3) *Conclusion*

    (3a) *Summarize the evidence presented and explains its significance.*

        Few papers have directly addressed perinatal bereavement, and so the scope of the review was broadened to include treatments used to treat psychological trauma post childbirth. Out of the 23 studies that reported on effectiveness of therapies used to treat psychological trauma post childbirth, only four focused upon treating *PTSD* post perinatal bereavement, with three therapies found to be effective and one ineffective. Two studies reported that CBT was effective at reducing *PTSD* symptoms post miscarriage, termination for medical reasons, and stillbirth. One study showed that four sessions of grief counselling reduced trauma symptoms post stillbirth ($n = 50$), and one other study showed that online yoga was ineffective at reducing symptoms of PTSD post experiencing a stillbirth.

    (3b) *Highlight gaps in the literature and indicate potential for a research project.*

        This paper found 23 papers that have reported treatments used to treat PTSD post childbirth. These papers were themed into 10 therapies, with only four reporting on therapies used specifically to treat perinatal bereavement. Three treatments were found to be effective and one ineffective. Out of the three effective therapies, one consisted of four grief-counselling sessions, and the other two effectiveness of CBT. All studies were low in participant numbers and consisted of only brief descriptions of the interventions. Hence, it is very important that new therapies are developed to test and treat PTSD that develops in the context of perinatal bereavement.

    (3c) *Suggest some practical applications along with implications and possibilities for future research.*

        Clearly, further research is required to develop and test therapies specifically designed to treat PTSD that develops in women who have experienced perinatal bereavement.

Source: Adapted from Hollins Martin and Reid (2022).

Having followed the processes involved in writing the Hollins Martin and Reid (2022) *scoping review*, it is important to note that there are many other types of literature reviews. The method (recipe) for each one of these varies slightly, with examples listed as follows:

- Scoping review

- Narrative review

- Systematic review.

- Meta-analysis

    When a researcher undertakes any form of literature review, the process involves four stages.

3.7 OUTLINE THE FOUR STAGES OF DEVELOPING A LITERATURE REVIEW

Learning how to determine the relevance and authority of a given resource for research is one of the core skills of the research process. Developing a literature review involves surveying scholarly articles, books, and other relevant sources (e.g. dissertations and conference proceedings) and providing a description, summary, and critical evaluation of each piece of work.

Four stages involved in developing a literature review
(STAGE 1) Clearly outline the topic being examined and its component issues.
(STAGE 2) Conduct the literature search, which involves a description of how you found the materials relevant to the subject being explored.
(STAGE 3) Carry out an evaluation of the literature and explain how it makes a significant contribution to understanding the topic.
(STAGE 4) Provide an analysis and discussion of the findings and conclusions of the most pertinent literature.

(STAGE 1) Clearly outline the topic being examined and its component issues.

The first stage in writing a research paper is deciding on a topic. Next, write down some ideas and keywords you might use to describe the topic. Then state your topic as a question. For example, if you are interested in finding out the drinking habits of student midwives and their effects upon attendance at university and clinical placements, you might ask the following question:

What are the drinking habits of student midwives and their related effects upon attendance at university and clinical placements?

It is important to have more than one idea. The topic of choice may narrow, broaden, or even change as the researcher progresses through the literature review.

3.7.1 SETTING THE TOPIC IN CONTEXT

A simple description of the relevant situation informs the reader of where the study intends to go. The main concepts under discussion should be described. Do not make assumptions that the reader understands work-related language used in midwifery practice, and therefore define all terms of language used and provide references to support. What follows is an example of how to generate a topic for your research study.

An example of how to generate a topic for your research study

(a) An area or topic of interest:
  e.g. Drinking habits of student midwives'
(b) Idea you wish to explore in detail:
  e.g. Drinking habits of student midwives' compared with other student groups
(c) Problem detected and requiring a solution:
  e.g. Drinking habits of student midwives' and their constructs of the effects of alcohol consumption on their health
(d) Question arising from experience or reading literature:
  e.g. Why do student midwives' drink alcohol?
(e) Clearly state the nature of the problem and its estimated extent:
  e.g. A literature review should be presented to answer your stated question.
(f) Locate the research question to the context studied:
  e.g. Are student midwives' drinking habits influenced by their knowledge of the negative effects of consuming alcohol?

(STAGE 2) Conduct the literature search, which involves a description of how you found the materials relevant to the subject being explored.

3.7.2 LOOKING AT INFORMATION SOURCES, E.G. SEARCH TOOLS

People looking for scholarly information may be confused about where to start. Relevant items are usually found in library catalogues, databases, and online journal subscriptions.

The university school librarian usually organizes sessions that teach the student midwife how to search for relevant research papers within the systems organized in your particular institution. Post writing the literature review question, it is necessary to identify:

3.7.3 WHAT DATABASES YOU ARE GOING TO SEARCH

Studies may be identified via electronic databases such as MEDLINE, CINAHL, APA PsycInfo, or the Cochrane Library. In addition, you can search reference lists at the back of research papers you have retrieved and through hand-searching relevant journals.

3.7.4 IDENTIFYING RELEVANT STUDIES USING PREDECIDED SEARCH TERMS

For example, a combined free text and thesaurus approach can be used to identify relevant papers for inclusion in your literature review. In relation to the Hollins Martin and Reid (2022) scoping review, the following search terms were used:

Search terms used in the Hollins Martin and Reid (2022) scoping review
('Post-traumatic stress disorder' OR 'stress disorders, post-traumatic' OR 'stress, psychological' OR 'complex post-traumatic stress disorder' OR 'complex PTSD' OR 'life change events' OR 'psychological trauma' OR 'psychotherapy events' OR 'psychological trauma' OR psychotherapy) AND (birth OR childbirth) (N5 trauma*) OR (birth OR childbirth) (N5 fear) OR (childbirth OR child birth OR labour OR 'delivery, obstetric' OR 'pregnancy complications' OR caesarean OR stillbirth OR bereavement OR 'perinatal death') AND SU (treatment or intervention or therapy). No date limit was selected, and 'clinical queries' was set to 'therapy-high specificity'. Studies required to be written in English.

(STAGE 3) Carry out an evaluation of the literature and explain how it makes a significant contribution to understanding the topic.

3.7.5 USING INFORMATION SOURCES

Begin evaluating the papers you have identified that relate to your literature review question. (e.g. research papers, books, and professional articles). Appraise the source by first examining the references cited. Reference citations characteristically have three main components: author, title, and publication information. These components can facilitate determining the usefulness of the source. In the same way as appraising a website by examining its home page. To help guide you through 'what' to appraise.

What to Appraise?

It is important to set out *inclusion criteria*. For example, in the Hollins Martin and Reid (2022) scoping review, the *inclusion criteria* for studies included research studies:

- That addressed therapies used to treat psychological trauma post childbirth.

- That addressed therapies used to treat psychological trauma post perinatal bereavement.

- That fit into the World Health Organization (WHO) definition of perinatal period, which is defined as an infant loss commencing at 22 completed weeks (154 days) gestation to seven completed days post childbirth (WHO 2021).

- That report on a therapeutic intervention used to treat women experiencing psychological trauma post perinatal bereavement or childbirth.

- That report on participants who have experienced *acute stress disorder (ASD)*, *post-traumatic stress syndrome* (PTSS), PTSD, and *Complex* PTSD.

- That are published in English, which is the international evidence-based language used.

- That are full-text paper and available for review.

    In addition, exclusion criteria are cited. In the Hollins-Martin and Reid paper, no exclusion criteria were applied. Next, the researcher *charts the data*, which involves citing the final number of selected papers in a table that reports the key themes identified. Papers identified as not fitting with the inclusion criteria are eradicated as illustrated in a PRISMA diagram (PRISMA 2020). The inclusion and exclusion criteria can be presented in a table, with a rationale provided. To view examples of inclusion and exclusion criteria and rationales (see Table 3.3).

Table 3.3 Inclusion and exclusion criteria.

Feature	Inclusion criteria	Exclusion criteria	Rationale
Year of publication	Studies post, e.g. 1990	Studies prior to 1990	Provide rationale
Language of publication	English	Any other languages	Author not fluent in any languages other than English
Language	English	Any other language	To enable understanding from an international perspective
Type of research	Primary research	Non-primary research	To only examine primary research in this field
Quality of study	Peer-reviewed	Non-peer reviewed	To ensure only quality primary studies are assessed
Study assessment of topic area	Meets a referenced criteria	Does not meet the referenced criteria	To examine research that uses consistent criteria for assessment of PTSD
Methodology	Any qualitative, quantitative, or mixed methods studies	No restriction	To identify a wide range of primary research
Focus of study			To focus on relevant research based on search question

3.7.6 RESULTS

Results are then reported. For example, a total of 801 papers were identified, with a further five found through hand-searching reference lists of selected papers. After 116 duplicate papers were excluded, 206 were screened, which resulted in 10 being identified for inclusion in the literature review. To view a PRISMA diagram which reports these figures (see Figure 3.1).

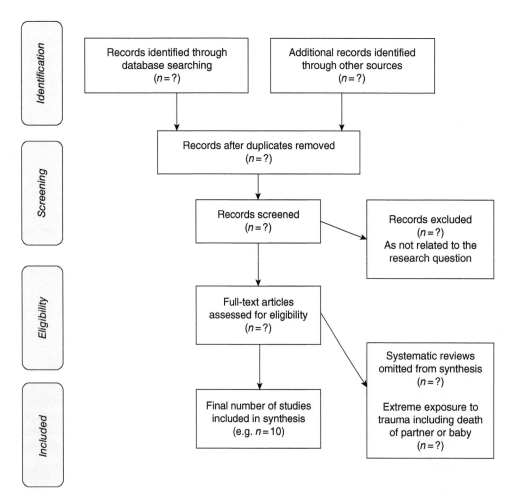

FIGURE 3.1 Prisma Flow Diagram (Moher et al. 2009) (*Source:* permission of Oxford University Press).

Table 3.4 Identified studies for inclusion

	Authors	Date	Method	Participant numbers	Theme 1	Theme 2	Theme 3	Etc.
1								
2								
3 etc.								

The final 10 selected papers are charted in a table. To view an example of how to list identified studies for inclusion (see Table 3.4).

These tables will vary between literature reviews, so take a look at a few examples to compare the differences.

3.7.7 VALIDATION

To validate the results, it is important that a minimum of two researchers undertake the task of including and theming papers independently, with final decisions negotiated and titles agreed upon. Any differences of opinion should be resolved through healthy discussion. These negotiations should lead to eventual consensus about final papers to be included in the literature review and themes that are identified and labelled.

3.7.8 USE OF APPRAISAL TOOLS

Appraisal tools are not used to assess quality of papers in a *scoping review*. However, they are used in systematic reviews. Examples of instruments to guide this process are critical appraisal skills programme (CASP) tools (2022). Two examples follow, with many more available at: www.casp-uk.net

CASP checklist for qualitative studies
(Answer Yes, cannot tell, or no to each of the following questions)

(1) Was there a clear statement of the aims of the research?
(2) Is a qualitative methodology appropriate? Consider
(3) Was the research design appropriate to address the aims of the research?
(4) Was the recruitment strategy appropriate to the aims of the research?
(5) Was the research collected in a way that addressed the research issue?
(6) Has the relationship between research and participants been adequately considered?
(7) Have ethical issues been taken into consideration?
(8) Was the data analysis sufficiently rigorous?
(9) Is there a clear statement of findings?
(10) How valuable is the research?

CASP checklist for Cohort Study
(Answer Yes, cannot tell, or no to each of the following questions)

(1) Did the study address a clearly focussed issue?
(2) Was the cohort recruited in an acceptable way?
(3) Was the exposure accurately measured to minimize bias?
(4) Was the outcome accurately measured to minimize bias?
(5a) Have the authors identified all important confounding factors?
(5b) Have they taken account of the confounding factors in the design and/or analysis?
(6a) Was the follow-up of subjects complete enough?
(6b) Was the follow-up of subjects long enough?
(7) What are the results of the study?
(8) How precise are the results?
(9) Do you believe the results?

(10) Can the results be applied to the local population?

(11) Do the results of this study fit with other available evidence?

(12) What are the implications of this study for practice?

(STAGE 4) Provide an analysis and discussion of the findings and conclusions of the most pertinent literature.

In relation to STAGE 4, there are many other factors that the researcher will focus upon when critiquing the list of finally selected papers for inclusion in the literature review.

3.7.9 THE AUTHOR

Biographical information located in the publication itself will help determine the author's affiliation and credentials. Questions to ask may include:

- What are the author's credentials, institutional affiliation (where he or she works), educational background, past writings, and experience?

- Is the book or article written on a topic in the author's area of expertise?

- Have your lecturers mentioned this author?

- Is the author's name referenced in other literature?

- Is the author associated with a reputable institution?

- What are the basic goals of the organization?

3.7.10 DATE OF PUBLICATION

Topic areas of continuing and rapid development, such as health sciences, demand more current information, whilst topics in the humanities often require material that was written many years ago. You need to provide a rationale for your chosen window of publications (e.g. 1990–present day). Questions to ask may include:

- When was the literature published?

- Is the literature current or out-of-date for your topic?

- Is this a keynote paper in relation to your topic of interest?

3.7.11 EDITION OR REVISION

Is this a first edition of this publication or not? Further editions indicate a source has been revised and updated to reflect changes and omissions in knowledge and synchronize with the reader's up-to-date needs. In addition, many printings or editions may indicate that the work has become a keynote standard source in the area.

3.7.12 PUBLISHER

Note the publisher. If the source is published by a university press, it is likely to be scholarly. Although the fact that the publisher is reputable does not necessarily guarantee quality, it does show that the publisher may have a high regard for the source being published. Objective reasoning is required to answer the following questions:

- Is the information fact, opinion, or propaganda?

Does the information appear to be valid and well-researched or is it questionable and unsupported by evidence?

- Is the author's point of view objective and impartial?

- Is the language free of emotion-arousing words and bias?

Coverage

You should explore enough sources to obtain a variety of viewpoints.

- Is the material primary or secondary in nature?

Primary research is standalone research studies reported in a single paper.

Secondary research is based on several primary research studies. What we are looking at in this chapter is how to write a literature review, which is a form of *secondary research*.

For example, a literature review is compiled of a viewing of primary studies and may follow the method (recipe) of a scoping review, narrative review, systematic review, or meta-analysis. A literature review is a summary of available research (*primary research*) on a given topic that compares studies based on design and methods. It summarizes the findings of each paper and points out selected aspects (e.g. low participant numbers) or confounding variables that may have been overlooked by the primary author.

Analysis and Discussions of the Findings and Conclusions of Pertinent Literature

Typically, there are three questions to ask about a given piece of research.

a. *Is the study relevant to the question/topic?*

b. *What are the conclusions?*

c. *How well do the findings carry over to settings of interest?*

It is helpful to look at the abstract as it summarizes the entire project. Ask whether the findings appear as though there is value to the paper's overall findings. Look at the tables and figures along with the study results. Consider how well the results relate to other studies on the topic of interest. Read the literature section of each paper and see how they link to the intended study.

3.7.13 CRITIQUING MODELS MAY BE USED TO ANALYSE PRIMARY PAPERS

Critiquing models are often used by researchers. These are guidelines which facilitate the reader to make sense of a paper. For example (see Box 3.1).

BOX 3.1   EXAMPLE OF A CRITIQUING MODEL

(1) What is the focus of the article?
(2) Does the author present a reason for undertaking the research?
(3) Are gaps highlighted within the literature review?
(4) What is the research question?
(5) What is the aim of the research?
(6) What is the research method and is it suitable for purpose?
(7) What tools have been used to collect the data?
(8) Did the study pass through an ethics committee?
(9) Who or what makes up the sample?
(10) Are those in the sample typical or are there elements of bias?
(11) Is the sample size large enough?
(12) Do the results make sense and/or could they have been presented better?
(13) What is the most important result of the study?
(14) What is the conclusion of the study?
(15) Has the research question been answered and the hypothesis accepted/rejected?
(16) What recommendations are made for practice and are they feasible?
(17) Was the study worth publishing?
(18) Are the author's arguments supported by primary material from the literature review?
(19) Is the author's perspective evenhanded or prejudicial (objective)?
(20) Are the author's arguments and conclusions convincing?

Organizing Information

Devoting serious time to planning the literature review is time well spent. An excellent review has a clear logical structure and tells a coherent story. This can be organized in a number of ways. For example:

a. Picking out important themes and listing them under headings.

b. Grouping studies that share the same research approach, i.e. qualitative followed by quantitative studies.

c. Placing the studies in chronological order, i.e. start with the earliest and show how knowledge has developed across time.

It probably requires a minimum of over 10 drafts before a writer has a finished product. A checklist may be used to facilitate the writing of a literature review.

Literature Review Checklist

Once you have completed, your literature review ask yourself the following questions:

I have identified gaps in current knowledge.	YES/NO
I have shown I am building on existing work.	YES/NO
I have shown I am aware of the most important topics and studies.	YES/NO
I have identified areas for future research.	YES/NO
I have identified different viewpoints.	YES/NO
The studies I have included are mostly from primary sources.	YES/NO
The studies I have included directly relate to my research question.	YES/NO
The studies I have included are well-conducted and robust.	YES/NO
The studies I have reported are from peer-reviewed journals.	YES/NO
I have written the literature review in a clear, concise style.	YES/NO
I have used an academic writing style.	YES/NO
I have checked spelling, punctuation, and grammar.	YES/NO

3.7.14 POSITIONING OF THE LITERATURE REVIEW

The literature review is placed after the introduction and before the methods section of the paper. It provides understanding of how existing literature supports, contradicts, and ignites the research question.

3.7.15 WRITING THE LITERATURE REVIEW

The intention is to provide a description, summary, and critical evaluation of each published primary study. The aim is to offer an overview of research studies that relate to the research question. A literature review consists of the following elements:

• An overview of the subject, issue, or theory being considered.

• Division of the retrieved studies into categories (e.g. those in support of a particular position, against those that offer an alternative viewpoint).

• Explanation of how the study is similar or varies from the others.

• A conclusion over how the study contributes to understanding the topic area of interest.

Once you have completed your literature review, the next step is to design your own primary study, which is captured in a research proposal. What follows now is a description of how to write a research proposal.

Designing your own primary research study

The template which follows directs the pathway to follow when designing a research proposal. Look at where the literature review is placed within it.

Template for writing a research proposal

Step (1): Give the research proposal a title.
This should accurately reflect the content of the research study.

Step (2): Provide relevant personal and professional details.
STAFF DETAILS 1 (see *Appendix 1 for Curriculum Vitae* [CV])
Name: (Principal Investigator)
Grade:
Professional certifications and academic qualifications, date obtained, and who awarded:
Employing organization: Named university or maternity unit:
Education:
Work experience, skills, and awards:
Contact information:
Prior projects delivered to completion:
Personal statement of why suitable to deliver the research project:
Publications:
Conference presentations:
STAFF DETAILS 2 (see *Appendix 2 for CV*)
Name: (Co-Investigator)

Step (3): Provide a short abstract or summary of around 300 words.
Abstract (Usually around 300 words).
Provide a clear summary of the proposed research study. Write the abstract at the end after completing the other sections of this form. The abstract should be structured to provide.

(a) *A brief background to the proposal –* ***Background***
(b) *Specific aim of the research (including research question and hypotheses if a quantitative method) –* ***Objective***
(c) *Study design being used –* ***Method***
(d) *Setting of the research (i.e. where and with whom the research will be carried out, including number of participants) –* ***Participants***
(e) *Proposed methods (including what you intend to collect data on and how you propose to collect it) –* ***Data collection***

Step (4): Supply six keywords to describe the research proposal.
Provide keywords to describe the research (e.g. childbirth, midwifery, and PTSD).

Step (5): Construct an introduction that contains a relevant literature review and rationale.
Title: **Introduction** (literature review citing key references)

(a) *Present a literature review that:*
  - *Summarizes and critically appraises previous research in the field.*
  - *Draws attention to gaps in present knowledge and cites key references. Where appropriate, the research method used in previous studies should be reviewed, making comments on its relative strengths and weaknesses.*

(a) *Give the background and justification for the research study.*

Step (6): State the objectives, aim(s), research question(s), sub-question(s), hypotheses, and null hypotheses of the proposed research study.
State the purpose of the proposed research, i.e. what you hope to achieve. Your introduction should provide some background that stands in support of your aim.

Objective(s)
Aim(s)
Research question(s)
Hypotheses (if a quantitative method)
Null hypotheses (if a quantitative method)

Step (7): Outline the research method.
Provide practical details of how answers will be obtained to answer the research question.

(a) **Method**
  Research method to be used. What type of study will be carried out, e.g. RCT, survey, grounded theory, and phenomenology. Provide a rationale for your choice of research method (recipe) and why it is appropriate to answer your research question.

Step (8): Select setting, participants, sampling method, inclusion and exclusion criteria, and method of recruitment.

(b) *Participants*
  Setting and participants to be included (or details of the data to be collected if no participants are being included). This should include numbers (n = ?), population, sampling method, inclusion/exclusion criteria (e.g. age, topic studying, and English speaker), method of recruitment, and justification for your choices.

Step (9): Describe data collection instruments.

(c) *Data collection*
  This section should provide details of the data collection method to be used (e.g. medical records review, questionnaire, interviews, observation, or apparatus being employed), how this method will be applied and the items of data that will be collected (e.g. demographic data and medical conditions). Justification for your choice of data collection should be provided. If existing, validated data collection tools are being used, these should be referenced. If new methods are being developed as part of the study, you should provide information on how you will establish the validity and reliability of these. The design should be described in sufficient detail to allow assessment of workload and timetable.

Step (10): Detail intended data processing and analysis.

(d) *Data analysis*

Data processing and analysis will be carried out. Outline how you intend to analyse the data. Steps in process need to be clearly outlined, e.g. thematic analysis or descriptive and inferential statistics you intend to produce. What comparisons might you make using your data, e.g. by age, sex, socioeconomic status, and variables. The analyses should relate to the aims/objectives / research questions for your study. For qualitative research, describe how you will go about analyzing interview transcripts and how you will code quotes. What soft wear you intend to use needs to be stated.

Step (11): Declare any ethical considerations and outline data protection procedures.

Detail ethical considerations that relate to your research proposal and how you will deal with these. Ensure confidentiality of participants in relation to any data collected. All research studies require ethical approval from the appropriate Ethics Committee. Particularize details of the intended ethics application.

Step (12): Produce a timetable and consider potential problems that may occur.

Provide a summary of the planned program of work (using a bar or Gant chart), which highlights significant phases of the project. For example, ethics approval, literature review, recruitment, data collection, and write-up for the study. Outline any potential organizational, practical, or methodological problems that might occur and how you might overcome these, (e.g. potential problems with recruiting participants or retaining them across a longitudinal study).

Step (13): Estimate resources that may be required.

Provide a summary of the estimated costs/requirements for the project including staff salaries, statistician, computers, software, steering group, public involvement, travel, consumables (e.g. stationery, postage, drinks, and food), equipment, and direct and indirect costs.

Step (14): Detail a public engagement plan

Provide a report from a group of public members of whether they think the study is worthwhile conducting, their perceived benefits, whether they themselves would take part in such a study, and problems or concerns identified.

Named members of the public have agreed to be involved in:

Design of the study	(YES / NO)
Management of the research (e.g. steering group)	(YES / NO)
Developing participant information sheets	(YES / NO)
Undertaking the project and/or analyzing the data	(YES / NO)
Contributing to reporting or writing of the study report	(YES / NO)
Dissemination of research findings	(YES / NO)

Step (15): Append a reference list

Provide a list of all the references used in your proposal and list them in alphabetical order and according to the requested referencing system.

Step (16): Appendix relevant additional material.

Appendix materials that are indicated in text (i.e. Appendix 1, 2, and 3). These will include participant information sheets, example consent form, study protocol, and data collection instruments (e.g. questionnaires, recording sheets, interview schedule, and diagrams of equipment).

Appendices (provide a list):

Participant information sheets	☐	*Consent form*	☐
Study protocol	☐	*Data collection instruments*	☐
Interview schedule	☐	*Diagrams of equipment*	☐
Other, etc.	☐		

Now undertake a literature review and during process respond to the questions asked in Activity 3.2.

Activity 3.2

(1) In relation to an area of midwifery practice that you think requires to be researched, begin your literature review by responding to the questions below.

  (a) What databases and journals yielded relevant research papers?

  (b) How many articles did you retrieve?

  (c) List these in the appropriate referencing style.

  (d) Divide the papers into themes and subthemes.

  (e) Write a skeletal framework for your literature review.

(2) Highlight gaps in the literature that could lead to a potential research project.

3.8 WHAT IS A RESEARCH CRITIQUE?

For a midwife to decide whether an individual study from the literature review is useful in clinical practice or otherwise, they require to critically appraise the content for trustworthiness and rigour. This activity is called '*research critiquing*' and must be carried out before the findings from a research paper can be implemented to alter or introduce a new professional midwifery practice. Critiquing a research paper involves detailed evaluation and critical comment of the research method employed.

To be successful at critiquing a research paper, the midwife requires to have practical understanding of research methods (recipes), which is the main reason a research methods module is taught in every UK midwifery degree program. Knowledge of the research process equips midwives to ask appropriate critical questions about the way in which the research was conducted and its value towards making changes to clinical practice. However, no research study is perfect, with each method a compromise between the ideal and what is practical to carry out in practice. In essence, the way, the study is conducted will greatly influence its validity, reliability, and the extent to which findings can be applied to other populations. Without thorough critiquing, changing professional practice from direct interpretation of a study's results could be hazardous for childbearing women or neonates. Additionally, when writing academic essays, it is simply not good enough to simply 'cut and paste' results and present them 'as is'. Hence, midwives require to scrutinize (critique) the research paper and formulate an evaluation of its worth before implementing its findings into clinical midwifery practice.

3.9 STAGES INVOLVED IN CRITICAL READING OF RESEARCH ARTICLES

LoBiondo-Wood and Haber (2016) propose four levels of understanding when critically appraising (critiquing) research. These include:

Four levels of understanding when critically appraising (critiquing) research

Stage	Purpose	Activities or critical questions:
Preliminary understanding (skimming)	Skimming or quickly reading to gain familiarity with the content and layout of the paper	• Highlight or underline main steps in the research process • Make notes (comments and questions) • Note down key variables • Highlight new or unfamiliar terms and significant sentences • Look up unfamiliar terms and write in definitions
Comprehensive understanding	Increasing understanding of concepts and research terms	• Review all unfamiliar terms before second reading • Clarify any additional terms • Read additional sources as necessary • Identify how the main concepts relate to each other and the context of the study • Write a brief summary of the main idea or themes of the article in your own words • Identify any further questions or areas that need further clarification
Analysis understanding (breaking into parts)	Break the study into parts; understand each aspect of the study. Relate to steps in the research process At this point, you can start to critique the study using a critiquing framework or criteria, applying them to each step in the research process	• What is the purpose of this article? • Am I clear about the specific design used, so I can apply appropriate critiquing criteria? • How are the major parts of the article related to the research process? • How was the study carried out? Can I explain it step by step? • What are the researchers' main conclusions? • Can I say I understand the parts of the article and summarize them in my own words?
Synthesis understanding	Pulling the above steps together to make a (new) whole, making sense of it, and explaining relationships.	• Review notes on how each step compared with the critiquing criteria • Briefly summarize the study in your own words, identifying the main components, and the overall strengths and weaknesses • This is a critical commentary on the study rather than a description or précis of it

(*Source:* adapted from LoBiondo-Wood and Haber 2016).

To assist with critiquing a published research paper, there are a variety of models that consist of questions that address each part of the research process. The student midwife can use these questions to prompt their process of critiquing. These models are tools to direct the midwife through the process of critiquing the selected research article and not a rigid prescription of how critiquing should proceed.

3.10 RESEARCH CRITIQUING MODEL

What follows is an example of a research critique model.

Research critiquing model (Source: Adapted from Rees 2011)

(1) *Focus*
   What is the focus of the article?
   What keywords would you file this article under?
   Does the title reflect content?
   How do findings relate to practice?
   Tell us about the authors and their credibility?

(2) *Background*
Does the author present a reason for undertaking research?
Do local problems or changes justify the study?
Is there a review of previous relevant related research?
Are gaps highlighted within this literature review?
Is a research question placed?

(3) *Terms of reference*
What is the aim of the research?
Is there a hypothesis?
If there is a hypothesis, what are the dependent and independent variables?
Are key concepts defined?

(4) *Study design*
Is the study experimental? descriptive? action research/ or audit?
Is it qualitative or quantitative?
Is the methodology appropriate for purpose?

(5) *Data collection method*
Which tool has been used for data collection?
Has more than one method been used to collect data?
Has the author addressed reliability and validity of measuring tool?
Has a pilot study been conducted?
Have any limitations of the measuring tool been suggested by the author?

(6) *Ethical considerations*
Are issues of informed consent and confidentiality addressed?
Was harm or discomfort which may be caused considered?
Did the study pass through an ethics committee?

(7) *Sample*
Who or what makes up the sample?
Are there clear inclusion and exclusion criteria?
Was a method of sampling used?
Are those in the sample typical or is there elements of bias?
Is sample size large enough?

(8) *Data presentation*
How are results presented; tables, bar graphs, pie charts, and percentages?
Does the author explain and comment on these?
Has the author used a correlation to establish association between variables?
Have tests of significance been used to establish differences between groups?
Can you make sense of results or could they have been presented better?

(9) *Main findings*
What is the most important result?
What is the second most important result, etc.?

(10) *Conclusion and recommendations*
What is the conclusion of the study?
If relevant, is the hypothesis accepted or rejected?
Do results support the conclusion?
What recommendations are made for practice?
Are the recommendations relevant and feasible?

(11) *Readability*
How readable was this article?
Is it clear or difficult to read?
Was it interesting?
Does it assume technical language about subject and research procedures?

(12) *Practice implications?*
What is the answer to the research question placed?
Was the study worth publishing?
How can you relate it to practice?
Who might find it relevant?
What questions does this study raise for practice and further study?

Activity 3.3

Select a primary research study that relates to the area of midwifery practice you think requires further research. Following the questions asked in the Rees (2011) critiquing model appraise this paper.

Earlier on in this chapter, we discussed in detail the processes involved in a *scoping review*. Let us take this one step further a look at the purpose of a *systematic review*.

3.11 SYSTEMATIC REVIEWS

A systematic review is a summary of research that uses explicit methods to perform a thorough literature search and critical appraisal of individual studies to identify the worth and applicability of the evidence. Systematic reviews can facilitate midwives to keep up to date with research that relates to a specific research question. A systematic review provides a summary of the evidence and assesses its quality in terms of a grading system. A *systematic review* is a literature review that focuses on a single question and appraises the evidence in a formal sequence of steps. In other words, a *systematic review* is a scientific investigation that follows a series of preplanned steps designed to assemble the original primary studies as 'participants' in the recipe The aim is to reduce bias and limit error through identifying, appraising (using tools such as CASP), and synthesizing all available research that is relevant to a particular review question (Temple University Libraries 2022).

A *systematic review* is a comprehensive search of all relevant primary research papers, which is explicit in the steps of its method (recipe) and reproducible were it to be repeated by a different researcher. During process, primary papers are appraised, data are synthesized, and results interpreted. Findings can be used for evidence-based midwifery practice guidelines, with an example rationale for selecting a *systematic review* provided below.

Example rationale for conducting a systematic review:
Midwifery researchers are inundated with unmanageable amounts of information on the topic of ... Consequently, a *systematic review* is required to efficiently integrate existing study findings to inform rationale evidence-based decision-making. *systematic reviews* establish whether research findings are consistent across studies and can be generalized over populations. A *systematic review* has been selected because it takes a scientific approach, with rationale for choice of method grounded in the need for large quantities of information to be reduced into evidence-based facts that midwives can use to inform their clinical practice in relation to the topic of ...

Many health and social care journals publish systematic reviews. The most renowned source is *The Cochrane Collaboration*, which is a group of over 15 000 specialists in health care who systematically undertake systematic reviews. Cochrane reviews are published in *The Cochrane Database of Systematic Reviews*, which can be accessed in *The Cochrane Library* (available at: https://www.cochranelibrary.com/search).

Activity 3.4

Enter *The Cochrane Database of Systematic Reviews*, which can be accessed in *The Cochrane Library* at: https://www.cochranelibrary.com/search. Enter in the search box the words 'Maternity Care' and you will observe that there are over 300+ Cochrane Reviews in this subject area. Download number 41 and read:

Barrrowclough, J.A., Lin, L., Kool, B., et al. (2022). Maternal postures for fetal malposition in labour for improving the health of mothers and their infants. *Cochrane Database of Systematic Reviews* 8 (8): CD014615. https://doi.org/10.1002/14651858.CD014615.

Have a browse through the 300+ Cochrane Reviews that relate to maternity care and see if any are in your chosen area of interest. This could be of great use to you when writing the forwarding literature review for your research proposal.

3.11.1 TYPES OF SYSTEMATIC REVIEW

There are different sorts of Systematic Review:

- *Cochrane Collaboration* (see https://www.cochranelibrary.com/search).

- *Joanna Briggs Institute* (see https://joannabriggs.org/).

- A personal *Systematic Review* as part of a research study (Tawfik et al. 2019).

The *Cochrane Collaboration* and the *Joanna Briggs* Institute have specific methods and handbooks listing the rigorous procedures involved. In contrast, a personal *systematic review* permits more flexibility and allows the reviewer to evaluate what they perceive the value of the paper is in relation to their research aims, objectives, and questions. The free-of-charge open access Tawfik et al. (2019) paper clearly outlines a step-by-step guide for conducting a systematic review and meta-analysis with simulation data. These steps include, how to develop the research question, forming criteria, search strategy, searching databases, protocol registration, title, abstract, full-text screening, manual searching, extracting data, quality assessment, data checking, statistical analysis, double data checking, and manuscript writing (Tawfik et al. 2019).

3.12 THE HOLLINS MARTIN RESEARCH CRITIQUING TOOL

Earlier we discussed the use of research paper critiquing tools ordinarily used in *systematic reviews*, such as the *critical appraisal skills programme* (CASP) toolkit (available at: www.casp-uk.net) and also the *Joanna Briggs Institute* (available at: https://jbi.global/critical-appraisal-tools). In addition, and for purpose of assessing papers for potential inclusion in a personal *systematic review, The Hollins Martin research critiquing tool* was developed by the author. This tool can be used to help you systematically grade the rigour of selected research papers for inclusion in the literature review that precedes your research proposal. *The Hollins Martin research critiquing tool* is a survey instrument that employs a systematic and explicit means of critically appraising and scoring selected research papers for inclusion in your personal *systematic review*.

The Hollins Martin Research Critiquing Tool (needs encased in a text box)
The Hollins Martin Research Critiquing Tool consists of 18 items and is scored using a 5-point Likert scale based on level of agreement with each statement. The possible range of scores is 18–90, with a score of 18 representing the lowest possible quality rating and 100 the highest. The statements on this questionnaire are structured as follows:

Reference of research paper being critiqued

Reviewer's name(s)   Number of reviewers involved

TOTAL SCORE   /90

Please do not miss out items on this questionnaire as this will have consequences for total score.

Please respond to the following statements:

(17)   The focus of this research paper is decidedly clear.

Strongly Agree	Agree	Neither Agree or Disagree	Disagree	Strongly Disagree
5	4	3	2	1

Comments:

(18)   The rationale for conducting the research study has been well explained by the author.

Strongly Agree	Agree	Neither Agree or Disagree	Disagree	Strongly Disagree
5	4	3	2	1

Comments:

(19)   The literature review is of a high standard (e.g. details databases searched, includes relevant studies, acknowledges limitations, uses a scoring system, and has employed more than one assessor).

Strongly Agree	Agree	Neither Agree or Disagree	Disagree	Strongly Disagree
5	4	3	2	1

Comments:

(20)   The key concepts have been clearly defined (e.g. technical language about subject and research procedures).

Strongly Agree	Agree	Neither Agree or Disagree	Disagree	Strongly Disagree
5	4	3	2	1

Comments:

(21)   The aim, research question, and objectives are present and comprehensible.

Strongly Agree	Agree	Neither Agree or Disagree	Disagree	Strongly Disagree
5	4	3	2	1

Comments:

(22)   The research method has been clearly stated and is appropriate for answering the research question.

Strongly Agree	Agree	Neither Agree or Disagree	Disagree	Strongly Disagree
5	4	3	2	1

Comments:

(23)   Data collection methods have been suitably described (e.g. reliability, validity, and limitations discussed).

Strongly Agree	Agree	Neither Agree or Disagree	Disagree	Strongly Disagree
5	4	3	2	1

Comments:

(24) **Ethical considerations have been addressed (e.g. consent, confidentiality, harm, data protection issues, and system of gaining ethics approval appropriate).**

Strongly Agree	Agree	Neither Agree or Disagree	Disagree	Strongly Disagree
5	4	3	2	1

Comments:

(25) **Population sampling has been clearly defined (e.g. participants (who, what), inclusion/exclusion criteria outlined, sampling method described, adequate, and justified participant numbers).**

Strongly Agree	Agree	Neither Agree or Disagree	Disagree	Strongly Disagree
5	4	3	2	1

Comments:

(10) **Data has been clearly presented (e.g. tables, graphs, and charts).**

Strongly Agree	Agree	Neither Agree or Disagree	Disagree	Strongly Disagree
5	4	3	2	1

Comments:

(11) **Method of data analysis is appropriate for the method and informative for answering the research question (e.g. apt descriptive and inferential statistics and/or thematic analysis).**

Strongly Agree	Agree	Neither Agree or Disagree	Disagree	Strongly Disagree
5	4	3	2	1

Comments:

(26) **The results section is unambiguous and clearly presented.**

Strongly Agree	Agree	Neither Agree or Disagree	Disagree	Strongly Disagree
5	4	3	2	1

Comments:

(27) **A comprehensive discussion of the findings has taken place (e.g. a conclusion presented, if relevant hypotheses rejected/accepted, results and relationship to research question discussed).**

Strongly Agree	Agree	Neither Agree or Disagree	Disagree	Strongly Disagree
5	4	3	2	1

Comments:

(28) **Relevant recommendations for practice have been considered (e.g. who might value the results and relationship of evidence produced to current practice).**

Strongly Agree	Agree	Neither Agree or Disagree	Disagree	Strongly Disagree
5	4	3	2	1

Comments:

(15) **Appropriate recommendations for future research have been proposed from the research findings.**

Strongly Agree	Agree	Neither Agree or Disagree	Disagree	Strongly Disagree
5	4	3	2	1

Comments:

(29) **Overall, this research paper is easy to read and understand.**

Strongly Agree	Agree	Neither Agree or Disagree	Disagree	Strongly Disagree
5	4	3	2	1

Comments:

(30) **This paper is a worthwhile contribution to the body of research.**

Strongly Agree	Agree	Neither Agree or Disagree	Disagree	Strongly Disagree
5	4	3	2	1

Comments:

(31) **This research paper is an engaging and interesting read.**

Strongly Agree	Agree	Neither Agree or Disagree	Disagree	Strongly Disagree
5	4	3	2	1

3.13 META-ANALYSIS

Meta-analysis is a statistical technique which amalgamates, summarizes, and reviews results from primary quantitative studies. The appeal of meta-analysis is that it combines all the findings on a topic into one large study. A *Meta-analysis* combines the sum total of all participants accumulated and applies statistical tests to the amassed global data. The resultant overall averages of results are more powerful estimates of the true effect size than those derived from one single primary study. The results from each of the selected primary studies are entered into a database, and the consequent 'meta-data' is 'meta-analyzed' to test an overarching hypothesis. Descriptive and inferential statistics are then used to test this hypothesis. One possible danger from conducting a *meta-analysis* is that amalgamating a large set of data from accumulated studies can reduce legitimacy of the construct definitions and thus produce imprecise results that are difficult to meaningfully interpret.

3.13.1 ADVANTAGES OF META-ANALYSIS

There are many advantages from conducting a *meta-analysis*. These include:

1. Its objectivity.

2. Its helpful insight into overall effectiveness of interventions (e.g. treatments, medications, and education).

3. Strengths of relationships between variables are calculated, e.g. meta-analysts report findings in terms of effect sizes. There are different ways that effect sizes can be explained, e.g. Cohen's (d), Hedges (g) or Pearson's correlation coefficient (r). Meta-analysts convert one effect size into another, with each offering scaled measures with different and complementary insights. Tests of statistical significance are also conducted on effect sizes.

3.13.2 STEPS INVOLVED IN A META-ANALYSIS

There are five steps involved in undertaking a *meta-analysis*.

1. A literature search of relevant primary quantitative research studies that pertain to the research question is carried out.

2. Inclusion criteria for study selection is clearly defined, e.g. randomization and blinding in a clinical trial are necessary for the primary study to be included in the *meta-analysis*.

3. Decide which dependent variables are relevant across studies.

4. Use a standardized method to eliminate differences in measurements, e.g. means or Hedges (g), which incorporates an index of variation between groups:

$$\delta = \frac{\mu_t - \mu_c}{\sigma},$$

μ_t = treatment mean
μ_c = control mean
σ^2 = pooled variance.

5. Chose a model. There are three main ones to select from.

   a. <u>Simple regression</u>

   Represented by the equation:

   $$y_j = \beta_0 + \beta_1 x_{1j} + \beta_2 x_{2j} + \cdots + \varepsilon$$

   b. <u>Fixed effects meta-regression</u>

   Represented by the equation:

   $$y_j = \beta_0 + \beta_1 x_{1j} + \beta_2 x_{2j} + \cdots + \eta_j$$

   c. <u>Random effects meta-regression</u>.

   Represented by the equation:

   $$y_j = \beta_0 + \beta_1 x_{1j} + \beta_2 x_{2j} + \cdots + \eta + \varepsilon_j$$

Meta-analysis combines effect sizes of a set of primary quantitative studies. Processes test whether the study outcomes show more variation than expected, because of sampling differences between research participants. Study characteristics, e.g. measuring tools and population sampled are coded and used as predictor variables to analyse the excess variation in the effect sizes. Method weaknesses in incorporated studies can be corrected statistically. In summary, meta-analysis removes the emphasis from single studies to multiple studies. Effect size is emphasized from the whole group of studies, as opposed to a single statistical significance from one single primary paper.

If you are completely confused by these equations, it is important to mention that ordinarily *meta-analysis* is carried out by statisticians who have studied at university for a minimum of three years. Therefore, if you are interested and want to learn more about mathematics, further reading and training are advised.

3.13.3 CHAPTER CONCLUSION

Chapter 3 has addressed the concept of writing a standalone literature review paper and an abridged version to frontload your research proposal. During process, we outlined the purpose of a literature review, the different research methods (recipes) involved, and the concept of using critical appraisal tools. *Chapter 3* has also introduced you to the concept of critiquing primary research papers to evaluate their rigour. *Chapter 4* now moves on to introduce you to the role and procedures involved in gaining ethical approval and its importance. Again, to test and develop your understanding, we now list some more *Self-assessment questions (SAQs)*.

Activity 3.5

Consider the area of midwifery practice which you think merits research attention

    (*Chapter 1 Activity 1.1 and Chapter 2 Activity 2.3*). Write an **Introduction** to your research proposal, which contains in sequential order:

(a) A description of the area or topic of interest (NB to add references and start a headed reference list (**References**) at the back of the research proposal).

(b) Conduct a literature search (NB to name the literature review method, e.g. scoping review).

(c) At the end of the literature search, describe the gap in the literature OR the problem identified.

(d) Provide a rationale for exploring this area/topic and carrying out your proposed research study.

(e) List the **aim**(s), **research question**(s) (if a quantitative study add **hypotheses/null hypotheses**), and state **objectives** (Chapter 5 addresses this in more detail).

    What will follow from this introduction to the research proposal is a heading titled **Method** (Chapter 5 addresses this).

3.14 SELF-ASSESSMENT QUESTIONS (SAQs)

3.1   **A literature review:**

    (a)   Is a list of publications relevant to a specified area of research interest.

    (b)   Should discredit research that disagrees with the study aims.

    (c)   Should only critically review research that agrees with the aims.

    (d)   Should be a critical review of all research related to the study.

3.2   **When conducting a literature review, the reason the researcher should evaluate all primary research studies that address the same topic is to:**

    (a)   Condense results from related papers into themes and subthemes.

    (b)   Evaluate the cost-effectiveness of related interventions.

    (c)   To identify gaps in the literature with a view to advancing theory.

    (d)   To measure the size of a therapeutic effect.

3.3   **The most directly important information reported in a literature review will ordinarily come from:**

    (a)   Professional articles.

    (b)   Research papers published in journals and databases.

    (c)   The World Wide Web.

    (d)   Books.

3.4 **Which of the following is not one of the steps involved in a literature review?**

   (a) Ignoring secondary sources.

   (b) Define the research problem as precisely as possible.

   (c) Select and peruse appropriate general reference works.

   (d) Obtain and read relevant primary sources.

3.5 **Which of the following best describes how a primary research study should be reported in the literature review section of a paper:**

   (a) The major findings of the study should be briefly reported.

   (b) Most of the details of how the study was conducted should be carefully described.

   (c) The abstract of the study should be paraphrased.

   (d) Only the reference of the study should be reported.

3.6 **A systematic review is a method researcher's use to:**

   (a) Validate the accuracy of personal results.

   (b) Obtain a complete set of references about a topic.

   (c) Evaluate the cost-effectiveness of a particular intervention.

   (d) Estimate the size of a therapeutic intervention.

ANSWERS TO CHAPTER 3 SAQs

3.1 **d**

3.2 **c**

3.3 **b**

3.4 **c**

3.5 **a**

3.6 **d**

Stating the Objectives, Aim(s), Research Question(s), Sub-Question(s), Hypotheses, and Null Hypotheses of the Proposed Research Study

STEP (6): State the objectives, aim(s), research question(s), sub-question(s), hypotheses, and null hypotheses of the proposed research study.

Research is an organized and systematic way of finding answers to specified research questions.

SYSTEMATIC

Research is systematic because there is a defined set of steps that the researcher follows, which are clearly laid out in the research proposal.

ORGANIZED

Research is organized through following a sequential structure of processes, which are planned and not spontaneous. Hence, your research proposal should follow headings that outline these chronological processes: (i) *Introduction (STEP 5)*, (ii) *Background (STEP 5)*, (iii) *Literature review (STEP 5)*, (iv) *Identification of a problem or gap in the literature (STEP 5)*, and the *Rationale (STEP 5)* for the proposed study. It is a good idea to place these as subheadings in your research proposal. It is a good idea to develop a template, which includes the subheadings (v) *Objectives (STEP 6)*, (vi) *Aim(s) (STEP 6)*, (vii) *Research question(s) (STEP 6)*, (viii) *Sub-question(s) (STEP 6)*, (ix) *Hypotheses (STEP 6)*, and *Null hypotheses (STEP 6)* if quantitative research. All of these are in front of the (x) *Methods* section (STEP 7–11), which will be discussed in the subsequent chapters. A crucial task in any research proposal is clearly defining the goals of your proposed research study. In other words, what area does the study precisely intend to address, and why? To capture this,

Research Recipes for Midwives, First Edition. Caroline J. Hollins Martin.
© 2024 John Wiley & Sons Ltd. Published 2024 by John Wiley & Sons Ltd.

Chapter Four outlines the process of defining the objectives, aim(s), research question(s), sub-question(s), and hypotheses/null hypotheses (if a quantitative study).

STEP (6): State the objectives of the proposed research study.

4.1 WHAT IS AN OBJECTIVE?

The objective(s) describe what the researcher expects to achieve by carrying out the research study. In essence, its purpose. The objectives define the direction and content of the investigation yet to be conducted. Without written objectives, the research proposal will be in disarray, akin to a builder with no plans to build a house. Hence, the researcher must be clear about what they intend to achieve from conducting their research study. The best objectives are written in a SMART format (Doran 1981).

Specific: Your objectives should be clearly written, with no room for confusion. Keep them narrow and focused.

Measurable: Make your objectives measurable, so you can gauge your progress.

Achievable: Create objectives that are realistically achievable, with a budget and resources to make this possible.

Relevant: Make your objectives relevant to what you want to achieve.

Time-based: Establish deadlines.

What follows is an example of STEP 6 presented in an example research study. We will walk through the relevant parts of STEP 6 one-by-one, but first, let us give the research proposal a title.

STEP (1): Give the research proposal a title.

TITLE: What are the effects of antenatal preparation upon women's levels of birth satisfaction, pain experience, birth trauma, and perceived levels of control during labour and childbirth: a quantitative experimental study.

Post completion of STEPS (2–5) (not discussed here), STEP (6) involves describing what you intend your research project to accomplish captured in objective(s). These objectives will capture and summarize the purpose of the research proposal, which will help the researcher to focus their own research study. Your objectives should appear after the (i) *Introduction*, (ii) *Background*, (iii) *Literature review*, (iv) *Identification of a problem or gap in the literature*, and the *rationale* for the proposed study. It is a good idea to place these as subheadings in your research proposal. It is a good idea to develop a template, which includes the subheadings (v) *Objectives,* (vi) *Aim(s)*, (vii) *Research question(s)*, (viii) *Sub-question(s)*, (ix) *Hypotheses*, and *null hypotheses* if quantitative research. All of these are in front of the (x) **Methods** section. In relation to the study example, the objectives that follow are applicable.

Objectives

Objective 1: Publish a *narrative systematic literature review* that captures what research already reports about the effects of antenatal preparation classes upon women's levels of birth satisfaction, pain experience, birth trauma, and perceived levels of control during labour and childbirth.

Objective 2: Develop an evidence-based guideline for midwives, which details the effects of specified antenatal preparation classes upon women's levels of birth satisfaction, pain experience, birth trauma, and perceived levels of control during labour and childbirth.

Objective 3: If effective, host the eight finalized antenatal education classes on a website designed to teach women how to improve their birth satisfaction and perceived levels of control during labour and childbirth and reduce their pain experience and risk of birth trauma.

STEP (6): State the aim(s) of the proposed research study.

4.2 WHAT IS AN AIM?

The aim of a research study is the overall purpose for carrying out the study. For example, the aim could be to:

- Add knowledge to the area of interest.
- Address a current gap in knowledge.
- Develop and test a solution for an existing problem.

In relation to the study example, the aim that follows is applicable.

Aim: To investigate whether attending antenatal preparation classes effects women's levels of birth satisfaction.

STEP (6): State the research question(s) of the proposed study.

4.3 WHAT IS A RESEARCH QUESTION?

Research questions are at the heart of the research proposal. If there are no question(s), then there are no answer(s). Also, the research proposed should be focused on relevant, useful, and important research questions to give it focus, drive, and purpose. It is the question that you are trying to answer when you do research on a topic or write a research report. The research question is the most crucial part of the study since it guides the process of enquiry and what type of research method (recipe) may be selected. If the research question is not clear and comprehensible to the reader, the proposal is unlikely to be successful at being passed by a supervisor or the ethics committee. For this reason, the researcher requires to spend time capturing precisely what they want to find out in an unambiguous and understandable overarching research question. A strong research question is relevant, clear, and explorable. Quality research questions are ones that catch and hold the interest of the reader, and which entice them to continue reading. Clear questions tend to be short, conceptually uncomplicated, and jargon-free. Sources of ideas for the research question may include:

a. Theory-confirmation/refutation of intuitive knowledge.

b. Practical problems: defining, solution seeking, and validating.

c. Dispelling practitioners' myths/assumptions.

d. Finding answers to conflicting findings, causes, and alternative explanations.

There are three aspects to think about when formulating the research question.

4.3.1 REFINING A BROAD TOPIC INTO A SPECIFIC RESEARCHABLE QUESTION

Choose a Topic of Personal Interest

Progress will be rapid and more fulfilling when the researcher is genuinely interested in the subject matter. A study often requires persistence, with the researcher more likely to persevere when they really care about finding the answer.

Select a Topic with a Moderate Amount of Published Information

If the topic is too broad, the researcher may find more published information than they can assimilate in the time available. In contrast, if the topic is too specific, they may discover that there is not enough available information.

Should a Research Question Be General or Specific?

It should be as specific as possible. In some cases, the researcher may need to write two or more research questions to completely cover a complex topic.

The Research Question Must Be Relevant

Questions which demonstrate their relevance to the profession are likely to be given more weight by proposal reviewers. As a rule, a research project is more likely to be considered acceptable when it is seen to answer a firm question and not merely as a means for the doer to gain a qualification. There are two ways of achieving this recognition:

1. Propose a question, which if answered will fill the missing link in the literature review.

2. Make the relationship between the question and the literature review crystal clear.

To achieve these points, a rationale for the chosen research question and an appropriate research method is provided within the research proposal.

The Research Question(s) Must Be Researchable

Research questions need to be clearly 'doable'. A common reason for rejecting a research proposal is because the question is simply too 'expansive' or 'expensive'. The researcher should therefore consider the limitations of their research question(s), post formulation of the research proposal, and the following practical questions should be asked:

How long will the project last?

1. Do I have the appropriate skills to collect and interpret the data?

2. Are there possible moral constraints that could prevent approval from being granted by the ethics committee?

3. Will I be able to gain the cooperation necessary to conduct the study from relevant individuals?

4. Do I have appropriate funding to cover the costs of carrying out the study?

Example of a Research Question?

What follows is an example of a research question that is derived from the aim in this particular example. The aim informs us that you are interested in studying the effects of attending antenatal education classes and their effects upon women's experiences of labour and childbirth. Hence, you might formulate the following research question:

Research question: What are the effects of attending eight antenatal preparation classes upon women's levels of birth satisfaction?

OR

Research question: Does eight birth preparation classes affect women's birth satisfaction?

OR

Research question: Are women's levels of birth satisfaction improved by attending eight antenatal birth preparation classes?

At the end of the (3) *Literature review* and post (4) *Identification of a problem or gap in the literature*, the researcher formulates the (7) *Research question(s)* to answer this void. In essence, the goal of the research proposal is to find the answer to the stated research question(s).

As a reminder, before developing an appropriate research question, the researcher must first ask themselves:

(a) Do I know the field and its literature well? (Action: Conduct a literature review)
(b) What are other principal research questions in the field? (Action: view final papers)
(c) What areas require more exploration? (Action: identify gaps in literature)

(d) Has a lot of research already been carried out in this topic area? (Action: list papers)

(e) Has this study been conducted before in another environment, country, or population, and is there room for improvement here? (Action: specify)

(f) Is the timing right for the question to be answered? Is it a hot topic or is it obsolete? (Action: check applicable social policy documents)

(g) Would funding bodies be interested in providing a research grant? (Action: e.g. charities or NHS if UK based)

(h) If proposing a service improvement, are the target population interested? (Action: carry out some public involvement work)

(i) Will the study have a significant impact on the body of knowledge? (Action: ask relevant people to rate the value of your proposed findings)

(j) Could my research proposal fill this gap OR lead to better understanding of the problem? (Action: write a justification/rationale for your research proposal)

Post answering these questions, it is important to consider the potential impact of your findings on your proposed population. This is a good time to ask a *public involvement* group about their perceived value of your proposed study before you continue designing your research proposal.

STEP (6): State the research sub-question(s) of the proposed research study.

Formulating the Research Sub-questions

The research focus should be narrow. For instance, in relation to the following research question:

Research question: What are the effects of attending eight antenatal birth preparation classes upon women's levels of birth satisfaction?

Perhaps this question is too large to answer, so let us narrow it down into three more focused sub-questions. Please note that intensity of pain and trauma experienced will affect levels of control felt during labour, and hence overall birth satisfaction.

Research sub-questions

(1) What are the effects of attending eight antenatal birth preparation classes upon women's perceived levels of pain during first stage of labour?

(2) What are the effects of attending eight antenatal birth preparation classes upon women's perceptions of how traumatic labour and childbirth were?

(3) What are the effects of attending eight antenatal birth preparation classes upon women's feeling of being in control during labour and childbirth?

For many researchers, choosing a workable topic is a daunting hurdle. The most common problem is that the topic selected is too broad, with the researcher faced with an overwhelming amount of published material. To make a broad subject more manageable, it is essential to focus on narrower aspects of the global topic, with the larger picture in this case 'birth satisfaction'. There are a few collective ways to narrow and sub-divide a selected area of research interest.

Common ways to narrow a selected area down

(a) By *time period* (e.g. only include women with a term pregnancy)

(b) By *place* (e.g. city, region, country, or specific maternity unit).

(c) By a specific *characteristic* (e.g. age, gender, ethnicity, education, marital status, and stated medical problem).

(d) By a specific *viewpoint* on the topic (e.g. wishing a waterbirth)

Applying these characteristics can help towards creating more narrow research sub-questions.

Research sub-questions

(1) What are the effects of attending eight antenatal birth preparation classes upon primiparous women's perceived levels of pain during first stage of labour in Scotland (United Kingdom)?

(2) What are the effects of attending eight antenatal birth preparation classes upon teenage women's perceptions of how traumatic labour and childbirth were?

(3) What are the effects of attending eight antenatal birth preparation classes upon women with diabetes feelings of being in control during labour and childbirth?

Characteristics of a Good Research Question

A good research question should capture a problem that is worth solving. The hallmarks of a good research question follow.

A good research question:

(a) Is clear, straightforward, and comprehensible.
(b) Is 'researchable', with information available to provide an answer.
(c) Is clear enough for other people to understand what it is asking.
(d) Identifies an important confusion or ambiguity, which relates to a problem.
(e) Is narrow in focus, which permits deeper exploration.
(f) Identifies new information.
(g) Will sustain the researcher's interest for the duration of the project.
(h) Is of interest to an audience.
(i) Forces a different view on the issue.
(j) Addresses a problem of significance to the researcher's field.

To help you identify where the research question is placed within a published paper, please undertake Activity 4.1.

Activity 4.1

Scan a high-impact research journal in a field of midwifery practice (e.g. *midwifery* or *woman and birth*) and identify five primary papers. The purpose of undertaking this task is to help you develop an awareness of research questions that are within the scope of midwifery practice. The research question is normally placed immediately before the *methods* section. The researcher may have captured the question as an *aim* or *objective*, which is often because the paper is addressing only one part of a larger study.

Activity
List the research aim, objective, or research question on each paper, and reference the publications from which they came.

STEP (6): State the hypotheses (if quantitative research) of the proposed research study.

4.4 WHAT IS A HYPOTHESIS?

A *hypothesis (singular)* and *hypotheses (plural),* within a quantitative research context, is a testable statement that represents a possible relationship between two or more variables (e.g. antenatal birth preparation classes and levels of pain). Alternatively, a *hypothesis* could be described as a proposed explanation for some observed event or change in an observation. In other words, a *hypothesis* is a statement that is supported or unsupported by the findings of the research study. As such, *hypotheses* are associated with quantitative research methods (recipes), which postdelivery of a measured intervention, the researcher will have measured a YES or NO answer about whether the hypothesis has been supported (YES) or rejected (NO). If YES, then antenatal birth preparation classes are effective at reducing levels of pain ($p = <0.05$). If NO, then antenatal birth preparation classes are ineffective at reducing levels of pain ($p = >0.05$). A research question can be made into a *hypothesis* by changing it into a statement. For example, the research question that follows can be converted into the following *hypotheses*. In relation to the example that is being developed, which intends to study the effects of attending antenatal education classes and their effects upon aspects of birth satisfaction, the following *hypotheses* could be written.

Hypotheses

Research question 1: What are the effects of attending eight antenatal birth preparation classes upon women's perceived levels of pain during first stage of labour?

Hypothesis 1: Attending eight antenatal preparation classes reduces women's perceived levels of pain during first stage of labour?

Research question 2: What are the effects of attending eight antenatal birth preparation classes upon women's perceptions of how traumatic labour and childbirth were?

Hypothesis 2: Attending eight antenatal preparation classes reduces women's perceptions of how traumatic labour and childbirth were?

Research question 3: What are the effects of attending eight antenatal birth preparation classes upon women's feelings of being in control during labour and childbirth?

Hypothesis 3: Attending eight antenatal birth preparation classes improves women's feelings of being in control during labour and childbirth?

STEP (6): State the null hypotheses (if quantitative research) of the proposed research study.

4.5 WHAT IS A NULL HYPOTHESIS?

A *null hypothesis* (singular) and *null hypotheses* (plural) is a statistical supposition that supports NO statistically significant difference between a pair of observations (e.g. antenatal birth preparation classes and levels of pain ($p > 0.05$). Essentially, a *null hypothesis* is the opposite statement to the *hypothesis*. This means that were the *hypothesis* to be supported by the results of the research study ($p < 0.05$), the *null hypothesis* would be rejected.

In contrast, were the *hypothesis* to be rejected by the results of the research study ($p > 0.05$), the *null hypothesis* would be supported. To be able to report the result either way, both the *hypothesis* and *null hypothesis* require to be stated in the research proposal prior to quantitative data collection. Whilst *hypothesis testing* assesses the trustworthiness of the hypothesis through use of sample data, the *null hypothesis* is used to:

- Reject the hypothesis.

- Demonstrate an alternative to the *hypothesis,* which proposes that there is a difference between the two sets of data (e.g. mean scores of participant's perceived benefits of attending eight antenatal birth preparation class, compared against their mean birth satisfaction scores).

- Speculate using statistics that there is no significant difference between two specified characteristics of a pair of mean observations (data) (p value >0.05).

- *Hypothesis* testing provides a method to reject the *null hypothesis* within a specified level of confidence.

In our example, the stated *hypothesis* can be turned into a working *null hypothesis*:

Null Hypotheses

Research question 1: What are the effects of attending eight antenatal birth preparation classes upon women's perceived levels of pain during first stage of labour?

Null hypothesis 1: Attending eight antenatal preparation classes makes no difference to women's perceived levels of pain during first stage of labour?

Research question 2: What are the effects of attending eight antenatal birth preparation classes upon women's perceptions of how traumatic labour and childbirth were?

Null hypothesis 2: Attending eight antenatal preparation classes makes no difference to women's perceptions of how traumatic labour and childbirth were?

Research question 3: What are the effects of attending eight antenatal birth preparation classes upon women's feelings of being in control during labour and childbirth?

Null hypothesis 3: Attending eight antenatal birth preparation classes makes no difference to women's feelings of being in control during labour and childbirth?

There are other ways of expressing these *null hypotheses*.

Null Hypotheses

Null hypothesis 1: Women's perceived levels of pain during first stage of labour are unaffected by attending eight antenatal preparation classes?

Null hypothesis 2: Women's perceptions of how traumatic labour and childbirth are unaffected by attending eight antenatal preparation classes?

Null hypothesis 3: Women's feelings of being in control during labour and childbirth are unaffected by attending eight antenatal birth preparation classes.

OR

Null Hypotheses

Null hypothesis 1: Attending eight antenatal preparation classes has no effect upon women's perceived levels of pain during first stage of labour.

Null hypothesis 2: Attending eight antenatal preparation classes has no effect upon women's perceptions of how traumatic labour and childbirth were.

Null hypothesis 3: Attending eight antenatal preparation classes has no effect upon women's feelings of being in control during labour and childbirth.

In summary, the researcher carries out experiments which are designed to disprove the *null hypothesis*. If this does not happen or the researcher wants to see an improved result from ($p < 0.05$) to ($p = 0.01$), or even better ($p = 0.001$), then the experiment could be repeated to improve the outcome measures, which will require that the hypotheses be redefined.

Redefined Research Questions and Hypotheses

Research question 1: What are the effects of attending twelve antenatal birth preparation classes upon women's perceived levels of pain during first stage of labour?

Hypothesis 1: Attending twelve antenatal preparation classes reduces women's perceived levels of pain during first stage of labour?

Null hypothesis 1: Attending twelve antenatal preparation classes makes no difference to women's perceived levels of pain during first stage of labour?

Research question 2: What are the effects of attending twelve antenatal birth preparation classes upon women's perceptions of how traumatic labour and childbirth were?

Hypothesis 2: Attending twelve antenatal preparation classes reduces women's perceptions of how traumatic labour and childbirth were?

Null hypothesis 2: Attending twelve antenatal preparation classes makes no difference to women's perceptions of how traumatic labour and childbirth were?

Research question 3: What are the effects of attending twelve antenatal birth preparation classes upon women's feelings of being in control during labour and childbirth?

Hypothesis 3: Attending twelve antenatal birth preparation classes improves women's feelings of being in control during labour and childbirth?

Null hypothesis 3: Attending twelve antenatal birth preparation classes makes no difference to women's feelings of being in control during labour and childbirth?

Activity 4.2 affords you the opportunity to turn two research questions into hypotheses and null hypotheses.

Activity 4.2

Attempt to turn the following research questions into hypotheses and null hypotheses:
- Does immersion in warm water during the first stage of labour reduce the pain experience of childbearing women?
- Are women's attitudes towards breastfeeding altered through having personal experience of feeding this way?

4.6 RELATIONSHIP BETWEEN THE NULL HYPOTHESIS AND THE THESIS STATEMENT

The *hypothesis* (not the *null hypothesis*) is used as a thesis statement. For example, if our hypothesis is supported by a significant difference ($p < 0.05$), three research statements can be stated by the researcher.

Thesis Statements

Thesis statement 1: Maximum levels of pain reduction during first stage of labour are achieved by the woman attending 12 antenatal birth preparation classes.

Thesis statement 2: Maximum levels of birth trauma are achieved by the woman attending twelve antenatal birth preparation classes.

Thesis statement 3: Maximum levels of perceived control during labour and childbirth are achieved through the woman attending twelve antenatal birth preparation classes.

Alternatively, the researcher may capture the thesis statement as follows.

Thesis Statements

Thesis statement 1: The investigation demonstrated that woman who attends twelve antenatal birth preparation classes experience reduced pain during first stage of labour.

Thesis statement 2: The investigation demonstrated that woman who attends twelve antenatal birth preparation classes experience reduced levels of birth trauma.

Thesis statement 3: The investigation demonstrated that woman who attends twelve antenatal birth preparation classes experience higher levels of perceived control during labour and childbirth.

It is a good idea to capture all that has preceded in a template, which includes the subheadings *objectives, aim(s), research question(s), sub-question(s), hypotheses,* and *null hypotheses*. An example outline follows, which is ordinarily placed immediately before the **Methods** section of your research proposal.

Objectives

Objective 1: Publish a *narrative systematic literature review* that captures what research already reports about the effects of antenatal preparation classes upon women's levels of birth satisfaction, pain experience, birth trauma, and perceived levels of control during labour and childbirth.

Objective 2: Develop an evidence-based guideline for midwives, which details the effects of specified antenatal preparation classes upon women's levels of birth satisfaction, pain experience, birth trauma, and perceived levels of control during labour and childbirth.

Objective 3: If effective, host the eight finalized antenatal education classes on a website designed to teach women how to improve their birth satisfaction and perceived levels of control during labour and childbirth, and reduce their pain experience and risk of birth trauma.

Aim

To investigate whether attending antenatal preparation classes effects women's levels of birth satisfaction.

Research questions

Research question (1): What are the effects of attending eight antenatal birth preparation classes upon women's levels of birth satisfaction?

Research sub-questions

Research question (1a): What are the effects of attending eight antenatal birth preparation classes upon women's perceived levels of pain during first stage of labour?

Research question (1b): What are the effects of attending eight antenatal birth preparation classes upon women's perceptions of how traumatic labour and childbirth were?

Research question (1c): What are the effects of attending eight antenatal birth preparation classes upon women's feeling of being in control during labour and childbirth?

Hypotheses

Hypothesis (1): Attending eight antenatal preparation classes reduces women's perceived levels of pain during first stage of labour.

Hypothesis (2): Attending eight antenatal preparation classes reduces women's perceptions of how traumatic labour and childbirth were.

Hypothesis (3): Attending eight antenatal birth preparation classes improves women's feelings of being in control during labour and childbirth.

Null hypotheses

Null hypothesis (1): Attending twelve antenatal preparation classes makes no difference to women's perceived levels of pain during first stage of labour?

Null hypothesis (2): Attending twelve antenatal preparation classes makes no difference to women's perceptions of how traumatic labour and childbirth were?

Null hypothesis (3): Attending eight antenatal birth preparation classes makes no difference to women's feelings of being in control during labour and childbirth?

4.7 THE METHODS SECTION OF THE RESEARCH PROPOSAL WILL FOLLOW

The methods section should contain a clear statement of the research method (recipe) to be used. This is followed by a methodological argument that justifies your choice of research method (recipe). An outline of the *method* is now presented.

Method

A quantitative experimental study will be used to find out whether attending antenatal preparation classes improves women's levels of birth satisfaction, noting that pain experienced, birth trauma, and control during labour are all components of birth satisfaction (Hollins-Martin and Martin 2014). This method was chosen because a quantitative experimental study is a highly rigorous and robust research method for determining the cause-and-effect relationships between an intervention and the outcomes. In this case, the intervention involves eight antenatal preparation classes and their effects upon birth satisfaction, which is subdivided into the three outcome measures of pain experienced, birth trauma, and perceived levels of personal control during labour and childbirth (Hollins-Martin and Martin 2014).

In this example, a *quantitative experimental study* will be carried out, during which the researcher attempts to *cause* an *effect,* instead of passively observing behaviours or recording data. For example, the researcher will compare the effectiveness of an intervention (eight antenatal preparation classes) and their effects upon *participants* (childbearing women):

- Pain experiences during first stage of labour.
- Perceptions of how traumatic labour and childbirth were.
- Perceived levels of control during labour and childbirth.

The next step is to design the study, and as this is a quantitative experimental design in which participants will be assessed using four measures.

STEP (8): Select setting, participants, sampling method, inclusion and exclusion criteria, and method of recruitment.

Setting

This study will be carried out at the *Ayrshire maternity unit* (AMU) at Crosshouse hospital in Kilmarnock Scotland (United Kingdom).

Participants

SAMPLE: A convenience sample of informed and consenting nulliparous childbearing women will be recruited from the antenatal clinic at the AMU ($n = 100$) (see data analysis section for rationale supporting sample size). Initially, 120 participants will be recruited to allow for a withdrawal rate due to complications. The rationale for only recruiting nultiparous women is that the labouring process differs considerably between nulliparous and multiparous women, with this limitation an attempt to reduce variables that influence outcome.

INCLUSION CRITERIA:

Primigravids
Occipito anterior position at commencement of data collection
<2cms dilated and uneffaced at commencement of data collection
Healthy
Uncomplicated pregnancy
Term (3–42 weeks)
Spontaneous onset of labour
Age range = 16–40 years
Have arrived in the labour ward still in latent phase of labour
Singleton pregnancy

EXCLUSION CRITERIA:

Multiparous
Foetal postion other than occipito anterior at start of data collection
>2cm dilated
Presence of a medical diagnosis

Premature (<37 weeks)/postmature (>42 weeks)

<16 years or >40 years of age

Waterbirth (as monitors not waterproof)

Stillbirth, perinatal/neonatal death

Have arrived in the labour ward in active phase of labour

Physical disability

METHOD OF RECRUITMENT: At the first clinic booking, a leaflet (see *Appendix 1*) will be given to interested participants providing an overview of the study and a contact point for interested parties. Substantive explanations will be provided, with time for questions and answers afforded. Potential participants will be given the opportunity of opting out at any point with assurance of continuation of quality care provision. To view participant information sheet and consent form (see *Appendix and Number*). If the woman's interest in participating is secured, she will be given a two-week window to consider and after a question-and-answer session asked to sign a consent form. A research midwife will be employed to undertake these activities, which will provide continuity of care.

STEP (9): Describe data collection instruments.

Intervention

Develop content of the antenatal education classes based upon evidence produced from the literature review that supports what aspects of learning and teaching are effective at improving childbearing women's:

- Pain experiences during first stage of labour.
- Perceptions of how traumatic labour and childbirth were.
- Perceived levels of control during labour and childbirth.

The *Steering group* and *public involvement group* will inform the development of these sessions, which will be piloted on ($n = 5$) women and altered in line with comments. To review outline of *DRAFT 1* of these evidence-based classes (see *Appendix and Number*).

Data Collection

(a) *Birth satisfaction measured using the Birth Satisfaction Scale-Revised (BSS-R)*

At two to four postnatal weeks, participants will respond to the Birth Satisfaction Scale-Revised (BSS-R) (Hollins-Martin and Martin 2014), which consists of 10 items that participants respond to on a five-point Likert scale based on level of agreement or disagreement with the statement placed. The possible range of scores is 0–40, where a score of zero represents least satisfied and 40 most. To view many references of validation papers, see Hollins-Martin and Martin 2014 and https://www.bss-r.co.uk/. To view the BSS-R, see *Appendix and Number*.

(b) *Pain experience will be measured using the Wong-Baker Pain Scale (WBPS)*

The WBPS is represented by faces with expressions that indicate intensity of pain, accompanied by a numerical participant response Likert scale (https://wongbakerfaces.org/) (see *Appendix and Number*). Zero is represented by a smiley face, whilst 10 corresponds to a distraught crying face. Scores of 1–10 will be used to measure pain experience of women at three points during labour (3, 6, and 9 cm cervical dilatation), based upon cervical dilatation on a partograph. The numbers are appended on the card and the woman will be facilitated by the attendant midwife with process of completion. Visual analogue scales have been extensively used and validated in pain research and are considered to produce consistent measurements of pain (Keck et al. 1996). Unlike numeric scales, the WBPS does not need magnitude or seriation and can therefore be used by compromised women in labour. The WBPS Scale has been extensively studied and its reliability and validity confirmed (Garra et al. 2010).

(c) *Perceptions of trauma will be measured using the International Trauma Scale (ITQ)*

The ITQ is a valid and reliable scale (Cloitre et al. 2018) that focuses upon the core features of post-traumatic stress disorder (PTSD) and Complex PTSD (CPTSD) according to the ICD-11 (WHO 2018), which defines PTSD (code6B40) and CPTSD (code6B41) as two distinct sibling conditions situated under one parent category of trauma-related disorders (https://www.traumameasuresglobal.com/) (see *Appendix and Number*). Participants respond to ITQ items on a five-point Likert scale, ranging from zero (Not at all) to four (Extremely). Thus, PTSD and *disturbances in self-organization* (DSO) scores range from 0 to 24 (the total of six items from each subscale), and CPTSD symptom scores range from 0 to 48 (i.e. the sum of the 12 ITQ items).

(d) *Perceived levels of control will be measured using the Support and Control in Birth (SCIB) scale*
The SCIB scale will measure perceived support and control during childbirth (see *Appendix and Number*). The SCIB is a 35-item scale, which the participant responds to on a Likert Scale that ranges from 'completely agree' to 'completely disagree', with good reliability and validity reports to support its use (Liu et al. 2020). The SCIB is available at:
https://cpb-eu-w2.wpmucdn.com/blogs.city.ac.uk/dist/b/1267/files/2015/06/SCIB-English-version-1rdhrcv.pdf

STEP (10): Detail intended data processing and analysis.

Data Analysis

Descriptive statistics
We will describe the sample in terms of important patient characteristics. A descriptive analysis will be used to explore the nature and extent of the effects of antenatal preparation classes upon women's levels of birth satisfaction, pain experience, birth trauma, and perceived levels of control during labour and childbirth. We will report descriptive statistics for these four primary outcome measures for the sample.

Inferential statistics
Will be used to relate the type and duration of effect of antenatal preparation classes upon the outcomes of women's levels of birth satisfaction, pain experience, birth trauma, and perceived levels of control during labour and childbirth. Multilevel modelling will be used where repeated observations are recorded. Regression models will be employed, appropriate to the type of outcome variable (nominal, ordinal, or continuous). The primary analysis will explore the relationship between nature and duration of effect upon each outcome. Ancillary analysis will explore the effects of the education program, taking into account important environmental and clinical characteristics.

STEPS (11–16) continue here, with examples from another study provided in Chapter 1
STEP (11): Declare any ethical considerations and outline data protection procedures.
STEP (12): Produce a timetable and consider potential problems that may occur.
STEP (13): Estimate resources that may be required.
STEP (14): Detail a public engagement plan.
STEP (15): Append a reference list.
STEP (16): Appendix relevant additional material.

Activity 4.3 provides you with the opportunity to consider the objectives, aim(s), question(s) and sub-questions, and if relevant the hypotheses relevant to the research proposal you are developing.

Activity 4.3

In relation to the area of midwifery practice that you are writing a research proposal to address:
- State your objectives.
- State your aim(s).
- State your research question(s) and sub-question(s).
- State your hypotheses and null hypotheses (if a quantitative study).

4.7.1 CHAPTER CONCLUSION

This chapter has addressed STEP (6) of writing a research proposal (recipe), which involves stating the objectives, aim(s), research question(s), sub-question(s), hypotheses, and null hypotheses of the proposed research study. The next chapter will now address STEP (7), which involves outlining the proposed research method; it is important for the researcher to apply an appropriate recipe to answer the selected research question(s). At this stage, it is important to set up a *public involvement group,* who will be asked to provide their perceived value of the study proposed and whether they themselves would be willing to participate in such a study and why. In research terms, to embrace *public involvement* means that the research is done '*with*' or '*by*' the public, not '*to*', '*about*' or '*for*' them. This means that childbearing women, partners, and family with relevant experience, contribute towards designing the research proposal and how the content is designed, conducted, and disseminated. Writing a *public involvement report* of members of the public contributions made towards designing and planning of the project is important. Also writing a further plan for future public participation during project delivery is presented in a *public engagement plan*. Together these reports are discussed in text and elaborated on in the Appendices, all of which is *STEP (14): Detail a public engagement plan.*

4.8 SELF-ASSESSMENT QUESTIONS (SAQs)

4.1 **The objectives in a research proposal:**

    (a) Describe the selected research method.

    (b) Help you write your data protection plan.

    (c) Appear in the conclusion of your research proposal.

    (d) Describe what your research is trying to achieve.

4.2 **A research question must be one of the following:**

    (a) Supported by a grant.

    (b) Presented at the end of an experiment.

    (c) Clear and answerable.

    (d) Is placed in the methods section of a research proposal

4.3 **Hypothesis testing involves:**

    (a) Deciding whether the data supports or rejects a hypothesis.

    (b) An ethnographic approach.

    (c) Deciding whether differences between groups are significant.

    (d) Using a testing kit.

4.4 **If the null hypothesis is supported:**

    (a) The hypothesis is also supported.

    (b) The hypothesis is rejected.

    (c) The experimental question remains unanswered.

    (d) The drug administered makes a difference to the condition of the participant.

ANSWERS TO CHAPTER 4 SAQs

Question Answer

4.1 **d**

4.2 **c**

4.3 **a**

4.4 **b**

Choosing an Appropriate Research Method (Recipe) to Answer the Question

CHAPTER 5

STEP (7): Outline the research method.

'What research method (recipe) do I select?'

5.1 SELECTING AN APPROPRIATE RESEARCH METHOD (RECIPE) TO ANSWER YOUR RESEARCH QUESTION

Research methods are simply ways of answering research questions. They do not have a life of their own and are purposely selected because they will give you the answer to your research question. In other words, the research method (recipe) selected is only as good as the answer; it will provide to your research question (s). Hence, deciding upon an appropriate research method (recipe) happens after you have clearly decided upon your research question. The research method (recipe) selected should use appropriate data collection methods (STEP 9) to answer that question, and if a quantitative deductive study is proposed, test the hypothesis. As has already been established, research studies may be either *quantitative* or *qualitative*, although it is possible to use both approaches in the same research project (mixed methods or triangulation). Now let us visit some research methods (recipes), from which you can decide if one would be suitable to answer your research question.

Research Recipes for Midwives, First Edition. Caroline J. Hollins Martin.
© 2024 John Wiley & Sons Ltd. Published 2024 by John Wiley & Sons Ltd.

5.2 CHOOSING A QUANTITATIVE METHOD

In quantitative research, the data collected takes the form of measurements that can be statistically analysed. Quantitative research follows standard procedures and reporting of results. In other words, each quantitative method (recipe) follows a set recipe. This standardization maximizes objectivity. Quantitative methods (recipes) are used to compare groups and/or measure things and analysis is conducted using statistics. As such, quantitative research methods (recipes) are based on meanings derived from numbers, and hence results are presented in numerical form.

The general sequence:

1. A measuring tool is used to record something (e.g. birth satisfaction or effectiveness of a treatment on say postnatal depression).

2. Numerical scores are attached to the findings.

3. Data is analysed using statistical procedures.

4. Results are generated in numerical form.

5. Conclusions are drawn.

6. Recommendations for clinical practice are made.

   Now let us compare the differences in approach of quantitative verses qualitative research.

5.3 CHOOSING A QUALITATIVE METHOD

In contrast, qualitative research methods (recipes) offer insight into participants' thoughts and feelings and aim to study people in naturally occurring situations and non-biased ways. In qualitative research methods, findings are instead presented as narratives, as opposed to numbers. Also, unlike quantitative research methods (recipes), which deduce findings down to one answer, qualitative research induces many answers to the research question. Methods of data collection in qualitative methods include for example structured and unstructured interviews. During these interviews, open-ended questions are asked, discussions are recorded, transcribed, and analysed to induce themes and subthemes to answer the research question. As such, and in contrast to deductive quantitative research methods, results are individualized to participants who may provide a variety of answers. In contrast to quantitative research methods, the qualitative approach is typically interested in the way people experience, perceive, understand and interpret their lives, and the nature or reality of the world around them. Factors that influence or impact upon people's lives are also important components of qualitative research, e.g. culture, race, class, gender, ethnicity, age, power, knowledge, material possessions, wealth, groups, and social structures. Researchers are often also interested in those who are privileged, marginalized, or represent 'atypical' members of a group. As such, this indicates that qualitative research methods (recipes) may address ethical challenges or political issues. When studying the experiences of people and what these experiences mean, qualitative researchers usually find themselves addressing concepts and questions like:

- What is reality . . . or whose reality?

- What is truth . . . or whose truth?

- What is knowledge . . . or whose knowledge counts?

- What does it mean to be a person?

- What is experience?

   Qualitative researchers aim to gather in-depth understandings through investigating the '*why*' and '*how*', instead of the '*cause*' and '*effect*' explored by quantitative researchers. In a qualitative approach, participant's thoughts, feelings, and emotions are assessed, and an in-depth analysis of discussions take place. Far less, participants are recruited in qualitative methods (recipes) compared with quantitative research methods (recipes), with the general sequence of steps including:

1. Observing or asking open-ended questions.

2. Recording what is said.

3. Interpreting individual participants transcribed quotes.

4. Inducing themes (categories) and subthemes (subcategories) from all data gathered.

5. Theorizing about what underpins participants' narratives (quotes).

6. Discussing identified themes (categories) and subthemes (subcategories) and their overall meaning.

7. Drawing conclusions and recommendations for clinical practice.

Questions to ask yourself when selecting the right research method

1. Is it a research method (recipe) that will generate the answer to the research question?

2. Is a qualitative (inductive) or quantitative (deductive) the best approach?

3. Is the selected research method (recipe) straightforward and easy to implement?

4. Does the chosen research method (recipe) allow access to the desired participant group?

5. Is triangulation of research methods (recipes) appropriate, which will involve more than one research method).

Now that we have looked at the differences between qualitative and quantitative research methods, undertake Activity 5.1 and consider whether a quantitative or qualitative approach is most suited to answer the research questions placed.

Activity 5.1

Select whether a quantitative or qualitative approach would be most suited to answer the research questions that follow.

(Q1) How many women with back pain postdelivery have been waiting more than six weeks for an appointment to see a physiotherapist?
(Q2) What is the quality of canteen food at your local maternity unit?
(Q3) What are women's experiences of breastfeeding?

5.4 SELECTING WHICH RESEARCH METHOD (RECIPE) TO USE

Once you have decided whether you are going to take a quantitative or qualitative approach to answer your research question, the next step (STEP 7) is to select and outline the research method (recipe). When writing a research proposal and considering what is the best research method (recipe) to use, the researcher first requires to consider the following points.

1. *Establish why you are undertaking the research study?*

   Possible reasons might include:

   a. To explore what is working well and what is not, in order to decide whether the project or program should be continued in its present form, altered, improved, expanded, or abandoned.

   b. To establish outcomes and impacts.

2. *Set the research question*

   Think specifically about the research question and what answer is required.

3. *Consider who the participant group will be*

   Typically, research participants are likely to include:

   a. Beneficiaries of the project or program, e.g. women, neonates, and student midwives.

   b. Project managers and deliverers of care (midwives/obstetricians).

   c. Decision makers and policy makers (e.g. government).

   d. Individuals who are affected by the process and/or outcome of the proposed project.

4. *Choose the most appropriate research method (recipe) to answer the research question*

   The method selected will depend on:

   a. The type of question needed answered.

   b. The size of budget allocated to the study.

   c. Deciding whether the method should be qualitative or quantitative.

5.4.1 CONSIDERING USING A QUANTITATIVE METHOD (RECIPE)

As a reminder, a quantitative approach involves collecting numerical data to explain, predict, or control the phenomena of interest. Data analysis is mainly statistical (deductive in process). As such, quantitative research is a formal, objective, systematic process in which numerical data is used to obtain information about the world (Burns and Grove, 2001).

5.4.2 FEATURES ASSOCIATED WITH THE QUANTITATIVE APPROACH

There are significant differences between quantitative and qualitative research approaches, with both systematic and following (STEPS 1–16) for writing a research proposal (see Table 5.1).

Before we move on, it is important that you clearly understand the meanings of the terms stated in Activity 5.2.

Activity 5.2

Cleary articulate the meanings of the following terms:
- Objective measures
- Subjective measures
- Deduction
- Induction

Both quantitative and qualitative research methods (recipes) are methodical in their approach. The main difference being that quantitative research methods are *objective* and qualitative *subjective*. The term *objective* means that the steps involved are mechanical and involve minimal amounts of human interpretation. That is when collecting, analyzing, and

Table 5.1 Differences between quantitative and qualitative research methods (recipes).

Quantitative research	Qualitative research
Objective in approach	Subjective in approach
Deductive	Inductive
Generalizable	Not generalizable
Numbers	Words

interpreting quantitative data, the researcher remains detached and is goal-directed. Also, if another researcher were to deliver the same research proposal again, they would simply be repeating the exact same systematic process, along with providing a similar result.

In stark contrast, the subjectivity of the qualitative approach involves a substantial amount of human interpretation. For example, a woman's *subjective* accounts of pain she experienced during labour, as opposed to *objective* ratings of labour pain on a numerical data collection tool. In this context, qualitative spoken words give rich depth to the symptomatic experience. Another example of the differences between *objective* and *subjective* meaning can be viewed in Table 5.2.

As such, quantitative research methods (recipes) are *deductive* and test a theory captured in a *hypothesis*. Whereas and in contrast, qualitative research is *inductive* and generates theories that capture many responses. To view another example of a difference between *objective* and *subjective* research methods (recipes), see Table 5.3.

Quantitative research methods (recipes) produce results that are deduced to one answer that supports or refutes the hypothesis. In contrast, qualitative research methods (recipes) produce several findings that are induced by clustering participants' similar viewpoints. Thoughts about waiting times contrast between people, dependent upon their personalities, responsibilities, and circumstances. For example, one participant may meet a friend or feel lonely, and consequently, they are quite happy to sit and enjoy others' company within the maternity clinic waiting room. In contrast, another participant may view the same situation quite differently. For instance, they have purchased a washing machine that is due to be delivered at 3 o'clock and require to be home for its arrival. The point made here is that researchers do not reduce findings to

Table 5.2 Example of one difference between an *objective* and *subjective* method.

Consider a research proposal designed to assess waiting times in a maternity clinic.

Objective research method (recipe)

A quantitative research method (recipe) would measure in minutes how long women waited to see their midwife, which is a numerical *objective* measure calculated in numbers (e.g. 45 minutes).

Versus

Subjective research method (recipe)

A qualitative research method (recipe) would address how women experienced waiting to see their midwife, which is described in *subjective* accounts that differ between individuals (e.g. '*I used the time to quietly meditate, which was a calming experience after a busy day*' OR '*I felt angry because I was as a consequence late in collecting my daughter from school*'.

Table 5.3 Example of another difference between an *objective* and *subjective* method.

Objective research method (recipe)

A quantitative research method (recipe) tests the following hypothesis:

Childbearing women who attend the maternity clinic do not have to wait more than 30 minutes to see their midwife.

If the answer is YES, the data supports the hypothesis, and if NO the data does not support the hypothesis. Findings are based upon statistical group numerical means and ranges.

Versus

Subjective research method (recipe)

A qualitative research method (recipe) has collected data that explored women's experiences of waiting in the maternity clinic to see their midwife. Data analysed is subdivided into four themes:

Theme 1: Anxiety aroused

Theme 2: Time to rest

Theme 3: Being late

Theme 4: Time to chat

one answer when using a qualitative research method (recipe). In comparison, when a quantitative research method (recipe) is used, the researcher deduces findings to one answer, which supports or refutes their hypothesis.

The clearest difference between the two approaches is that quantitative data is structured in numbers and qualitative data is captured in words. That is, *objective* numbers are associated with quantitative research and *subjective* interpretation with qualitative research. Quantitative research methods (recipes) produce solid, generalizable, and repeatable results, whilst qualitative research methods (recipes) construct varied, creative, and differing outcomes. With qualitative research methods, a story is constructed to help the reader empathize with a situation, e.g. what it is like to experience an event (e.g. waiting to be seen by a midwife in an antenatal clinic).

Whether a researcher selects a quantitative or qualitative research method (recipe), depends upon the topic of interest. Researchers select an appropriate research method (recipe) to answer their own unique research question. When the researcher wants to know whether a particular treatment works or not, then a quantitative research method is appropriate (i.e. to clarify the cause (treatment) and its effect (measured). If the research question is about women's experiences of having the treatment, then a qualitative research method (recipe) is appropriate. We are now going to move forward and look at some examples of research methods (recipes), starting with descriptive research method which is quantitative in approach.

5.5 DESCRIPTIVE RESEARCH METHOD

A *descriptive research method* (recipe) is a quantitative approach, which collects information without changing the environment (i.e. nothing is manipulated). In some published research papers, *descriptive research method* is instead called a *correlational* or *observational* research method. During a quantitative *descriptive method* (recipe), data is gathered about a population and is described using statistics. The results are factual, accurate, and systematic, and show the effect that one *variable* has upon another. A *descriptive research method* uses descriptive statistics that calculate a coefficient that summarizes a dataset, which represents a similar sample population, or entire population. Descriptive statistics subdivides its findings into measures of central tendency and measures of variability (spread of the data). Measures of central tendency include calculating the mean, median, and mode. In contrast, measures of variability include calculating the standard deviation, variance, minimum and maximum variables, kurtosis, and skewness. A further branch of the *descriptive research method* is epidemiology.

5.5.1 EPIDEMIOLOGY

Epidemiology investigates factors that determine presence or absence of diseases and disorders within a population. Data that epidemiologists collect can come from self-report measures and from answers provided by women participating in a study. For example, an epidemiological study may collect data on the number of women who answer YES to having excessive morning sickness. Each woman providing an answer may interpret 'extent of vomiting' differently. This means that the results of one study may be quite different from another in which midwives are in fact measuring 'extent of vomiting'. In this case, the epidemiologist attempts to determine how many pregnant women are affected by the disorder and how this changes across time. Key terms to understand include:

Incidence: The number of new cases of a disease/disorder in a population over a stated time period.

Prevalence: The number of existing cases of the disease/disorder in a stated population at a specified time.

Cost of illness: Calculating expenditures on maternity care provision, which includes work-related costs, educational costs, the cost of support services required, and costs of prevention.

Within maternity care, the goal is to identify factors that have an impact on childbearing women's and neonates' lives. For example, finding the most frequent problem (Variable 1) that affects childbearing women in a city such as Edinburgh (Scotland, United Kingdom), and what causative factor in the environment provokes the problem (Variable 2). One purpose is to find ways of reducing the incidence of the disease or problem and help childbearing women and neonates live healthier lives. Part of the analysis involves calculation of the correlation between two stated variables.

5.5.2 CORRELATIONS

Correlations determine relationships between variables. The main difference between *descriptive method* compared with *experimental method* is that causality cannot be established because variables in *descriptive method* because 'cause' and 'effects' are not being manipulated by the researcher (e.g. giving a dose of treatment and measuring the effects on symptoms). In other words, a correlation does not prove causation. Correlations point out an association (relationship) between two variables (e.g. smoking and bronchitis). The researcher identifies a sample of people diagnosed with the disease (e.g. bronchitis) and a matched sample who do not have the disease. The statistician then looks for differences between the two groups in antecedents, behaviours, or related conditions. Correlations demonstrate the strength and direction of relationships between two variables (e.g. smoking and bronchitis), and when there is a high correlation the researcher can predict the effects of one variable (e.g. smoking) upon the other (e.g. bronchitis). In this example, there is a positive correlation between bronchitis and smoking. There are two types of correlations:

1. *Positive correlation*: With a *positive correlation*, as the value of one variable increases the value of the other variable also increases (e.g. the more a person smokes [Variable 1] the more likely they are to develop bronchitis [Variable 2]).

2. *Negative correlation*: With a *negative correlation*, as the value of one variable increases the value of the other variable decreases (e.g. as the value of a car decreases [Variable 1] its age increases [Variable 2]).

When two variables are completely unrelated, there is no correlation. An example of two variables with no correlation is shoe size (Variable 1) and intelligence scores (Variable 2). To view visual graphs of correlations, see Figure 5.1.

A researcher may also conduct mathematical calculations to determine a *correlation coefficient*. As a student midwife, you need to understand what a correlation coefficient is, so you can appraise the value of reporting within a published research paper. A *correlation coefficient* is a number between (-1 and 1), which tells you the direction and

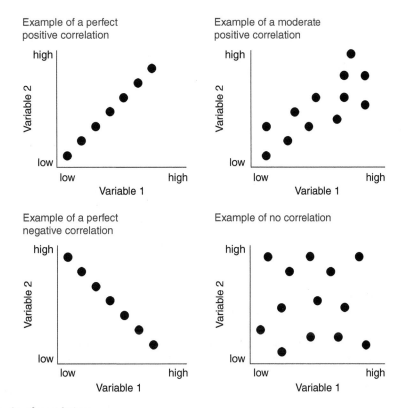

FIGURE 5.1   Visual graphs of correlations.

strength of the relationship between two variables (e.g. smoking and bronchitis). The values of a *correlation coefficients* are illustrated in (Table 5.4):

Table 5.4 Values of correlation coefficients.

(+ or −)	0.8–1.0	Very high
(+ or −)	0.6–0.8	High
(+ or −)	0.4–0.6	Moderate
(+ or −)	0.2–0.4	Low
(+ or −)	0.0–0.2	Insignificant

Epidemiologists study and analyse the distribution, patterns, and causes of health conditions in defined populations, which within midwifery practice involves childbearing women, partners, and neonates. Epidemiology is the cornerstone of public health. Epidemiology is used to identify risk factors for developing diagnosed conditions, and what factors are preventive towards reducing incidence of the disease or medical condition. Some examples of topics examined by epidemiologists include hypertension, mental illness, and obesity. Before moving on from *descriptive research method* to discuss *experimental research method* (recipe), first carry out Activity 5.3.

Activity 5.3

Access and read the following descriptive method study:

Rishard, M., Fahmy, F.F., Senanayake, H. et al. (2021). Correlation among experience of person-centered maternity care, provision of care and women's satisfaction: cross sectional study in Colombo, Sri Lanka. *PLoS One* 16 (4): e0249265. https://doi.org/10.1371/journal.pone.0249265

We are now going to move forward and look at *experimental research method* (recipe), which is quantitative in approach.

5.6 EXPERIMENTAL RESEARCH METHOD

An *experimental research method* is a quantitative approach that involves manipulating variables to determine 'cause' and 'effect' relationships between two factors (variables). For example, measuring improvement in symptoms of *postnatal depression* (PND) (Variable 1) in response to receiving a set number of sessions of *cognitive behavioural therapy* (CBT) (Variable 2). There are three primary properties of an *experimental research method*.

The three primary properties of an experimental research method

1. *Manipulation:* The researcher issues an intervention to half of the participants in the study.

2. *Control*: The experimenter introduces a control over the experimental situation (e.g. the *control group* do not receive the treatment, with the results compared against an *experimental group* who do receive the treatment).

3. *Randomization*: The experimenter assigns participants to different groups on a random basis (e.g. Group 1: *control group* who do not receive the intervention and Group 2: *intervention group* who receive the treatment).

Experimental research method involves comparing pre-test scores with post-test scores, which allows the researcher to evaluate how effective the treatment was in the given situation (e.g. Group 2). During any *experimental research method*, a hypothesis is tested through issue of an *independent variable* or intervention (e.g. CBT), and the *dependent variable* or measured effect (e.g. using the *Edinburgh Postnatal Depression Scale* [EPDS]) (Cox et al. 1987). For example, depression scores (*dependant variable*) are measured using a valid and reliable scale (e.g. in this case using the EPDS) before and after the manipulation (*independent variable*) (e.g. CBT). The matched *control group* do not receive any treatment for their depression. Differences in EPDS scores between the *intervention group* and *control group* are then statistically analysed by comparing group means and establishing significance through calculating 'p' values (e.g. $p = 0.05$; 0.01, or 0.001). The gold standard of *experimental research method* (recipe) is a *randomized controlled trial (RCT)*.

5.6.1 RANDOMIZED CONTROLLED TRIAL (RCT)

The architype gold standard of *experimental method* is an RCT, which is designed to maximize control so that causality may be determined through reducing sources of error. The key feature of an RCT that differs from an experiment, involves random allocation (*randomization*) of participants into either the *control group* (Group 1) or *intervention group* (Group 2). During process, the *intervention group* receives the intervention (e.g. antidepressants), and the matched in characteristics *control group* receive no intervention. During an RCT, potential *extraneous variables* are controlled to reduce sources of error. An *extraneous variable* is an eternal influence that may affect findings (e.g. attending an additional postnatal support group). In an RCT, two virtually identical experiments are conducted at the same time and having a *control group* helps the researcher to study one variable at a time. In one of them, the *treatment* being tested is given to the *intervention group* participants, and in the other *control group,* the variable being tested is not given. This allows for a comparison to be made between *the intervention group* who receive the treatment, and the *control group* who did not. To reduce experimenter influence or bias, it is important to verify that effects of the drug are produced only by the medication itself and not by some other influential factor (e.g. trying to please the researcher or *Hawthorne effect*). What makes the RCT gold standard different to an experiment, is the effort the researchers make to achieve bias reduction. For example, conducting a *double-blind* trial in which two matched groups of women are compared. Instead of receiving the drug, the *control group* receive a placebo (e.g. a sugar pill), and they are randomly allocated to a group and oblivious to whether they have received the antidepressant or otherwise. During the RCT, neither the woman nor researcher knows which participant received the real drug. Such an approach reduces the chance of a *Hawthorne effect*, which involves the participant providing reporting's designed to please the researcher. In summary, an RCT is the *experimental method* most used for testing maternity or neonatal services or technologies (e.g. drugs, devices, or surgery). RCT's involve random allocation of different interventions (or treatments) to participant groups. Medical companies must convince their consumers that the medicine or treatment works, with all new medicines and surgical treatments undergoing RCT's before being approved for use in the maternity services. Before moving on, take a look at the published paper which describes an RCT carried out within the maternity services (Activity 5.4).

Activity 5.4

Access and read the following Randomized Controlled Trial:

Buran, G. and Aksu, H. (2022). Effect of hypnobirthing training on fear, pain, satisfaction related to birth, and birth outcomes: a randomized controlled trial. *Clinical Nursing Research* 31 (5): 918–930. https://doi.org/10.1177/10547738211073394

Now let us look at another example of an *experimental research method* (recipe) called *quasi-experimental research method*

5.6.2 QUASI-EXPERIMENTAL RESEARCH METHOD

A *quasi-experimental research method* is a structured recipe that does not involve:

1. A *control group* who does not receive the variable (e.g. the drug, treatment, or intervention).

2. Random assignment of participants to the *intervention group.*

Quasi-experimental research method was developed to provide an alternate recipe of examining causality in situations in which the researcher cannot eliminate the influence of extraneous influences (*variables*) (e.g. outside influences like a postnatal women having support networks), which is an incorporate part of individual participants' living conditions. For example, a childbearing woman's living conditions may affect her development and recovery from PND. In experimental terms and for this reason, it is difficult to set up a *control group*. There are many types of quasi-experiments, with most adaptations of the *experimental method*, with one of the following three elements missing.

1. Manipulation

2. Randomization

3. Control group

BOX 5.1	AN EXAMPLE OF A QUASI-EXPERIMENTAL METHOD

The researcher sets a table with a variety of foods. Some of the foodstuffs are high fat, high cholesterol, and full of sugar (e.g. sausage rolls, quiche, crisps, pizza, cheese, and muffins). Other foodstuffs are low fat, low cholesterol, and reduced in sugar (e.g. lentil soup, salmon, chicken breast, fish, brown bread, fresh fruit, yoghurt, and salad). The researcher invites ($n = 100$) people in for lunch and observes what each naturally selects to eat. The researcher then proceeds to record the calorie and fat units' that each participant has consumed. What the researcher is studying, is the weight and Body Mass Index (BMI) of participants who naturally select healthy or unhealthy foodstuffs. On the way out, the researcher weighs participants and assorts them into one of three groups. Those who are underweight (Group 1), middle range (Group 2), or overweight (Group 3) according to their BMI index. In essence, the researcher is examining the relationship between calorific and fat unit intake against body BMI. Statistical analysis of numerical data collected is then carried out.

An example of a *quasi-experimental research method* could involve the researcher creating groups (*control group* and *intervention group*) that have evolved naturally in some way, as opposed to participants being randomly selected. To view an example of a *quasi-experimental research method,* see Box 5.1.

Take a look at the published paper which describes a quasi-experimental research method carried out within the maternity services (Activity 5.5).

Activity 5.5

Access and read the following quasi-experimental research method:

Gadappa, S.N., and Deshpande, S.S. (2021). A quasi-experimental study to compare the effect of respectful maternity care using intrapartum birth companion of her choice on maternal and newborn outcome in tertiary care centre. *The Journal of Obstetrics and Gynecology of India* 71 (Suppl 2): 84–89. https://doi.org/10.1007/s13224-021-01587-7.

To conclude, *experimental research methods* strictly adhere to the scientific research design, which includes having a hypothesis, a variable that can be manipulated by the researcher, and variables that can be measured, calculated, and compared. Excluding *quasi-experimental research method*, *experimental research methods* include a control group against which measures can be statistically compared. We will now move on to look at processes involved in *survey research method*.

5.7 SURVEY RESEARCH METHOD

Survey research method involves collecting data through use of an *instrument, scale, questionnaire,* or *tool*. A survey *instrument, scale, questionnaire,* or *tool* consists of a series of items designed to gather *outcome measures* from participants. Surveys can be quantitative, qualitative, or both. For example:

- Surveys with closed-ended items and scores attached are designed for statistical analysis and are deductive and quantitative in nature.

- Surveys with open-ended questions are designed to collect individualized answers and are inductive and qualitative in nature.

- Surveys with both closed-ended and open-ended items are both quantitative and qualitative in nature.

Survey research method presents advantage over other research methods, given that it is a cheap way to collect data, and does not require as much effort from the researcher as carrying out face-to-face, telephone, or computer-based interviews. A second advantage is that survey questions generate standardized answers that are often easier to analyse. Nevertheless, such uniformity of answers on a survey tool may frustrate some researchers, due to lack of richness in terms of providing enough data to interpret full meaning. A third advantage of *survey research method* is that questionnaires can be sent both extensively and geographically to increase participant numbers. At the same time, *survey research method* is sharply limited by the fact that respondents are required to write in a written language, which may exclude important demographic and population groups or require an interpreter. Also, the response rates are often low and often require second or third survey resends (Kongsved et al. 2007). As mentioned earlier, surveys can be organized to be either quantitative, qualitative, or both.

5.7.1 QUANTITATIVE SURVEY RESEARCH METHOD

Quantitative survey research method (recipe) is probably the most common recipe used by researchers. Since data collected is quantitative, the data collection instrument consists of closed-ended questions that the participant responds to on a Likert scale. Participant responses are scored and post-study data collection is statistically analysed. To view an example item taken from a validated quantitative survey instrument, see Table 5.5.

When designing the 'data collection' section of a *quantitative survey research method*, you are required to consider several points.

a. The types of questions that will answer your research question (e.g. quantitative closed-ended items and their response scales).

b. Are you going to develop your own quantitative survey instrument or use one that has already been psychometrically validated (e.g. the BSS-R (Hollins Martin and Martin 2014) OR the EPDS (Cox et al. 1987))?

c. If you are designing your own survey instrument, is the wording of items comprehensive? To answer this, you will need to pilot your newly developed survey instrument and speak about how you did this in your research proposal. If this is a PhD, you may need to gather data and carry out psychometric statistical testing on your newly developed quantitative survey instrument.

d. What sort of response format will you use (e.g. Likert scales)?

e. The question sequence and providing a sense of appropriate order.

f. The length of your quantitative survey instrument, in terms of number of items needed to answer the research question and sustain participant interest in terms of full completion.

g. A method of collecting data that will maximize participant response rates. If you want high numbers of participants, it is important to persuade managers to encourage your strategy of participant engagement.

Styles of Survey Data Collection

Survey data collection can take several forms, with possibilities including:

a. Administering survey instruments to groups of participants (e.g. midwifery staff meetings OR support groups.).

b. Sending your quantitative survey instrument by post, email, or face-to-face in an interview, which may require two to three rounds.

The subsequent section is designed to help you design item for a quantitative survey instrument.

Processes Involved in Designing Items for a Quantitative Survey Instrument

You are interested in finding out midwives' attitudes towards wearing high-heeled shoes. An attitude is a person's degree of favourability or un-favourability towards the topic of interest. The items formulated on such a scale should relate to beliefs, thoughts, intended behaviour, or actual self-reported behaviour in relation to wearing of high heels. For example:

Table 5.5 Item 5 taken from the Birth Satisfaction Scale-Revised (BSS-R).

	I felt well supported by staff during my labour and birth.				
	Strongly agree	Agree	Neither agree or disagree	disagree	Strongly disagree
Scores	4	3	2	1	0

Source: Adapted from Hollins Martin and Martin (2014).

I believe that extended wearing of high-heeled shoes will damage the wearer's feet.

Notice that this item is not a question, but a statement. Such items will measure participants' attitudes towards wearing high-heeled shoes, with the person responding by indicating whether they 'agree' or 'disagree'. It is usual to ask participants not just to 'agree' or 'disagree', but also indicate the strength of this conviction across a point on a scale that corresponds to their thoughts for or against the statement. For example:

	I believe that extended wearing of high-heeled shoes will damage the wearer's feet.				
	Strongly agree	Agree	Neither agree or disagree	Disagree	Strongly disagree
Scores	5	4	3	2	1

The scores are absent on the actual measuring tool, with the participant straightforwardly asked to respond on the 5-point Likert scale. Such Likert scales allow for measurement that is more sensitive. Hence, the researcher can measure how favourable or unfavourable the participant's attitude is towards the item. Half of the statements on a quantitative survey instrument identify attitudes in one direction and the other half in the opposite direction. For example, scoring in the opposite direction may be presented as:

	I believe that extended wearing of high-heeled shoes is harmless for the wearer's feet.				
	Strongly agree	Agree	Neither agree or disagree	Disagree	Strongly disagree
Scores	5	4	3	2	1

Quantitative survey research method includes definitive objective items used to gain insight about a clearly defined research topic. Post-data collection, the answers to the items are statistically analysed and a research report is written from the quantitative data produced. Help evolve your ability to develop a survey measuring tool. In efforts to help you evolve your ability to develop a survey measuring tool, see Activity 5.6.

Activity 5.6

Develop a quantitative survey instrument

Design a six-item quantitative survey instrument to answer the following research question:
What are midwifery students' attitudes towards breastfeeding?

Now take a look at the published paper which describes a *quantitative survey research method* carried out within the Croatian maternity services (Activity 5.7).

Activity 5.7

Access and read the following quantitative survey research method paper:
Nakić Radoš, S., Martinić, L., Matijaš, M. et al. (2021). The relationship between birth satisfaction, posttraumatic stress disorder and postnatal depression symptoms in Croatian women. *Stress & Health* 2021: 1–9. https://doi.org/10.1002/smi.3112

5.7.2 QUALITATIVE SURVEY RESEARCH METHOD

In contrast to objective quantitative survey data collection, qualitative researchers aim to gather greater in-depth understandings of participants' thoughts about the object of interest, and by doing so investigate in larger detail their individual subjective attitudes and opinions. As such, *qualitative survey research method (recipe)* involves asking *open-ended* questions, which involve the respondent supplying their own answers without being constrained by a fixed set of possible responses. This open expression allows the participants to answer the item in their own words and provide an opinion. An *open-ended* question is designed to encourage full and meaningful answers that tap into the participant's individual knowledge and feelings about the object of interest. This approach provides the opposite of a *closed-ended question*, which asks for a short answer with a numerical value attached. *Open-ended* questions typically begin with words such as *why* and *how*, or phrases such as *tell me about* . . . Examples of *open-ended* questions can be viewed in Table 5.6.

Closed Versus Open-Ended-Questions

A *closed-ended* question is a form of request that can be answered by the participant by supplying a simple 'yes' or 'no' response. Alternatively, a *closed-ended* question may ask the participant for a specific simple piece of information or to select from multiple-choice responses. For example:

(Q) Do you know your weight?
Answer: Yes / No
(Q) What is your weight?
Answer: 8 stone 13 pounds

An *open-ended* question is a form of question that should be answered with a more elaborate and convoluted answer. A simple 'yes' or 'no' is not an appropriate response. For example:

How do you feel about breastfeeding?
What types of food do you prefer to eat and why?
What types and amounts of exercise do you undertake in a week?

Table 5.6 Examples of open-ended survey questions.

What do you think about .... ?

What could you do about .... ?

How could we fix .... ?

Is there another way of .... ?

What is your opinion about .... ?

What would happen if .... ?

What else could we do to .... ?

What is it like to have .... ?

What if we .... ?

Why do you think this happened .... ?

How did you .... ?

How could you .... ?

How do You Feel?

The most notorious *open-ended* question is: *How does this make you feel?* or some variation thereof. Stories are about people and how they are affected and effected by events. Researchers want to understand the participant's emotions, thoughts, and feelings in relation to a clearly defined context (e.g. breastfeeding OR labour).

The Benefits of Asking Open-Ended Questions

Asking *open-ended* questions permits participants to articulate a wide range of responses.

For example, participants:

- Can be invited to tell you what they consider to be important about a topic.
- Have maximum latitude to speak freely.
- Are invited to share more than straightforward facts.

Listening to the answers to *open-ended* questions helps the researcher to:

- Gather information about the person's agenda.
- Clarify understanding of what is being discussed.
- Connect with and understand the person better.

Summary to Survey Research Method

In summary, *survey research method* involves the researcher using or devising instruments that consist of a set of items or questions designed to gather information from respondents in ether a qualitative, qualitative, or mixed methods fashion. As such, a research questionnaire can be typically a mix of closed-ended and open-ended questions. Questionnaires have advantages over other research methods (recipes), given that they are cheap to administer and require limited effort from the researcher compared with conducting interviews. Also, the directed and standardized answers on a survey instrument make it easier for the researcher to analyse the data. Nonetheless, one criticism that can be made of *survey research method*, is that the nature of standardized responses can frustrate respondents, simply because the answers they provide may not accurately represent their individualized and elaborated responses. Another limitation of *survey research method* is that questionnaires require respondents to be able to read the items and respond to them appropriately, which may not be possible if they cannot read or write or do not know the relevant language. Thus, for some populations, a questionnaire may not be the best choice. Now take a look at a published paper which describes a *qualitative survey research method* that has explored partners experiences of childbirth (see Activity 5.8).

Activity 5.8

Access and read the following qualitative survey research method paper:
   Daniels, E., Arden-Close, E., and Mayers, A. (2020). Be quiet and man up: a qualitative questionnaire study into fathers who witnessed their partner's birth trauma. *BMC Pregnancy Childbirth* 20: 236. https://doi.org/10.1186/s12884-020-02902-2

To conclude*, survey research method* involves collecting information from a sample of participants through gathering their responses to questions or items on a preprepared questionnaire, tool, or instrument. As such, this approach creates flexibility for the researcher to use a wide variety of styles of recruitment and data collection. Having discussed *survey research method* in some detail, we will now move on to explore the processes involved in *action research method*.

5.8 ACTION RESEARCH METHOD

Action research method (recipe) can be qualitative or quantitative in nature and involves reflecting upon and problem-solving issues surrounding an implementation into clinical midwifery practice. The process is led by a researcher who is working as part of a team, which intends to improve the way a problem in clinical practice is being addressed. Overall, the aim of *action research method* within the maternity services is to improve strategies, practices, and knowledge about the environment in which midwives work and in relation to how childbearing women, their partners, and neonates are cared for. *Action research method* is geared towards improving the quality of an organization and its performance, and in this case is carried out by midwifery practitioners who analyse data to improve their own clinical practice. Within a maternal health context, *action research method* is carried out by individual midwife's or in teams with colleagues. As such, *action research method* gives midwifery practitioners new opportunities to:

- Reflect on and assess midwifery clinical practice.

- Explore and test new ideas and methods of undertaking tasks.

- Assess how effective new approaches to midwifery care are.

- Share feedback with fellow team members.

- Make decisions about what new approaches may be included in treatment, care, social provision, and assessment plans used by a midwifery team.

Action research method may take a quantitative approach, which incorporates hypotheses that are formed and tested through data collection using quantitative measures. Since *action research method* is conducted in the field of clinical midwifery practice, the variables measured are not as rigorously controlled as they would be in an *experimental method*. The global aim of an *action research method* is to improve clinical midwifery practice through solving issues, snags, and problems in a circular and repeating process. As such, *action research method* involves a systematic cyclic series of steps that comprise a circle of planning, which together involve fact-finding about delivery and results from a clearly named and defined action. Hence, *action research method* includes a methodical, orderly, and organized set of steps, which include:

1. A circle of planning

2. An action

3. Fact-finding about the results of this action

Action research method essentially is a cyclical process of change, which commences with planned actions initiated by the participants and researcher. Data are not returned in the form of a written report. Instead, results are fed back in open sessions with the team, during which the participant(s) and researcher(s) collaborate to identify and rank identified issues, snags, and problems. The purpose is to find causation and develop practical plans for coping with what has been identified as the issue, snag, or problem. During the cyclic steps of *action research method*, measurable data is gathered to support or reject clearly defined hypotheses. As such and during each cyclical round, *action research method* is self-correcting and finds practical solutions to issues, snags, and problems identified. The cyclical process of *action research method* includes specified steps (see Figure 5.2).

During *action research method,* the research team may elect to go around the cycle in Figure 5.2 several times, or at least until there are minimal and ideally no further issues, snags, or problems identified. As each cycle is completed, the following steps are taken.

1. *Collective cooperative method*
   Faced with an issue, problem, or snag, the clinical midwifery team become aware of a need for change. This should include a preliminary diagnosis and an action plan of change to be implemented into clinical midwifery practice.

2. *Observation and data gathering*
   The new change is implemented into clinical midwifery practice, and observations, interviews, and/or data collection tools are used to identify and measure the effects of each implemented change. The researcher is looking for evidence to support a clearly defined hypothesis of predicted change.

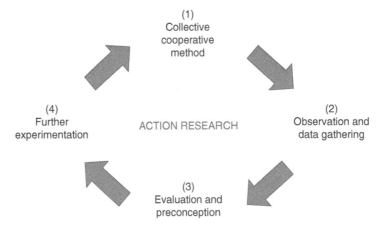

FIGURE 5.2   Cyclical process of *action research method.*

3. *Evaluation and Preconception*

   Application of the action plan of change is evaluated and if perceived to be successful, the implemented change is adopted. If there have been two or more action research cycles, this process will include all the changes that have resulted from each round of corrective steps. At the end of the third stage in Figure 5.2, team discussions take place surrounding issues, problems, or snags. Data are not just returned in the form of a written report but are also fed back into a research forum, which may take the form of open joint sessions with participants (childbearing women and/or partners), and the change agents (researcher(s) and midwifery team). In discussions, specific problems are ranked and methods are devised for dealing with appropriate issues raised.

4. *Further experimentation*

   Implementation of the tweaked changes and solutions occur in a further action research cycle, during which data are again gathered, analysed, and necessary adjustments made. Post evaluation, the team will decide whether or not it is worth repeating the whole action research cycle again.

   Adjustments are implemented with each completed action research cycle. Hence, as the team make changes and reevaluations during each round, a repetitive cycle of planning, action, and measurement is undertaken. Each full cycle encompasses implementation of new changes, which involves trying out new forms of action. The overall process involves the team creating new improvements, which are evaluated on the job and if successful become part of the system's repertoire. There are inevitable overlaps between each action research cycle, which makes it a continuous process that does not have clear-cut boundaries. As such, *action research method* is problem centred and action oriented.

   To view a published paper that describes an *action research method,* which has been implemented into clinical midwifery practice, see Activity 5.9.

Activity 5.9

Access and read the following action research method paper:

   O'Brien, D., Butler, M.M., Casey, M. (2021). The importance of nurturing trusting relationships to embed shared decision-making during pregnancy and childbirth. *Midwifery* 98: 102987. https://doi.org/10.1016/j.midw.2021.102987

In summary, *action research method* creates knowledge surrounding inquiry into practical midwifery contexts. Hence, *action research method* permits midwives to learn through their actions, for the purpose of promoting and developing a specified area of professional practice. Due to its participatory landscape, the processes involved in *action research method* make it a distinct method that midwives can use to improve their clinical practice.

Having discussed *action research method* in some detail, we will now move on to explore the processes involved in *clinical audit research method.*

5.9 CLINICAL AUDIT RESEARCH METHOD

Clinical audit research method (recipe) focuses upon improving care provided to childbearing women and neonates, through structuring a systematic review of clinical midwifery practice. During process, *clinical audit research method* involves the researcher taking measurements, which are then compared against explicit preexisting criteria or standards. The principle of *clinical audit research method* within the context of midwifery practice is to review midwives' clinical performance and audit it against the standard, guideline, or protocol that directs how care should be provided. The audit results provide a framework against which improvements in care can be implemented and measured. A notorious example of a historic audit can be viewed in (Box 5.2).

Box 5.2 illustrates that *clinical audit research method* is a method of investigating whether or not care provided is in line with the standard, guideline, or protocol, which will inform midwives and childbearing women of their service performance, and where improvements could be made. Similar to *action research method*, *clinical audit research method* also involves a cycle of stages.

5.9.1 CYCLE OF STAGES INVOLVED IN CLINICAL AUDIT RESEARCH METHOD

Stage 1: Identify the Problem or Issue

Stage 1 involves selection of the topic to be audited. This topic needs to be clearly defined (e.g. organization and delivery of antenatal care).

Stage 2: Define Criteria and Standards

Identify the relevant standard, guideline, or protocol that prescribes best practice (e.g. see NICE: www.nice.org.uk). NICE guidance in the United Kingdom is evidence-based and prescribes health care professionals with key points for practice that have proved to produce best outcomes. There is a whole section of NICE guidance that relates to maternity care provision (e.g. see NICE guideline [NG201]), which prescribes evidence-based delivery of antenatal care: https://www.nice.org.uk/guidance/ng201). In response, the clinical audit method should be written as a series of tasks to be carried out by the researcher, which collectively are called the audit criteria and define aspects of care that are to be measured objectively. An example of a measurable outcome of care follows.

> **An Example of a Measurable Outcome of Care:**
>
> Have childbearing women been involved in negotiations and planning of their care?

A standard will state a threshold of expected success relative to each criterion, which is ordinarily captured as a percentage. An example of application follows.

> **For Example, an Appropriate Standard Would Be:**
>
> There is evidence of childbearing women having been involved in negotiations and planning of their care in 90% of cases.

BOX 5.2   A NOTORIOUS CLINICAL AUDIT CARRIED OUT BY FLORENCE NIGHTINGALE

During the Crimean War, upon arriving at the hospital barracks in Scutari in 1854, Sister Nightingale was dismayed by the unhygienic conditions and high mortality rates of sick and injured soldiers. Sister Nightingale's team of 38 nurses applied stringent organized sanitation routines to raise standards of care and produce more positive outcomes, which were compared against fastidiously measured and recorded variables of morbidity and mortality. Because of improvements made, mortality rates fell from 40% down to 2%. Sister Nightingale's methodical research records made this example one of the first ever-recorded *clinical audit research method*.

Source: Adapted from Aravind and Chung (2010).

Stage 3: Data Collection

Certain details of what is to be audited must be established from the outset. These include:

a. The user group to be included.

b. The health care professionals to be involved.

c. The time span over which the audit data will be collected.

Considerations need to be given to:

a. What data will be collected?

b. Where data will be collected?

c. Who will collect the data?

Ethical issues are considered:

a. The data collected must relate only to the objectives of the audit.

b. Staff and participant confidentiality must be respected.

c. Sensitive topics are discussed with the research ethics committee.

Stage 4: Compare Performance Against Standards

Analysis concludes how well the standard was met and if not why. Reasons are scrutinized and improvement measures are considered. When standard results are close to 100%, it is likely that further improvement will be difficult. Low percentage returns are considered to be priority targets. Such decisions are dependent upon the topic area. For example, in life-or-death scenarios, achieving 100% is important. Whilst for other standards, lower levels of compliance might be considered acceptable.

Stage 5: Implementing Change

Once the results of the audit have been discussed, an agreement is reached about recommendations for change in clinical practice. An action plan of how to improve practice is devised and decisions are made about who is responsible for organizing each improvement. Each point is clearly defined, a named individual agrees to take responsibility and the timescale for reevaluation is agreed.

Reaudit: Sustaining Improvements

After an agreed period-of-time, the audit should be repeated. The same method (recipe) for identifying the sample, method, and data analysis is utilized to guarantee comparability with the first audit. The reaudit should demonstrate that changes have been implemented and improvements made. With each round of audit, further changes may be required, which leads to reoccurring audits of the same standard. Reports of each audit should be written and disseminated to relevant and appropriate strategic health authorities, and ideally published in research journals. Two types of *clinical audit research method* will now be discussed, which includes: (i) *standard-based audit method* and (ii) *critical incident audit method*

5.9.2 STANDARD-BASED AUDIT METHOD

This preceding type of *clinical audit research method* is also called *standard-based audit*. Like all other research methods, the recipe is systematic, independent, and documented through the 16-step model to determine the extent to which the audit criteria are met (i.e. guideline, protocol, or standard). In summary, *standard-based audit method* (recipe) involves defining the specified standard of expected steps of maternity care provision, which forms a baseline against which care provided can be assessed (e.g. see NICE intrapartum guidance: https://www.nice.org.uk/guidance/health-and-social--care-delivery/maternity-services/intrapartum-care). Data collection methods (STEP 9), such as interviews, surveys, and measuring tools, are used to gather data from women and maternity care professionals about their perceptions of actual care provided. The data collected is analysed and compared against the prescribed standard of care (STEP 10). Writing a report, which is placed in the public domain (e.g. see NMPA Project Team. National Maternity and Perinatal Audit Clinical Report 2022: https://www.hqip.org.uk/wp-content/uploads/2022/06/Ref.-336-NMPA-annual-report-FINAL.pdf). In response, the maternity unit is expected to implement strategies to improve the care provided, which is remeasured against the standard to assess whether appropriate changes in care have been provided. As such, *standard-based audit method* is an essential part of clinical governance. The purpose of clinical governance is to ensure that the maternity unit has a system in place to ensure accountability towards continuously monitoring and improving the quality of care provided. In this context, clinical governance ensures a systematic approach is taken towards maintaining and improving the quality of maternity and neonatal care provided within the given unit, which involves repeated data collection and analysis of maternity care user and staff views about the quality of care provided. The six pillars of clinical governance include:

1. Constantly striving to improve clinical effectiveness.

2. Supporting research and development.

3. Openness.

4. Risk management.

5. Education and training.

6. Clinical audit.

7. Public involvement.

The maternity unit audit lead has a clear role in creating the strategy for embedding clinical audit into the organization. To view a published paper that describes a *clinical audit research method* designed to improve intranatal care provision, see Activity 5.10.

Activity 5.10

Access and read the following standard-based audit research method paper:

Minooee, S., Simbar, M., Sheikhan, Z., and Alavi Majd, H. (2018). Audit of intrapartum care based on the national guideline for midwifery and birth services. *Evaluation & the Health Professions* 41 (3): 415–429. https://doi.org/10.1177/0163278718778095

Having discussed *standard-based audit method* (recipe) in some detail, we will now move on to explore the processes involved in *critical incident audit method*.

5.9.3 CRITICAL INCIDENT AUDIT METHOD

Another *clinical audit method* is *critical incidence audit,* which is used to review near miss or critical maternity care incidents that have aroused serious concern. As part of process, the research team includes a range of maternity care professionals and researchers, who gather to reflect upon the specified 'critical incident', so that prevention strategies can be organized to reduce chances of reoccurrence. In accordance with maternity unit procedures, the acknowledged incident is reported to the senior midwife and medical officer using the appropriate documentation system. To view processes involved in recording a critical incident, see Table 5.7.

When there has been a series of critical incidences reported from one maternity unit, the health minister may commission an enquiry. One example of such a *critical incident review* is the Ockendon Report (2022), which reports 250 fully assessed *critical incident reviews* that occurred within the maternity services at Shrewsbury and Telford Hospital NHS Trust in the United Kingdom. The researchers independently assessed the quality of investigations of maternal and infant harm that occurred at the trust. The Ockendon Report (2022) outlines the findings, conclusions, essential actions, and system-wide learnings that took place from this series of critical incidents. To view the Ockendon Report (2022), see Activity 5.11.

Table 5.7   Summary of processes involved in recording a *critical incident*.

When writing the report, it is important to provide as much detail as possible about the critical incident. The following questions should be answered.

- When (date) and where the incident occurred.
- Names, addresses, and status of staff involved.
- A factual account of the incident.
- Action taken to resolve the situation.
- The names of people bearing professional responsibility for the *critical incident* and their role(s).
- Observations made of the situation and its context (e.g. mental states of those involved).
- An account of injury or damage that has occurred.
- Any additional comments.
- Signatures of staff involved, and the document dated and signed.

Activity 5.11

Access and Read the Ockendon (2022) Critical Incident Report

　　Independent Maternity Review. (2022). *Ockendon report: final: findings, conclusions, and essential actions from the independent review of maternity services at the Shrewsbury and Telford Hospital NHS Trust* (HC 1219). Crown. https://assets.publishing.service.gov.uk/government/uploads/system/uploads/attachment_data/file/1064302/Final-Ockenden-Report-web-accessible.pdf

---

　　In summary, *clinical audit research method* is the process whereby real clinical midwifery practice is compared against explicit standards of best practice. Once a topic for investigation has been identified, valid evidence-based standards are selected that relate to stated aspects of maternity care that are measurable. This allows researchers to strive to improve midwifery care provided. We will now move on to look at the processes involved in *grounded theory method*.

5.10 GROUNDED THEORY RESEARCH METHOD

Grounded theory research method is a systematic qualitative recipe, which involves construction of hypotheses and generating theories through analysis of gathered data (Strauss and Corbin 1997). As such, a *grounded theory research method* begins with a research question or merely from a collection of qualitative data. In essence, as the midwife researcher reviews their collected data, gradually ideas or concepts begin to 'emerge' which are labelled as themes. During this process, the researcher tags these 'emerged' 'ideas' or 'concepts' with codes and labels that reflect the content. As the researcher gathers and reviews more data, these codes and labels are then grouped into higher-level ideas or concepts and finally overarching themes or categories, which become the underpinning of a new hypothesis or theory. Hence, *grounded theory research method* differs from quantitative deductive research, because instead of deducing answers to one numerical finding, the researcher builds a theoretical framework from which they derive one or more hypotheses. Subsequent to generating these hypotheses, the researcher collects more data from more participants, for purpose of generating more hypotheses and to assess the validity of each preexisting hypothetical concept or idea.

　　In other words, *grounded theory research method* categorizes collected data to build a general theory to fit the data, rather than the other way around. In summary, *grounded theory research method* is a qualitative recipe that uses a systematic set of procedures to develop an inductively derived *grounded theory* about a phenomenon of interest. The objective is to expand upon an explanation of a stated phenomenon, by identifying its key elements and categorizing relationships of these elements to the context and process. That is, the aim is to go from the general to the specific, without losing sight of the object of the study. Consequently, the research question is general and not specific, and an emerging theory is generated to explain the phenomenon under question. *Grounded theory research method* contains many unique characteristics that are designed to maintain the '*grounded-ness*' of the recipe. Data collection and analysis are combined and conducted simultaneously, with each enquiry generated used to shape continuing data collection. The purpose of *grounded theory research method* is to increase insight and clarify parameters of the emerging theory. There are four primary requirements for judging an emerged theory:

1. Fitting the phenomenon.

2. Providing understanding and being comprehensible.

3. Providing generality.

4. Providing control which involves stating the conditions under which the theory applies and describing the basis for action.

    Grounded theory research method begins with a research situation. Within this prescribed situation, the researcher's task is to understand what is happening and how the players manage their roles. The researcher achieves this understanding through observing and interviewing the participant, and after each bout of data collection, they write down the key issues in an event called 'note-taking'. *Constant comparison* is at the heart of process, with new interview data compared with prior gathered data, and from this process, a new theory 'emerges'. Once a theory begins to surface, new data is compared against this 'emerging' constructed theory. As the researcher progresses analysis of data, the results of each 'constant comparison' are written in the margin of their note-taking as coding. The researcher's task is to identify categories (themes) and their subcategories (subthemes).

    As the researcher repeats similar codes, certain theoretical propositions will become evident. These theoretical propositions may involve links between a core category (theme) and one of its subcategories (subthemes). As subcategories (subthemes) and their properties emerge, each is linked to the core category to provide the theory. As data collection continues and coding proceeds more codes and memos accumulate. When the core categories (themes) and their linked subcategories (subthemes) become *saturated*, data collection ceases because the researcher can find nothing new to add to the story. *Saturation* is the signal that it is time to move to the next stage in *grounded theory research method*, which is called *sorting*. The researcher groups the memos, like with like, and sequences them in an order which makes the theory most clear. It is important to acknowledge that with *grounded theory research method*, the literature review happens post generation of a core category (theme) and its linked subcategories (subthemes). The order of the sorted memos, which are usually laid out on a table by the researcher, provide the skeletal framework for the write-up of the research study. To illustrate the overlapping phases of *grounded theory research method* (recipe) (see Figure 5.3).

    Figure 5.3 illustrates, how *data collection, note-taking, coding,* and *memoing* all occur simultaneously and at the beginning of *grounded theory research method* (recipe). *Sorting* occurs when all the categories (themes) have become saturated, which means there is nothing new participants can add to the data pool. *Writing up* of findings occurs after *sorting* of data, with ideally a new theory emergent and discovered in the data. In response to each newly developed theory, literature

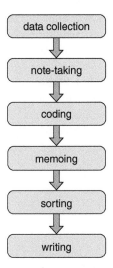

FIGURE 5.3   Illustration of the overlapping phases of *grounded theory research method*.

reviewing takes place to find out more about the concept and justify its discovery, which is very different from other research methods (recipes) where the literature review takes place at the beginning of the study.

What differentiates *grounded theory research method* from other research methods (recipes), is that it is explicitly *emergent*. *Grounded theory research method* does not test a hypothesis, but instead sets out to identify a theory that accounts for the research situation as it is found. Hence, theory develops gradually and as data interpretations accumulate. In essence, *grounded theory research method* involves a continued search for evidence to confirm the emerging theory, with the final shape of the theoretical concept providing a good fit to the situation.

5.10.1 WRITING A METHODOLOGY FOR GROUNDED THEORY

In relation to writing the philosophy that underpins your choice of research method, which in this case is *grounded theory research method*. First, the researcher must provide a rationale for their choice of research method (recipe), which explains why they have specifically selected *grounded theory research method* (STEP 7) to answer the research question they proposed in STEP 6 of how to write a research proposal. When writing up a doctorate, a whole methodology chapter will be written to explain and justify the postgraduate student's choice of research method. This methodology chapter should conscientiously provide justification for all the choices that have been made, which will include the type of approach you have selected (quantitative or qualitative) (STEP 7), your selected research method (recipe) (STEP 7), who (participants) and where you will collect data from (setting) (STEP 8), how you intend to collect your data (data collection) (STEP 9), and how you intend to analyse the data gathered (data analysis) (STEP 10). An example philosophy for grounded theory follows, which in a research proposal is placed in STEP 7.

5.10.2 EXAMPLE PHILOSOPHY UNDERPINNING GROUNDED THEORY RESEARCH METHOD

Grounded theory includes a variety of slightly differing approaches, all of which are based upon positivist philosophy, sociology, and symbolic interactionism. Positivism is an empirical approach which endorses that all information is genuine knowledge. Grounded theorists reject the idea that facts are derived through reasoning, applying logic, and/or sensory experience. Instead, the theory of symbolic interactionism has been developed from practical deliberations, such as from communications and interactions between people, which cause them to create images and deduce meaning (Hall 2016). Ralph et al. (2015) viewed grounded theory as not being a complete methodology, but rather a means of constructing methods to aid understanding of specified situations (Ralph et al. 2015). Together, Glaser (1967) view grounded theory as methodologically dynamic (Glaser 1967). In part derived through Glaser having a background in positivism, which helped him develop a system of labelling for the purpose of coding interviewees' qualitative narratives. In essence, Glaser recognized the significance of systematically analyzing qualitative research, which as part of the method requires generation of codes, categories, and properties (Aldiabat and Navenec 2011). In contrast, Strauss had a background in symbolic interactionalism, which focuses upon aiming to understand how humans interact with one another using symbolic worlds that in turn shape behaviour. Straus viewed people as active participants who form their own comprehensions of their world, which underscores the richness of qualitative research in terms of learning about social processes and convolution of life (Aldiabat and Navenec 2011). Hence and according to Glaser, the methodology of grounded theory is to interpret meaning within the context of the social interaction (Glaser 1992). Within this context, when undertaking *grounded theory research method,* symbolic codes based upon categories emerge from the recorded qualitative data, from which the researcher explains the phenomenal world of participants in the specified context (Aldiabat and Navenec 2011). In essence, Milliken and Schreiber explain how the grounded theorist's task is to comprehend socially shared meaning that underpins the behaviour and reality of the individual studied (Aldiabat and Navenec 2011). To view an example of how STEP 7 of the research proposal could be written, see Activity 5.12.

Activity 5.12

Access and read the following Grounded theory research method paper.

Ismaila, Y., Bayes, S., and Geraghty, S. (2021). Midwives' strategies for coping with barriers to providing quality maternal and neonatal care: a Glaserian grounded theory study. *BMC Health Services Research* 21: 1190. https://doi.org/10.1186/s12913-021-07049-0

NOTE that STEP 7 explains the research method, the rationale for choice of method, and the underpinning methodology

Method

Glaserian (classic) grounded theory (GT) methodology was employed in this study (Glaser 1967). The methodology was chosen for this study because it provides a way to explain ongoing behaviours of participants and the way they solve issues of concern (Glaser 2002). The first author (YI) collected all the data for the study and led the analysis. In Glaserian GT, it is important that the researcher keeps theoretical sensitivity low at the beginning of the study to allow the data analysis to augment it, therefore, it is recommended that the researcher discerns and purges his or her prior assumptions on the phenomenon under study as much as possible at the inception of the study (Glaser 1967). Accordingly, similar to what happens in bracketing, YI noted all prior assumptions he had as someone with direct and vicarious personal and professional experience of the Ghanaian maternity system and discussed it with SB and SG (Speziale et al. 2011). The participants' narratives were thus heard and analysed objectively without being obscured by any prior assumptions.

To view a summary of the specific approaches involved in a *grounded theory research method,* see Table 5.8.

Table 5.8 Specific processes involved in a *grounded theory research method.*

(1) The midwife develops a researchable question that is flexible enough to allow for in-depth investigation (e.g. Why do women stop breastfeeding?) (STEP 6).

(2) The literature review is carried out post inducing themes (categories) and subthemes (subcategories) from the data, with evidence used to ground the developing theory (STEP 5). *NOTE: Grounded theory is the only research method that does the literature review post developing categories (themes) and subcategories (subthemes), with papers retrieved used to evidence developing grounded theories.*

(3) In relation to the 'methods' section of the research proposal, clearly outline the philosophy that underpins the selected *grounded theory research method* (recipe). For example, Strauss and Corbin (1997) who developed grounded theory in practice, or Charmez (2014, 2017) who established *constructivist grounded theory method.* (STEP 7).

(4) The researcher does not predecide on a fixed number of participants and instead keeps recruiting until no new viewpoints are offered, which is the point called *saturation.* (STEP 8). An example follows:

Participant 1: Informs you that they stopped breastfeeding because they wanted to return to work. This reason is written down and formed into a *mini hypothesis* to be tested on subsequent participants. The researcher has called this category (theme) *Returning to work*, which is followed by a literature review to ground theoretical discussion in relation to the category (theme) identified (noted).

Participant 2: Informs you that they stopped breastfeeding because their partner felt embarrassed about them doing so in public. This reason is also written down and formed into a *mini hypothesis* to be tested against what subsequent participants say about why they stopped breastfeeding. The researcher has called this category (theme) *Partner influence*, which is followed by a literature review to ground theoretical discussion in relation to the category (theme) identified (noted). Once *participant two* has said their piece about why they stopped breastfeeding, the mini hypothesis is introduced and tested by the researcher (i.e. *Did going back to work play a part in your decision to stop breastfeeding?*). *Participant Two* will respond with a *'yes'* or *'no'* and their elaborated response is used to ground theoretical discussion in relation to this new category (theme) identified (noted), which the researcher has called *Returning to work*.

Participant 3: Informs you that they stopped breastfeeding because it was too painful to continue, with this reason also written down and formed into a *mini hypothesis* to be tested against what subsequent participants say. The researcher has called this category (theme) *persistent pain*, which is followed by a literature review to ground theoretical discussion in relation to the category (theme) identified (noted). Once *Participant Three* has said their piece about why they stopped breastfeeding, the mini hypothesis; *Did going back to work play a part in your decision to stop breastfeeding?* Followed by: *Did your partner feel embarrassed about you breastfeeding in public*? Again, *Participant 3* will respond with a *'yes'* or *'no'*, with these responses used to ground theoretical discussion in relation to the category or theme *Returning to Work* and *Partner Influence.*

As you can see so far three themes have been identified:

(1) *Returning to work.*

(2) *Partner influence.*

(3) *Persistent pain.*

The above process continues until no new reasons for discontinuing breastfeeding are provided by participants, which is the point of *saturation* and may occur at any number of participants. The literature review is conducted to ground theoretical discussion in relation to these categories (themes) identified (noted).

(5) *Data collection, note-taking, coding,* and *memoing* of this study occur simultaneously and are followed by *sorting,* and lastly *writing.* This is different to other research methods, which strictly adhere to the 16-STEP model (see Figure 5.3).

To summarize, *grounded theory research method* is a systematic methodology that has been largely applied to qualitative studies carried out by social scientists. The methodology involves the construction of hypotheses and theories through gathering and analyzing data collected. *Grounded theory research method* also requires the application of inductive reasoning. It is important to note that there are sub-recipes for *grounded theory research method*, which involve different philosophical approaches that effect how the method (recipe) is applied. Whatever the choice, the method (recipe) will still follow the general 16-step approach, except for STEP 5, which occurs within STEPS 9 and 10. If you decide to use grounded theory as your chosen research method, it is important to follow the philosophical path discussed by the underpinning author, which will require more reading (Birks and Mills 2023). For example, Strauss and Corbin (1997) who developed grounded theory in practice, or Charmez (2014, 2017) who established *constructivist grounded theory method*. Both of these qualitative *grounded theory research methods* are commonly used across many disciplines and professions, including midwifery (e.g. Cunen et al. 2022; Mirzaee and Dehghan 2020). We will now move on to look at a different qualitative approach, which is called *phenomenology research method*.

5.11 PHENOMENOLOGY RESEARCH METHOD

Phenomenology research method is essentially about the philosophy of experience, with definitive source of all meaning and value rooted within the lived experiences of humans. Phenomenology was founded in the early twentieth century by Husserl (Zahavi 2003, 2019). In Husserl's conception, phenomenology is primarily concerned with making the structures of consciousness and the phenomena, which appear in acts of consciousness, objects of systematic reflection and analysis. In other words, *phenomenology research method* involves the researcher studying the 'lived-in experiences' of a person operating in their social world, with data collection focusing upon the predefined area of interest (STEP 6). As such, aims and research question(s) are written, but no hypotheses. Hypotheses are not relevant because *phenomenology research method* sits at the opposing end of the research continuum to the quantitative approach, given that it philosophically values each participant's individual subjective experience. Acknowledging this point in relation to *phenomenology research method* is key, with quantification in terms of numbers utterly irrelevant. Instead, the phenomenologist attempts to capture each individual participant's conscious experience (e.g. judgements, perceptions, and emotions) in relation to the subject of interest, which is essentially the opposite of hardcore quantitative research (e.g. RCT or quantitative survey). When a participant pronounces their own account of what they 'really see', it is not an objective event, but a subjective one, which may or may not in part be shared by others. The goal of *phenomenology research method* is to understand how the participant's viewpoint is organized by the person experiencing it. Hence, *phenomenology research method* could be criticized for its first-person approach and its incompatibility with the scientific third-person approach. Nonetheless, *phenomenology research method* (recipe) is frequently used by midwifery researchers to make sense of experiences (e.g. Norris et al. 2020), and so its principles have been captured in (Table 5.9).

Table 5.9 Principles of *phenomenology method*.

(1) *Phenomenology research method* (recipe) produces a description of circumstances surrounding a participant's immediate experience, more often obtained through an interview.

(2) *Phenomenology research method* (recipe) involves an attempt to capture experience as lived through descriptive analysis. The focus is upon the way things appear to consciousness or are given in experience, and not how they are in themselves. For example, people who have experienced childbirth may experience subsequent fear for months or years post event. What does this fear mean? Where does it come from? How is it experienced? The answers provided bring the researcher closer to understanding the phenomenon that is lived.

(3) *Phenomenology research method* (recipe) focuses upon learning about another person experiences, through listening to their descriptions of what their subjective world is like. During process, attempts are made to understand that person's conditions as fully as possible, within a dialogue that is free from preconceptions and interferences.

5.11.1 WRITING A METHODOLOGY FOR PHENOMENOLOGY

In relation to writing the philosophy that underpins your choice of method, which in this case is *phenomenology research method* (recipe). First, the researcher must provide a rationale for their choice of research method (recipe), which explains why they have specifically selected *phenomenology research method* (STEP 7). As a reminder, when writing up a doctorate, a whole methodology chapter is written to explain the choice of research method and how the recipe is designed to answer the proposed research question (STEP 6) explicitly and appropriately. Within this methodology chapter, the doctorate student writes the philosophical underpinnings for choices made, which drive the research design. In other words, the purpose of the methodology chapter is to explain why the researcher has selected the specific research method and justify the design of their study. This methodology chapter should painstakingly provide justification for all choices made. Together, this will include the type of research you have selected (quantitative or qualitative), selected method (STEP 7), who and/or where you will collect data from (STEP 8), how you intend to collect your data (STEP 9), and a data analysis plan (STEP 10). If you plan to use *phenomenology research method* (recipe), it may be a good idea to obtain a written thesis from the university library and observe how the methodology chapter has been written up. An example philosophy for phenomenology follows.

5.11.2 EXAMPLE PHILOSOPHY UNDERPINNING PHENOMENOLOGY RESEARCH METHOD HUSSERL

As envisioned by Husserl, phenomenology is a method of philosophical inquiry, which rejects the rationalist bias that has dominated western thinking. It is a method of reflective attentiveness that discloses the individual's 'lived experience' (Tassone 2017). Husserl describes his position as 'descriptive psychology'. Husserl analyses the intentional structures of mental acts and how they are directed at both real and ideal objects. Husserl's method requests that the researcher suspend all judgment, which requires that they pay attention to what the participant relates with no presupposition or intellectualizing. Intentionality represents an alternative to the representational theory of consciousness, which proposes that reality cannot be grasped directly because perception is constructed by the mind with the researcher making sense of information by filtering it through their own personal templates of values and opinions (Husserl 1997). The direct approach of Husserlian *phenomenological research method* expects the researcher to analyse the participant's description of phenomena purely as it is given. During data collection and analysis, the researcher must suspend (bracket) their own theoretical explanation and advance with 'naïve' experience of the matter under discussion. In essence, the researcher is being asked to erase their experience of the feeling, idea, or perception. According to Husserl, this is suspension of belief in what we ordinarily take for granted.

5.11.3 HEIDEGGER

In contrast, Heidegger modified Husserl's (Husserl 1997) concept of phenomenology emersed in the belief that people cannot simply eradicate their subjectivist tendencies. Therefore, when the researcher takes a Heideggerian approach, they are expected to declare personal interest, preferences, and experiences (Heidegger 2005, 2010). This personal engagement with the research in action is called *reflexivity*, which involves the researcher acknowledging that their prior experiences, assumptions, and beliefs may influence the research process (Kingdon 2013). Hence and in response to this assumption, *reflexivity* refers to the researcher examining their own beliefs, judgements, and practices throughout the study and how these may influence the process (Burns et al. 2012). When writing a thesis, the researcher will thread *reflexivity* throughout the chapters, and write a standalone section or chapter which describes how they have achieved this. To view a short example of declaring *reflexivity,* see Table 5.10.

Table 5.10 Reflexivity.

The author has background and experience that assisted in the analysis and interpretation of the data. First, the author has been a registered practising midwife for 20 years. Over this time span, she has been employed as a midwife at grade 5, 6, 7, and 8 in a Scottish (United Kingdom) maternity unit. Second, the author has both a BSc and MSc in psychology. This variety of experiences afforded advantages in understanding and negotiation of the interview data.

If you plan to use a Heideggerian-informed *phenomenology research method* (recipe), it would be useful to obtain a completed thesis and read the *reflexivity* chapter and observe how *reflexivity* has been threaded throughout the chapters. There are tools for undertaking such reflexive analysis, with English et al. (2022) providing an example. One of the consequences of Heidegger's modification of Husserl's conception of phenomenology, is that it privileges the researcher to conceptualize the participants' encounters through their own experiences, knowledge, and awareness, which infers intentionality (Heidegger 2005, 2010).

5.11.4 INTENTIONALITY

Intentionality refers to the idea that people are conscious of whatever it is they are discussing (e.g. the childbearing woman's experiences with their midwife). Whether the woman's consciousness is a direct perception or fantasy is inconsequential. As such, *intentionality* means that the object of consciousness (e.g. the childbearing women's experiences of their midwife) can be either a fantasy or memory. These structures of consciousness, perception, memory, and fantasy are called *intentionality's*, with *intentionality* a cardinal principle of phenomenology.

To view a summary of the specific approaches involved in a *phenomenology research method,* see Table 5.11.

5.11.5 INTERPRETATIVE PHENOMENOLOGICAL ANALYSIS (IPA)

IPA is a *phenomenology method* which aims to produce generalized findings that offer insight into how the participant in a given context makes sense of the situation (e.g. childbirth, breastfeeding, and use of contraception) (Smith et al. 2009). As an approach, IPA is psychological, interpretative, and deals with concrete events, which are characteristics that distinguish

Table 5.11   Specific processes involved in a *phenomenology research method.*

---

(1) Identify a phenomenon of interest that relates to the midwifery profession.

(2) Develop a detailed description of this identified phenomenon.

(3) Carry out a literature review to find out what papers have already been published about the stated phenomenon (STEP 5).

(4) In relation to the 'methods' section of the research proposal, clearly outline the philosophy that underpins your selected *phenomenology research method* (recipe). For example, bracket personal prejudices and a priori assumptions if research is underpinned by a Husselarian philosophy (Husserl 1997), or not bracketing and declaring biases and prejudices (reflexivity) if Heideggerian in approach (Heidegger 2005, 2010). If Heideggerian philosophy is selected, acknowledge preconceptions, declare prejudices and biases, and state how you will thread reflexivity throughout delivery of the project (STEP 7).

(5) Small participant sample sizes are recommended, with Ellis (2016) suggesting 6–20. Such small numbers allow the researcher to undertake in-depth interviews that may be repeated across longitudinal time points (STEP 8).

(6) There are several ways of collecting data when a *phenomenology research method*. For example:

  • Interviews

  • Focus groups

  • Observation

  • Action research

  • Analyzing other forms of spoken text (e.g. documentaries).

Whatever type of data collection is selected, the researcher must stay focused upon the research question and seek to avoid influencing participant responses, precisely because it is their real experiences you are interested in. In addition, it is important to show empathy towards participants', and develop a good rapport to gain trust and achieve meaningful insight (STEP 9).

(7) Data analysis involves reading the transcribed data (e.g. interview), identify relevant content that describes participants' lived experiences of the phenomenon of interest, eliminate irrelevant data, coding quotes in a way that makes them anonymous and retrievable from the whole pool, group data into themes, and name these relevant themes and subthemes (STEP 10).

Outside of the above-stated characteristics of *phenomenology research method,* the researcher adheres to the 16-STEP model of writing a research proposal.

---

the recipe from the other *phenomenology research methods*. IPA involves the researcher taking part and closely examining and making meaning of each individual participant's experiences. With similarity to other *phenomenology research methods*, the researcher examines the experiences of a very small number of participants (three to five participants) (Reid et al. 2005). Participants are purposely sampled because they are in a position to offer some meaningful insight into the phenomenon under study. An IPA researcher gathers qualitative data from participants using techniques that are curious and facilitative, and not challenging or interrogative. Gaining deep, rich, and meaningful accounts are at the heart of IPA. Unlike *grounded theory research method*, data collection does not set out to test hypotheses and during data analysis, the researcher reflects upon their own preconceptions about what they think the data may report. As part of this process, the researcher attempts to suspend their acknowledged preconceptions, and instead apply focus upon seizing the experiential world of the participant. Hence, transcripts are coded in substantial detail, with attention shifting back and forth from the participant's key claims and the researcher's interpretation of the experience. The interpretive stance of IPA is one of inquiry and sense making of meaning (Larkin et al. 2006). As such, the researcher (interpreter) attempts to make sense of the participant's efforts to describe their personal experience, which is called a double hermeneutic. IPA analysis takes a 'bottom-up' approach, which involves the researcher generating codes, as opposed to using preexisting theory to identify enigma. Hence, IPA *phenomenology research method* does not test theories, but instead generates new concepts or adds to preexisting views. Along these lines, the IPA researcher encourages open-ended conversations, which leads to both parties viewing experiences in an altered light. To view an example of an IPA study that has focused upon an aspect of maternity care, see Activity 5.13.

Activity 5.13

Access and read the following phenomenology research method (IPA) report

Norris, G., Hollins Martin, C.J., and Dickson, A. (2020). An exploratory interpretative phenomenological analysis (IPA) of childbearing women's perceptions of risk associated with having a high body mass index (BMI). *Midwifery* 89 (2020): 102789. https://doi.org/10.1016/j.midw.2020.102789

In summary, *phenomenology research method* (recipe) is a qualitative research approach that pursues understanding and describes the universal essence of a particular defined phenomenon. During processes of data collection in a *phenomenology research method* (recipe), the approach investigates the in-depth everyday experiences of participants. Again, it is important to note that there are sub-recipes for *phenomenology research method*, which involve adapting the method used. Whatever the researcher's choice, the recipe still follows the 16-step method. If you decide to use phenomenology as your chosen method, it is important to follow the philosophical path of the underpinning author, which will require more reading (Birks and Mills 2023). For example, differing approaches to *phenomenology research method* have been philosophized by Husserl (1997), Heidegger (2005, 2010), or IPA (Smith et al. 2009). We will now move on to look at a different recipe called *ethnography research method*.

5.12 ETHNOGRAPHY RESEARCH METHOD

Ethnography research method (recipe) is a branch of anthropology, which involves using a systematic approach that is focused upon cultures and sub-cultures. More often, quantitative data collection methods are used, however, on occasion a qualitative approach may be taken or even mixed methods. In the main, *ethnography research method* is used to study clearly specified social situations for the purpose of gaining greater understanding of the specified population's interpretation of certain behaviours (e.g. breastfeeding, postnatal rituals, and managing childbirth). To gain true embedded comprehension of the underpinning values and behaviours of the culture of interest, the researcher may select to engage with the population either declared or undeclared, which is a standpoint called participant observation. As such, *ethnography research method* relies upon close-up personal experience and participation, as opposed to straightforward observation. It is important to note that if the researcher proposes the role of undeclared participation, this may arouse some ethical considerations that must be stated in the ethics application. The purpose of participant observation is to play a marginal role in the society of interest and document patterns of behaviour and social interaction from which conclusions are drawn.

Many social organizations have been studied using *ethnographic research methods,* with classic examples including religious organizations, such as cults (e.g. Souček and Karásek 2022) and youth behaviour (Briggs et al. 2015). *Ethnographic research method* has also been used to study social behaviours and values held in relation to maternal and child health (e.g. Flacking and Dykes 2013). If you elect to use this *ethnographic research method* to undertake a maternal or child health project, a book is available to instruct about application of the method (recipe) (e.g. Dykes and Flacking 2016).

Outside the researcher being present and observing a social situation, alternative methods of data collection can be used in *ethnographic research method.* For example, interviewing participants or searching documents, books, notes from meetings, or reading archived letters. In the modern world, netnography is a newer often used approach (Bartl et al. 2016). As such, netnography utilizes *ethnographic research method* to research and understand social interactions within a contemporary digital communications context (Dykes and Flacking 2016; Kozinets 2019).

5.12.1 FEATURES OF ETHNOGRAPHIC RESEARCH METHOD

The essential features of ethnography involve the researcher gathering data about a context or situation (Dewan 2018). Using *ethnography research method*, the researcher gathers data about what is available, what is considered normal, what people actually do, what they say, and how they work within the culture under study. Data collection aims to capture the social meaning and ordinary activities of participants under study within natural settings, which ethnographers call the field. During processes involved in *ethnography research method*, the researcher attempts to cause minimal contamination or personal bias to avoid data skew.

Multiple methods of data collection may be used in unison, all of which attempt to gain an in-depth picture of participants 'just being' within their own community. For example, interviews may be taped and transcribed, for purpose of allowing the researcher to progress conversation without interruption of writing notes. In addition, document analysis may play a part in generating further insights into the topic area of interest. During data analysis and to make interpretation transparent, the researcher carries out 'reflexivity', which explores ways in which their involvement may have influenced, effected, or informed findings. When recruiting participants, 'snowball sampling' is often used, with participants asked to identify other people who represent the community and have common cultural denominators connected to the topic of interest. *Ethnography research method* relies upon close-up personal experience and participation, as opposed to straightforward observation.

5.12.2 EXAMPLE PHILOSOPHY UNDERPINNING ETHNOGRAPHY RESEARCH METHOD

The ontological and epistemological assumptions that underlie *ethnography research method* range from the realist perspective of observing behaviour across to a constructivist standpoint that socially assembles cultural understandings of behaviour (Ybema and Kamsteeg 2009). As such, ethnographic fieldwork is a balancing act between distancing and immersing (de Jong et al. 2013). During process, researchers who work in the field require to come close to participants and their culture, for purpose of being able to meaningfully grasp and make sense of the concept they are looking at. de Jong et al. (2013) explain how immersion is often emphasized as paramount and a better approach to 'distancing' oneself. Selecting a philosophy requires the researcher to choose between 'familiarization' or 'defamiliarization'. If 'familiarization' is the choice, then the ethnographer is existing amongst the population of participants. Whilst in contrast, 'defamiliarization' involves the researcher using estrangement strategies, which permits development of a detached standpoint from which data is interpreted (de Jong et al. 2013). In summary, ethnography can take a position which ranges from an objectivist account of fixed observable behaviours to instead taking an interpretive narrative approach that involves describing the interplay of individual participants within their social structure.

A further form of understanding ethnographic data is through 'image', which involves the researcher gathering and sensemaking through their personal perspective and experience. For example, one midwife's account of an event (e.g. a birth) may differ to another's. In this instance, the 'image' encompassed within the physical world is interpreted and constructed from each midwife's past experiences of caring for women in labour. This accounted 'image' is based upon feelings, memories, and imagination. In essence, the 'image' presents the perspectives, experiences, and influences of a single person, with the researcher retaining this image within the group under study. 'Images' can be presented as case studies that join up to produce sociograms or participant-produced drawings, which are presented in a described and structured form. Fundamentally, a sociogram is an illustrative representation of the individual social links within a group, which are

Table 5.12 Five criteria to evaluate whether or not your *ethnographic research method* (recipe) will be effective.

(1) Will your study make a substantive contribution to understanding of social life? (e.g. home birth, postnatal rituals, and bereavement care).

(2) Will your study attract interest and is it appealing?

(3) Is *reflexivity* involved, with adequate self-awareness of what could affect the data collector's judgements when making sense of participants' points of view?

(4) Will your proposed research method affect you emotionally and intellectually (e.g. create a bias)?

(5) Will your proposed study specify a relevant situation, and will it produce a credible account of a cultural, social, individual, or communal sense of the 'real'.

Source: Adapted from Richardson (2000).

presented as a graph drawing that plots the assembly of interpersonal relations. The purpose is to discover visual and interactional representations that are difficult to translate into language (Ayala and Koch 2019). In summary, creating 'images' is about making sense of the social using a structured method (Ayala and Koch 2019).

5.12.3 QUESTIONS TO HELP YOU EVALUATE YOUR RECIPE

It is important to evaluate the *ethnographic research method* you design for your research proposal. This is because *ethnographic research method* does not follow such a clear-cut recipe as an RCT method or survey method does. Although predominantly a qualitative approach is used in *ethnographic research method*, you may elect to include some quantitative measures. Richardson (2000) suggests five criteria that you can use to evaluate whether or not your recipe will be effective (Table 5.12).

Activity 5.14

Access and read the following ethnography research method report

   Goldkuhl, L., Dellenborg, L., Berg, M., et al. (2022). The influence and meaning of the birth environment for nulliparous women at a hospital-based labour ward in Sweden: an ethnographic study. *Women and Birth* 35 (4): e337–e347. https://doi.org/10.1016/j.wombi. 2021.07.005

To view an example of an ethnographic study that has focused on an aspect of maternity care, see Activity 5.14.

In summary, *ethnographic research method* is a recipe that involves the systematic study of individual cultures. As such, *ethnography research method* essentially explores a cultural phenomenon from the standpoint of the study participant(s). It is important to note that there is adaptability in the sub-recipe design, which can accommodate both quantitative and qualitative methods. Whatever the choice, the recipe still follows the 16-step method. We will now move on to look at *case studies method*.

5.13 CASE STUDY RESEARCH METHOD

A *case study research method* (recipe) involves empirical inquiry that investigates a phenomenon of interest within its real-life context. It involves intensive study of a single group, incident, or community. Rather than using samples and following a rigid protocol to examine a limited numbers of variables, *case study research method* undertakes in-depth and longitudinal examination of a single instance or event (a case). Hence, a case study is a systematic way of:

1. Looking at events.

2. Collecting data.

3. Analyzing information.

4. Reporting results.

The goal is to sharpen understanding of why the instance happened as it did and identify what is important to examine more extensively in future research. *Case study research method* generates and tests hypotheses and should not be confused with qualitative research, given that it involves a mix of quantitative and qualitative evidence. A case study is helpful for generalizing. For example, if one observes that all sheep are white, then just one observation of a single brown sheep falsifies this proposition and stimulates investigation and theory-building. *Case study research method* is well suited for identifying brown sheep because of its in-depth approach. That is, what appears to be white often turns out on closer examination to be brown.

5.13.1 CASE SELECTION

When selecting an instance for a case study, researchers often use information-oriented sampling, as opposed to random sampling. This is because the average case is often not richest in information, with atypical cases revealing further information. Consequently, it is more appropriate to select a few cases, which are selected for their validity. Three types of information-oriented cases may be distinguished:

1. Extreme case study.

2. Critical case study.

3. Paradigmatic case study.

1. *Extreme case study*
   An *extreme case* study is well suited for transmitting a point in a dramatic way. What follows is an example of an *extreme case study* (Table 5.13):

Table 5.13 The extreme case study of Genie.

Genie was a child deprived and isolated from almost all social interaction and language development until adolescence. She spent her first 13 years locked inside a room until she was discovered in 1970. Psychologist, linguists, and other scientists took great interest in Genie's case due to its perceived ability to reveal insights into the development of language and linguistic development. Linguistic research attempted to answer the following questions using the *extreme case study* of Genie:

- Is there a critical period for language acquisition?

- If so, what kind of language development is possible beyond the critical period?

- What happens to cerebral organization when one of the brain's basic functions fails to develop?

In 1994, a book was published about Genie's case.

Source: Adapted from Rymer (1994).

2. *Critical case study*
   A *critical case study* has strategic importance in relation to a specified general problem. For example, a researcher wishes to investigate whether midwives who work with organic solvents suffer brain damage. Instead of selecting a representative sample of many enterprises in which workers are exposed to organic solvents, a specific enterprise is selected for study. That is, the maternity unit will represent all (or many) cases.

3. *Paradigmatic case study*
   A *paradigmatic case study* is a detailed analysis of a person or group that is selected for its qualities as medical, psychiatric, psychological, or social phenomena. For example, a detailed intensive *paradigmatic case study* of a unit, such as a company or corporate division, which identifies factors that contribute to success or failure.

To view an example of a case study that has focused on an aspect of maternity care, see Activity 5.15.

Activity 5.15

Access and Read the Following Case Study Method Report

Mehretie Adinew, Y., Kelly, J., Marshall, A., and Hall, H. (2021). 'I would have stayed home if I could manage it alone': a case study of Ethiopian mother abandoned by care providers during facility-based childbirth. *International Journal of Women's Health* 24 (13): 501–507. https://doi.org/10.2147/IJWH.S302208

Table 5.14   An example method STEP 7.

A qualitative *interpretative phenomenological analysis* (IPA) was used to identify women with a high BMI ($>35\,kg/m^2$) perceptions of risk and what this meant to them. Phenomenology is a philosophical approach to the study of experience and is concerned with the study of experience as it occurs for that individual person (Smith et al. 2009). There are two main different schools of thought in phenomenological philosophy, namely Edmond Husserl's (1859–1938) descriptive or eidetic phenomenology and Martin Heidegger's (1889–1976) hermeneutics or interpretative phenomenology. Husserl's own epistemological belief placed more emphasis on describing the '*essence*' or structure of that experience, rather than how it was experienced by the individual (Smith et al. 2009). In contrast, Heidegger was more concerned with the ontological question of being in the world embodied in the social world surrounded by people, language, and culture. Heidegger (1889–1976) rejected notion of separating consciousness from the lived world and as a result took a more interpretative stance and in effort s to answer the question of being (Smith et al. 2009). In recognition that risk is not a static objective phenomenon, with an assumption that perceptions of vulnerability may change across time, a longitudinal approach was taken (Lupton 1999). An IPA approach was selected because it places the individual at the heart of the experience and acknowledges how they can be influenced by culture, history, social interactions, and language (Smith et al. 2009). IPA provided an opportunity to uncover the embodied experiences of high-risk childbearing women with BMI's ($>35\,kg/m^2$) perceptions of risk, with a rich interpretative account uncovering beliefs surrounding level of obstetric risk (the phenomenon). IPA draws on three key areas of philosophy, which includes phenomenology, hermeneutics, and ideography. Phenomenology is made up of two parts is derived from the Greek '*phenomenon*' and '*logos*', and is about examining meaning that is perhaps not obvious (Smith et al. 2009). IPA methodology is idiographic given that it is committed to uncovering in-depth phenomena. Hermeneutics is the study of theory and interpretation, which involves generating a deeper understanding of the meaning of the phenomenon under study (Smith et al. 2009).

Source: Rymer (1994)/Elsevier.

In summary, *case study research method* is a research approach that involves in-depth, detailed examination of a particular case (or cases) within a real-world context. For example, case studies in maternal health may focus on an individual woman or neonate. It is important to note that the recipe still follows the 16-step method.

5.13.2 POSTSCRIPT

Within *Chapter 5*, we have covered many research methods that could be used as the recipe to underpin your research proposal (STEP 7). Some of these research methods (recipes) allow a degree of flexibility surrounding how they will be delivered, with any deviations from the main method justified. Please note that whatever recipe you decide to use, the methodology needs to be justified in terms of philosophy, which is presented under the heading **Method** within the proposal. An example follows (STEP 7), which is taken from (Norris et al. 2020) (Table 5.14).

Once you have selected a research method (recipe) to answer your selected research question, take a look at the example paper provided in the related activity box in this chapter. Download this paper or another using the same method (recipe) and read what the authors have written under each of the (STEPS 1–16). A hot tip is to use this selected paper as a template of the method (recipe), which you can use to populate your research proposal. I would recommend that you keep your research proposal straightforward, by selecting just one research method (recipe), especially if it is a word-limited research proposal for assessment for an undergraduate or postgraduate master's program. However, if you are writing a PhD or doctorate proposal for a potential supervisor to review, your research proposal will require to proposition a substantial and meaningful project, which may require triangulation of mixed methods (recipes).

5.14 TRIANGULATION

Triangulation is the application and combination of two or occasionally more research methods in the same proposal. You may ask yourself why and when would triangulation be necessary. By combining multiple observers, theories, methods, and empirical materials, researchers can hope to overcome the weakness or intrinsic biases and problems that come from using one single research method. Triangulation combines research methods (recipes) for the purpose of achieving a multidimensional view of the phenomenon of interest. There are four types of triangulations (Denzin 2012) (Table 5.15).

Triangulation is extremely valuable when the researcher has used a quantitative method, such as an RCT. Classically, the experimental approach supports or rejects a hypothesis, which states whether the intervention worked or not. This will inform the researcher of *cause* and *effect* supported with statistics, but will not explain how participants experienced the intervention. Triangulation of an RCT with qualitative narratives of staff or women's experiences of the intervention will inform the developer of whether the intervention is tolerable or otherwise. Triangulation is a component of mixed methods. To view an example of a mixed methods study, see Activity 5.16.

Table 5.15   Examples of types of triangulations.

(1) *Data* triangulation: refers to the use of different data sources, which should be distinguished from the use of different methods for producing data. Denzin (2012) proposes that it is useful to study phenomena from different dates, places, and from different persons.

(2) *Investigator triangulation:* engages different observers or interviewers to detect or minimize biases resulting from the researcher or person. This involves a systematic comparison of different researcher's influences on the issue and the results of the research.

(3) *Theory triangulation:* approaches data with multiple perspectives and hypotheses. Various theoretical points of view can be placed side by side to assess their utility and power. The purpose is to extend possibilities for producing knowledge.

(4) *Methodological triangulation:* is a strategy for validating results. A between-methods approach combines a questionnaire with a semi-structured interview. Methodological triangulation was first conceptualized as a strategy for validating results, with focus shifting increasingly towards further enriching and completing knowledge and transgressing the (always limited) epistemological potential of individual methods.

Source: Adapted from Denzin (2012).

Activity 5.16

Access and Read the Following Mixed Method Report

Nishimwe, A., Conco, D.N., Nyssen, M., et al. (2022). A mixed-method study exploring experiences, perceptions, and acceptability of using a safe delivery mHealth application in two district hospitals in Rwanda. *BMC Nursing* 21: 176. https://doi.org/10.1186/s12912-022-00951-w

---

5.15 A SUMMARY OF HOW PAPERS ARE WRITTEN

Having retrieved and reviewed a variety of published research papers which report different research methods (recipes) that you could use, which are from both qualitative and quantitative camps. If you make comparisons between these published research papers, regardless of the journal they are published in, you should observe the similar organizational structure between these reports. There are small variations in house style between journals, with a summary of the general sequence summarized in Table 5.16. Please note that the sequence in Table 5.16 follows the same pathway as a research proposal, with an additional findings report and discussion section precisely because the study has been completed.

5.15.1 CHAPTER CONCLUSION

This chapter has addressed (STEP 7) of writing a research proposal (recipe), which involves outlining the research method. The next chapter will address (STEP 8), which will guide you towards populating the **Participant** section of your research proposal. During the process, you will outline the setting, who the participants are to be, what sampling method you will use, inclusion and exclusion criteria for being eligible to participate, and method of recruitment.

Please note, that when you write a research proposal (STEPS 1–16), the study is called *primary research*. *Primary research* is a study that is not singularly based on a literature review or synthesis of prior published studies. Instead, the purpose of *primary research* is to produce original new work, as opposed to exploring an existing series of preexisting published primary research papers to summarize themes about total findings. The concept of originality of *primary research* is a key criterion for publication in peer-reviewed academic journals, with graduates commonly required to perform an original study. For a doctorate study (e.g. PhD; Prof Doc; Doc Ed) originality is an essential criterion.

Table 5.16   *General sequence that research papers follow.*

(1) *A title*: reflecting the content of the paper, which ordinarily also states the research method (recipe) followed (STEP (1): Give the research proposal a title).

(2) *Authors details*: with titles, universities, and often contact emails. STEP (2): Provide relevant personal and professional details.

(3) *An abstract*: which contains a summary of the research study, and ordinarily contains sub-headings. STEP (3): Provide a short abstract or summary of around 300 words.

(4) *Keywords*: that will facilitate a library search, which reflect the topic and research method. STEP (4): Supply six keywords to describe the research proposal.

(5) *An introduction*: which introduces the study and contains:

- *Back*ground: an explanation of the background to the study, with definitions of key terms used.

- *A literature review*: which accounts preexisting and relevant research that has paved the way for the study, which conveys to the reader what has already been established about the topic and what strengths or weaknesses of the findings are.

- *A rationale*: that justifies the reason why the researcher was interested in the topic and a projection of its worth for future mdwifery practice.

STEP (5): Construct an introduction that contains a relevant literature review and rationale.

(6) *The objective, aim, and research question*: which are abbreviated from the original research proposal and usually captured as one aim or research question, because more than one paper may be written from the global study. STEP (6) State the objectives, aim(s), research question(s), sub-question(s), hypotheses, and null hypotheses of the proposed research study.

(7) *Methods (section)*: which outlines whether the study is qualitative or quantitative and the research method used. This is followed by a referenced methodological justification for the choice of method and how it will achieve answering the research question. STEP (7): Outline the research method.

(8) *Participants (section)*: which consists of place study was carried out (e.g. Elgin House), number of participants (e.g. $n = 60$), method of sampling (e.g. convenience sampling), inclusion criteria (e.g. age and primigravids), exclusion criteria (e.g. teenage mothers and medical conditions), and an explanation of how participants were recruited (e.g. online). STEP (8): Select setting, participants, sampling method, inclusion and exclusion criteria, and method of recruitment.

(9) *Data collection (section)*: which consists of an explanation of how the data was collected, e.g. interviews, survey questionnaire, observations, physical measurements, and how the researcher gathered this information. If validated quantitative measuring tools have been used, these will be described in term of reliability and validity, and their scoring systems described. STEP (9): Describe data collection instruments.

(10) *Data analysis*: If a qualitative method, steps in process and coding will be described. If a quantitative, a statistical plan is outlined. STEP (10): Detail intended data processing and analysis.

(11) *Ethics (section)*: which may be part of the method or participant section, and will outline ethics approval and informed consent procedures. STEP (11): Declare any ethical considerations and outline data protection procedures.

PLEASE NOTE that STEPS (12), (13), and (14) of writing a research proposal are not included in the published research paper. In their place is a:

- *Findings (section)*: which will report statistics if quantitative data, and a table of themes and subthemes if qualitative.

- *Discussion (section)*: which makes sense of the meaning of the findings and how they advance the literature review, limitations of research, and recommendations for professional practice and future research.

- *Conclusion*: A summary of study and future intentions are presented, along with a summary of important points and their meaning. Also, where the researcher intends to go next.

- *Acknowledgements*: of participants, persons who have facilitated the study, and funders.

(15) *References*: An accurate list of references in the journal's house style will be listed. STEP (15): Append a full and accurate reference list

(16) *Additional information*: A website may be referenced that holds additional information, etc. When the paper is submitted to the journal, all the tables and figures are placed as appendixes at the end of the written paper. STEP (16): Appendix relevant additional material.

5.16 SELF-ASSESSMENT QUESTIONS (SAQs)

5.1   In an RCT the dependant variable is:

   (a)   The measuring tool (i.e. scale/questionnaire) used by the researcher.

   (b)   An ethical issue that must be addressed.

   (c)   A schematic diagram of themes.

   (d)   A clear-cut hypothesis.

5.2   A control group is:

   (a)   A researcher who keeps participants in order.

   (b)   A placebo.

   (c)   A matched group of participants who do not receive the intervention.

   (d)   A manipulation strategy.

5.3   Surveys involve data collection using questionnaires.

   (a)   Only when a treatment reduces participants' symptoms.

   (b)   False.

   (c)   True.

   (d)   Only when an intervention is given.

5.4   A researcher posts a questionnaire to ($n = 100$) postnatal women asking if they are happy with the midwifery care they have received. The research method used is?

   (a)   Phenomenology

   (b)   Grounded theory

   (c)   An RCT

   (d)   A survey

5.5   Phenomenology method is:

   (a)   A research method that studies an organization's culture.

   (b)   Involves writing hypotheses.

   (c)   An attempt to capture participants lived experience of the topic of interest.

   (d)   A research method that uses large numbers of participants.

5.6   Ethnography method:

   (a)   Involves constant comparison.

   (b)   Is a quantitative research method (recipe).

   (c)   Includes a control group.

   (d)   Has its roots in anthropology.

5.7   Ethnography method is a type of:

   (a)   Descriptive qualitative study of a person's lived experience.

   (b)   Quantitative study comparing two cultures.

    (c)   Descriptive qualitative study of how culture influences someone's experiences.

    (d)   Ethics approval.

5.8 **Grounded theory method involves:**

    (a)   The researcher conducting an extensive literature review in advance of data collection.

    (b)   Data collection stopping when saturation has been reached.

    (c)   Issue of drugs to matched groups.

    (d)   Issue of scored questionnaires.

5.9 **Triangulation:**

    (a)   Combines research strategies for the purpose of achieving a multidimensional view of the topic of interest.

    (b)   Is used to establish average efficacy of a treatment.

    (c)   Is a quasi-experimental design.

    (d)   Is a form of qualitative research.

5.10 **Which research method is suited to answer the research question?**

Does immersion in warm water reduce the pain experience of women in labour?

    (a)   An ethnographic study of the effects on lifestyle.

    (b)   An experiment which uses pain scales.

    (c)   A survey which uses open-ended questions.

    (d)   A grounded theory study.

5.11 **Which research method is suited to answer the research question?**

Are women's attitudes towards parenthood education altered through participation?

    (a)   An RCT.

    (b)   An experiment.

    (c)   A survey.

    (d)   A grounded theory study.

ANSWERS TO CHAPTER 5 SAQs

5.1   **a**

5.2   **c**

5.3   **c**

5.4   **d**

5.5   **c**

5.6   **c**

5.7   **c**

5.8   **b**

5.9   **a**

5.10 **b**

5.11 **c**

CHAPTER 6

Accessing Populations of Participants and Sampling Them

6.1 Identifying the Appropriate Participants to Answer your Research Question(s)

6.2 What is a Population?

6.3 What is a Sample?

6.4 Stages of the Sampling Process

6.5 Summary of the Sampling Process

6.6 Self-Assessment Questions (SAQs)

STEP (8): Select setting, participants, sampling method, inclusion and exclusion criteria, and method of recruitment.

6.1 IDENTIFYING THE APPROPRIATE PARTICIPANTS TO ANSWER YOUR RESEARCH QUESTION(S)

The first step in recruiting participants for your research study involves making a clear decision about what type of contributors you need to answer your research question. To achieve such, you require to define precisely what you want to uncover or discover. Your job is to create a profile of perfect participants, which could contain some of the following information:

- *Demographic data*: Years of age, parity, marital status, socioeconomic grouping, level of education, etc.

- *Setting of interest*: Country, city/town/village, health board, maternity unit, etc.

- *Social attitudes of interest*: Women's attitudes and/or intentions. For example, breastfeeding, attending parenthood education classes, type of desired birth, having a birth partner present during labour and delivery, pain relief preferences, being diabetic, etc.).

- *Personal behaviours*: Smoking, drinking, diet, medical conditions, etc.

Being very specific about such pointers will produce a very clear profiling picture. It is also important to be crystal clear about what participants you do not want to take part in your study. For example, if you plan to carry out a study with women who have never given birth before, then you do not want to include multigravidas. Having introduced some concepts surrounding participant selection, we will now define the terms *population*, *sampling*, and *sampling process*, but first undertake Activity 6.1.

Activity 6.1

Write a profile to identify appropriate participants to answer your research question.

You can adapt below to suit your agenda. For example, your participants may be neonates.

Demographic data

Years of age

Parity

Marital status

Research Recipes for Midwives, First Edition. Caroline J. Hollins Martin.
© 2024 John Wiley & Sons Ltd. Published 2024 by John Wiley & Sons Ltd.

Socioeconomic grouping
Level of education
Etc.
Setting:
Country
City/town/village
Health board
Maternity/neonatal unit
Etc.
Social attitude or behaviour of interest
What do you specifically want to find out?

6.2 WHAT IS A POPULATION?

Successful research is focused upon defining a problem and finding an answer to it and to answer the research question within the context of interest. Hence, the *population* of participants from which the data is collected needs to be applicable and clearly defined. A *population* includes people (or items) with the characteristics you want to study. For example, pregnant insulin-dependent diabetic women or women carrying a multiple pregnancy. Since it is impossible to gather information from all pregnant insulin-dependent diabetic women or all women carrying a multiple pregnancies, the goal of the researcher is to find a representative *sample* (or subset) from the *diabetic population of pregnant women* or the *multiple-pregnancy population* of women. From these select groups, you will require to clearly define *inclusion criteria* and *exclusion criteria* for your exact participants. Data is then gathered from your clearly defined and appropriate *population*, which will then be analysed, and a report produced. In the case of a quantitative study, if the findings are significant, results can then be extrapolated to the larger *diabetic population of pregnant women* or the *multiple-pregnancy population of women.*

As such, a research *population* is a selected group of participants about which the researcher wants to know something about and from which a select *sample* is drawn. In other words, a *population* is a collection of people who share similar characteristics that are of interest to the researcher. Within maternity care, relevant *populations* can be defined by several clearly defined characteristics. For example, pregnant woman diagnosed with a specific complication (e.g. preeclampsia, breech presentation, and placenta previa), or a specific physical, mental, or social problem. In quantitative research, the study of *populations* is regulated by the law of probability, which applies to most of the *population* the results are drawn from. However, it is important to note that post quantitative data analysis, the conclusion(s) drawn may not be relevant to the remaining small minority of participants, which is where triangulating the study with a qualitative method would enable deeper exploration of individual meaning(s). When designing a research study, the population must be specific enough to provide a clear understanding of applicability to the purpose of the study. Consequently, it is important to select study participants from an appropriate *population* using a specific method of *sampling.*

6.3 WHAT IS A SAMPLE?

Sampling is concerned with selecting participants who are appropriate to yield the desired information to answer the research question, which makes the selected participants the *population* of interest (e.g. *pregnant insulin-dependent diabetic women* or *women carrying a multiple pregnancy*). Taking a subset of the relevant whole *population*, with the support of inferential statistics, allows the researcher to make presumptions (inferences) about the whole *population*. In this case, *insulin-dependent diabetic women* or *women carrying a multiple pregnancy*. Within a written research proposal, the researcher requires to clearly outline the processes involved in *sampling* suitable participants from the clearly defined *population* of interest. What follows will now explain the processes involved in *sampling* a subsection of a clearly defined *population*.

6.4 STAGES OF THE SAMPLING PROCESS

There are six stages included in the sampling process (see Table 6.1).

6.4.1 (STAGE 1) DEFINE THE POPULATION OF INTEREST

In quantitative research, the *sampling frame* is a list of all the women (or items) within a *population* from which the researcher can attempt to select a subset sample from. As such, the *sampling frame* must be representative of the *population* you want to study. Once the data has been collected and analysed, inferential statistics will inform the researcher about the uncertainties in extrapolating findings from your selected *sample* (e.g. pregnant insulin-dependent diabetic women) to the whole *population* of pregnant insulin-dependent diabetic women. To start this process, the researcher selects a *sample* of participants who represent their clearly defined whole *population* of interest.

The Proposed Sample

It is impossible to identify and measure every person (or item) in a *population*. For example, it is difficult to interview all students that attend universities in the United Kingdom (UK). Hence and as a solution, the researcher selects a sample from the whole *sampling frame,* which involves identifying a group of students who become the *target population*. To select this *study population,* the researcher identifies one university (e.g. Edinburgh Napier University (ENU) and from the student population select a *sample* of the required numbers of participants (e.g. $n = 100$). When defining the size of the *sample*, practical, economic, ethical, and technical issues are considered. As part of process, *inclusion criteria* specify which participants are to be included or excluded from the study. These written *inclusion* and *exclusion criteria* will clearly profile and define what type of participants the study needs to answer the research question. To view examples of *inclusion* and *exclusion criteria*, see Tables 6.2 and 6.3.

To summarize, so far in developing the stages of your sampling process (Table 6.1), we have dealt with (i) *Define the population of interest*. The next stage in the sampling process is to (ii) *Specify a set of participants (or items) that are obtainable to investigate*.

Table 6.1   Stages of the sampling process.

(Stage 1)	*Define the population of interest*
(Stage 2)	*Specify a set of participants (or items) that are obtainable to investigate*
(Stage 3)	*Specify a sampling method for selecting participants from the population*
(Stage 4)	*Determine the sample size*
(Stage 5)	*Write the sampling plan*
(Stage 6)	*Practical sampling and data collection guidance*

Table 6.2   Examples of inclusion criteria.

- A specified age range (e.g. between 20 and 40 years old)
- Female
- Pregnant
- Primiparous
- Having insulin-dependent diabetes since childhood
- English as a first language
- Being Caucasian
- Absence of other health issues, e.g. ulcerative colitis and epilepsy.

Table 6.3 Examples of exclusion criteria.

- Out with specified age range (e.g. <30 or >40 years old)
- Being male
- Not being pregnant
- Multigravida
- Having diet or tablet-controlled diabetes
- Unable to read or write
- Born and raised outside the United Kingdom
- Having additional health problems, e.g. ulcerative colitis and epilepsy

6.4.2 (STAGE 2) SPECIFY A SET OF PARTICIPANTS (OR ITEMS) THAT ARE OBTAINABLE TO INVESTIGATE

A *sampling scheme* is one in which every unit in the *population* has a chance of being selected for the *sample*, with the specified *inclusion* and *exclusion criteria* making it possible for the researcher to produce an uncluttered pure *population* to take part in the study. In *experimental methods*, sampling involves selecting a subset of participants (or items) from a whole *population* who have the same clearly defined characteristics (see Table 6.4).

A variety of *sampling methods* may be employed individually or in combination to gain the prescribed number of participants required to undertake fruitful statistical analysis. When making such decisions, there are factors that will influence the researcher's choice of *sampling method* (see Table 6.5).

To summarize, so far in developing the stages of your sampling process, we have dealt with (i) *Define the population of interest,* and (ii) *Specify a set of participants (or items) that are obtainable to investigate.* The next stage in the sampling process is to (iii) *Specify a sampling method for selecting participants from the population.*

Table 6.4 Example of sample taken from a population.

As a midwifery researcher, you want to measure the amount of exercise pregnant insulin-dependent diabetic women undertake in one month in a named city. You attend the diabetic maternity clinic in this city and randomly select ($n = 5$) women every day over 20 consultation days (Total $n = 100$). Each participant selected must meet the stated inclusion criteria. Post gaining informed consent, you ask each participant to wear a wireless-enabled watch (e.g. Fitbit available at https://www.fitbit.com/global/uk/hom) to monitor their physical activity in terms of steps, quality of sleep, dietary, and fluid intake, which are measured and compared against maternal blood sugar levels across the month (i.e. 30 days). Within your study, you may also elect to conduct a triangulated qualitative component, which involves interviewing selected participants about their perceived lifestyle.

Table 6.5 Factors that influence choice of sampling method.

- The nature and quality of the *population* (i.e. total available number of participants who meet the inclusion criteria).
- Availability of supplementary information (e.g. participants understanding of calorie units to input into their Fitbit).
- Accuracy requirements for data analysis (i.e. does the Fitbit accurately measure steps).
- Whether detailed analysis of the sample is expected or just an estimate is good enough (e.g. if this was a drug trial accuracy would be mandatory).
- Cost (i.e. Is there funding to cover the cost of Fitbits, equipment, and salaries).
- Operational concerns (e.g. are staff on board with supporting this study).

6.4.3 (STAGE 3) SPECIFY A SAMPLING METHOD FOR SELECTING PARTICIPANTS FROM THE POPULATION

Under the participants' section of the research proposal, it is important to clearly specify your chosen sampling method and provide the reason for this choice (Berndt 2020). To view the main methods of population sampling, see Table 6.6.

An explanation of the central methods of population sampling now follows. Please note that the type of sampling you choose must match your choice of research method (i.e. either a qualitative or quantitative approach).

Types of Probability Sampling

Probability sampling methods involve randomly selecting a sample or part of the population you want to study. To qualify as being random, each participant must have an equivalent chance of being selected to take part in the study. Probability sampling utilizes tools to select samples from the entire population. For a participant to partake in a probability sample, they must be selected at random from the subset of *population* of interest. A crucial requirement is that all members of the population have an equal chance of being selected to participate in the study. For example, in a population of $(n = 1000)$ eligible participants, each one has the same chance of being selected to join *Group 1* and receive an intervention $(n = 500)$ or *Group 2* who acts as the control $(n = 500)$. By ensuring an equal chance of selection, probability sampling provides the highest prospect of obtaining a sample that is truthfully representative of the eligible population. Four main methods of random sampling or probability sampling include (a) *Simple random sampling*, (b) *Stratified sampling*, (c) *Cluster sampling*, and (d) *Purposive random sampling* (see Table 6.6).

Simple random sampling   *Simple random sampling* is a method of probability sampling ordinarily used in quantitative research, which places each participant in a position where they have equal probability of being selected to receive some sort of intervention (e.g. treatment, technique, and drug). The group of participants selected is chosen randomly from the elected subset of the *population* of interest and should represent an unbiased typification of the inclusion criteria. Randomization means that participants are assigned by chance to different research groups (e.g. *Group 1* who receive the intervention, or *Group 2* who are the matched control and do not receive the intervention). For ethical reasons, before random allocation to either *Group 1* or *Group 2*, the participant is informed that there is an equal chance of them becoming a member of the treatment group (*Group 1*) or the control group (*Group 2*). Where possible blinding is applied, so neither the researcher nor the participant is aware of which choice has been made. An example of how randomization can be achieved would be to toss a coin and 'tails' places the participant in the intervention group (*Group 1*) and 'heads' the control group (*Group 2*). Alternatively, participant names could be pulled out of a hat. More often to blind events to both the participant and researcher, allocation to a specific group may be achieved through the candidate selecting group membership through randomly selecting a preprepared sealed envelope or using a software computer program.

To reiterate, *random sampling* attempts to ensure that findings are the same as what would have been obtained had the whole population been measured. Consequently, and in advance of data collection, it is important to clearly estimate the number of participants required to produce a significant difference between the treatment group (*Group 1*) and the control group (*Group 2*). For example, take $(n = 10\,000)$ participants, and divide them randomly between the treatment group (*Group 1*) $(n = 5000)$ and the control group (*Group 2*) $(n = 5000)$. Power analysis may be carried out by a statistician in advance of deciding participant numbers for purpose of helping the researcher determine the smallest sample size that is suitable to detect the effects of the intervention at a desired level of significance (e.g. $p = 0.01$ or $p = 0.001$ or $p = 0.0001$). Now, we will link *random sampling* to *stratified sampling*, where the researcher divides the population into smaller subgroups based upon characteristics of clearly defined members.

Table 6.6   Types of probability sampling and non-probability sampling.

Types of probability sampling (also known as random sampling)	Types of non-probability sampling (also known as nonrandom sampling)
(a) Simple random sampling	(e) Convenience sampling
(b) Stratified random sampling	(f) Purposive sampling (also known as *criterion sampling*)
(c) Cluster random sampling	(g) Intensity sampling
(d) Purposive random sampling	(h) Homogeneous sampling
	(i) Snowball sampling

Stratified random sampling *Stratified random sampling* is a method of probability sampling ordinarily used in quantitative research, which involves a population being divided into nonoverlapping subareas. It is the process of selecting a *sample* in such a way that identifies subgroups in the population and ensures that they are represented in the participant group in near similar percentages. To achieve this, *random sampling* may be carried out more than once (i.e. for each subgroup). As with *simple random sampling*, once the population is defined and a sample size has been determined, all members of the selected *population* are classified into one of the identified subgroups of that *population*. Again, a random number of participants is selected (e.g. each sixth person is invited to participate in the study). As such, *stratified random sampling* basically uses the same processes as *simple random sampling*.

To summarize, *stratified random sampling* is a method of *sampling* a clearly defined *population*, which is then partitioned into subpopulations. For example, in quantitative research, when subpopulations vary within the overall population, it may be of benefit to sample each subpopulation separately. If you want to make this proportionate *stratified random sampling*, the sample size of each subpopulation is proportional to the share of the total population. For example, if one named subgroup out of five comprises of 20% percent of the total specified *population*, the sampling procedures must ensure each group makes up 20% of the total sample. To view an example of stratified sampling, see Table 6.7.

Stratified random sampling shares some similarities with *cluster random sampling*, given that both methods are probability sampling methods, in which every member of the *population* of interest has an equal chance of being selected from the total *sample* of the *population* of interest.

Cluster random sampling *Cluster random sampling* is a method of probability sampling ordinarily used in quantitative research, which involves random selection of 'groups of participants', as opposed to selecting individual candidates. For example, recruiting a support group of pregnant drug addicts from the total *population* of rehabilitation clinics across the United Kingdom. As such, *cluster random sampling* is a probability sampling method in which the researcher divides a total *population* into clusters and proceeds to randomly select some of these named clusters from the total *population* (in this case rehabilitation clinics across the United Kingdom). What is important, is that each cluster should characterize mini representations of the *population*. During process, the researcher devises a sampling plan, from which the total population is divided into homogeneous groups (known as clusters), and a *simple random sample* is sampled from this whole. Within these homogeneous groups, the researcher is looking for heterogeneous elements. A common reason for conducting *cluster random sampling* is to decrease the total number of participating clinics and reduce financial costs. For set sample size numbers, the expected random error is reduced when the majority of variation within the *population* is present within the groups and not between the groups.

Purposive random sampling *Purposive random sampling* or *random purposive sampling* is a method of probability sampling ordinarily used in quantitative research, which involves the researcher classifying a population of interest and then developing a systematic method of selecting participants that is not based on knowledge about how the outcomes would appear. As such, the *purposive random sampling* strategy increases credibility. An example involves the researcher purposely sampling a few participants from a larger purposeful group (e.g. purposely selecting ($n = 350$) pregnant diabetic women to participate out of the possible ($n = 3500$) that are available). This *purposeful sample* of ($n = 350$) participants is then *randomly* sampled to join either the intervention group ($n = 175$) or the control group ($n = 175$).

In total contrast to probability sampling (also known as random sampling) and its affiliated methods, non-probability sampling (also known as nonrandom sampling) involves methods of selecting participants based on factors that are biased and subjective in nature, which is the opposite to random chance.

Table 6.7 Example of stratified sampling.

Assume that a midwifery researcher wishes to estimate the average number of pregnant women who have insulin-dependent diabetes within three cities in the United Kingdom. City A has 1000 pregnant insulin-dependent diabetics, City B has 2000 pregnant insulin-dependent diabetics, and City C has 3000 pregnant insulin-dependent diabetics. The researcher sets out to gain a random sample of ($n = 60$) pregnant insulin-dependent diabetics across the whole *population*. Yet there is a chance that the resulting random sample is poorly balanced across these three cities, which would result in a bias and significant error in estimation. To resolve this situation, the researcher would elect to take a random sample of ($n = 10$) participants from *City A*, ($n = 20$) from *City B*, and ($n = 30$) from *City C*, which would produce the smallest error in estimation in terms of the whole sample size of ($n = 60$).

Types of non-probability sampling Non-probability sampling (also known as nonrandom sampling) encompasses various useful sampling methods, which are characteristically used in qualitative studies. As such, non-probability sampling encompasses selecting participants from a *population* using subjective and deliberate nonrandom processes. Since non-probability sampling or nonrandom sampling does not require a full survey framework, this makes it a quick and inexpensive method of gathering data. Non-probability sampling or nonrandom sampling involves the researcher using their own judgement and selecting participants based on convenience, experience, or judgement. Non-probability sampling or nonrandom sampling is totally inappropriate for use in quantitative experimental research. In contrast, it is used in qualitative research to gain deeper, more elaborate, and personal explanations and understandings of the phenomena of interest. For example, the researcher wants to gain a fuller understanding of participants' experiences of labour or breastfeeding. Recognizing that viewpoints vary, means the researcher will require to have discussions with participants either in a one-to-one interview or focus group. Four main methods of non-probability sampling or nonrandom sampling include (e) *Convenience sampling*, (f) *Purposive sampling*, (g) *Intensity sampling*, (h) *Homogeneous sampling*, and (i) *Snowball sampling* (Table 6.6).

Convenience sampling *Convenience sampling* is a non-probability sampling or nonrandom sampling method more often used in qualitative research and involves drawing participants from an opportune *population*. When applying *convenience sampling*, the researcher may go to places where appropriate participants will be found and invite them in a congenial way to participate in their study (e.g. a social club, pub, or shopping mall). This approach makes *convenience sampling* a quick and economical method of recruiting participants. A *convenience sample* is generally gathered from a place that is suitable and accessible to the type of required participant. However, it is important to note that *convenience sampling* does not involve extricating participants based upon their individual characteristics. For example, the data collector could stand in a shopping mall and ask accessible young women with prams who pass by questions listed on a preprepared questionnaire (e.g. market research). *Convenience sampling* is different from *purposive sampling*, with the main difference being that *purposive sampling* is less casual and focuses upon selecting participants who meet the detailed preorganized inclusion and exclusion criteria for the study. Consequently, an important point to note is that findings from data collected from a *convenience sample* can only be generalized to the relevant *(sub) population* from which the sample was taken, with findings not applicable to the whole *population*. In this example, the whole population of new mothers, precisely because no specified inclusion or exclusion criteria were applied.

Purposive sampling *Purposive sampling* (also known as *criterion sampling*) is a non-probability sampling or nonrandom sampling method ordinarily used in qualitative research, which focuses upon selecting participants who possess clearly defined characteristics that are associated with the aim of the research study (i.e. candidates meet the inclusion and exclusion criteria). As such, *purposive sampling* involves selecting participants who meet the inclusion criteria that have been agreed for the study. For example, all childbearing women within the *population* who have diabetes or have experienced perinatal bereavement. To access these goal-directed populations, the researcher could approach women with diabetes at an endocrinology clinic, or access those who have experienced perinatal bereavement through a specialized organization (e.g. 'Held in Our Hearts' available at: https://heldinourhearts.org.uk/). By approaching a dedicated perinatal bereavement charity, many of the attendant population will be eligible to participate in the study, which makes this approach towards recruiting participants *purposive sampling*. At such specialized organizations, the researcher can invite women to participate who meet the set inclusion and exclusion criteria for the study (e.g. perinatal death before or after 22 weeks). There are also other methods of non-probability sampling or nonrandom sampling, which includes *intensity sampling*.

Intensity sampling *Intensity sampling* is a non-probability sampling method or nonrandom sampling method ordinarily used in qualitative studies, which involves selecting participants in relation to strength of focus of the study. For example, the researcher's aim is to find out about pregnant women's alcohol consumption. One purpose of the study is to find out how many pregnant women continue to drink socially, or in terms of intensity fit into the category of heavy drinkers. As such, *intensity sampling* requires prior information and exploratory work to identify intensity of the prescribed categories, which are then clearly defined. *Intensity sampling* is usually conducted in conjunction with another sampling method.

For example, the researcher may collect ($n = 50$) participants who have affirmed that they are drinking alcohol whilst pregnant using *convenience sampling* (e.g. from a pub) or *purposive sampling* (from an addiction clinic), and then select a subset of participants based upon intensity of drinking from this number. *Intensity sampling* allows the researcher to hand-pick a small number of rich case participants who are then interviewed to gain in-depth knowledge about why they continue to consume alcohol during pregnancy. Data gathered from a subset of intense case (e.g. $n = 8$ out of $n = 50$) transcripts are then analysed to provide underlying themes for why women continue to drink alcohol during pregnancy. Another method of non-probability sampling or nonrandom sampling is *homogenous sampling*.

Homogeneous sampling *Homogeneous sampling* is a non-probability sampling or nonrandom sampling method ordinarily used in qualitative research, which involves the researcher focusing upon a similar and standardized *population*. For example, people who share similar circumstances or situations, such as age, gender, backgrounds, or occupations). An example that relates to midwifery practice is a researcher who wants to study leadership styles of senior midwives. In such a study, the population of interest to be *homogeneously sampled* is midwives who are in leadership positions. A final method of non-probability sampling or nonrandom sampling is *snowball sampling*.

Snowball sampling *Snowball sampling* is a non-probability sampling method or nonrandom sampling method ordinarily used in qualitative studies, which involves already participating women recruiting further candidates from amongst acquaintances who share similar characteristics (i.e. inclusion criteria). Hence, the sample number grows like a snowball rolling down a hill. *Snowball sampling* is extremely useful for finding concealed or difficult-to access *populations* (e.g. drug misusers or sex-workers). Alternatively, *snowball sampling* could be viewed as a 'bring your friends' approach, in which participants identify other women who meet the study requirements (e.g. women who have experienced perinatal bereavement and are members of the same support group). Such an approach to participant sampling brings with it a degree of bias, simply because friends customarily share characteristics of interest (e.g. shared interests, politics, religion, and hobbies). In contrast, this respondent-driven sampling method allows the midwifery researcher to make assessments of social networks that may underpin the issue of interest.

To summarize, we have looked at several diverse types of sampling methods and hope you are now equipped with knowledge to select one for use in your research proposal. In terms of placement within your research proposal, the proposed sampling method is placed under the 'participants' subheading. When you are documenting your proposed sampling method, please remember to stipulate a rationale for your choice and remember to provide a reference to support this decision. To conclude, so far in developing the stages of your sampling process, we have dealt with (i) *Define the population of interest,* (ii) *Specify a set of participants (or items) that are obtainable to investigate,* and (iii) *Specify a sampling method for selecting participants from the population.* The next stage in the sampling process is to (iv) *Determine the sample size,* which involves deciding upon an appropriate number ($n = ?$) of participants to take part in your study.

6.4.4 (STAGE 4) DETERMINE THE SAMPLE SIZE

Determining your sample size involves selecting participant numbers ($n = ?$) or observation points if your study does not include people (i.e. items). If a quantitative method has been selected, participants number size is about gaining enough people (or items) to allow for valid statistical calculations to be carried out that will support valid differences between the intervention group and the control group (i.e. p values that are smaller than $p = 0.05$, $p = 0.01$, and $p = 0.001$). The size of the sample selected must be large enough to permit the researcher to make inferences about the population of interest and to secure significant differences between groups ($p < 0.05$ at minimum and ideally smaller $p = 0.01$, $p = 0.001$). As such, the need is to offer sufficient statistical power, with the p value selected ($p = 0.05$, $p = 0.01$, or $p = 0.001$). This choice may be determined by cost, time, or availability of participants (items) and the need to offer sufficient statistical power. For example, if you are testing a new drug, then the statistical value needs to be very small (e.g. $p = 0.001$) to demonstrate that there is a 1 in a 1000 chance that any difference between group mean(s) against the control group happened by chance or accident. It is important to note that in an experimental method the numbers of participants (items) in each intervention group and the control group should be equal (e.g. *Group 1* ($n = 50$); *Group 2* ($n = 50$); *Group 3*: the control ($n = 50$), with a TOTAL of ($n = 150$) participants (or items) in the whole experimental study.

Table 6.8   How to determine sample size from a population.

N	S	N	S	N	S	N	S	N	S
10	10	100	80	280	162	800	260	2800	338
15	14	110	86	290	165	850	265	3000	341
20	19	120	92	300	169	900	269	3500	246
25	24	130	97	320	175	950	274	4000	351
30	28	140	103	340	181	1000	278	4500	351
35	32	150	108	360	186	1100	285	5000	357
40	36	160	113	380	181	1200	291	6000	361
45	40	180	118	400	196	1300	297	7000	364
50	44	190	123	420	201	1400	302	8000	367
55	48	200	127	440	205	1500	306	9000	368
60	52	210	132	460	210	1600	310	10000	373
65	56	220	136	480	214	1700	313	15000	375
70	59	230	140	500	217	1800	317	20000	377
75	63	240	144	550	225	1900	320	30000	379
80	66	250	148	600	234	2000	322	40000	380
85	70	260	152	650	242	2200	327	50000	381
90	73	270	155	700	248	2400	331	75000	382
95	76	270	159	750	256	2600	335	100000	384

Note: N = population size; S = sample size.
Source: Adapted from Krejcie and Morgan (1970).

Determining the *sample size* is important because participant numbers that are large can waste time, resources, and money. Particularly in situations where you can answer the research question(s) by means of smaller numbers of participants. In contrast, *sample sizes* that are too small may lead to underpowered results. The researcher can determine the minimum *sample size* required to estimate a process parameter (appropriate *p* value) through use of powering, which is more often calculated by a statistician. The question here is, how large does the sample need to be to infer findings back to the *population* of interest? A good maximum sample size is ordinarily approximately 10% of the total *population*. For example, in a population of around 4000, a sample of ($n = 400$) participants would cover this. It is usual not to have a participant number of over ($n = 1000$). Hence, in the case of the population being ($n = 1000000$), where 10% equals ($n = 100000$), it may be acceptable to recruit ($n = 1000$) participants. A statistician can apply formulas to inform the researcher what their sample size requires to be. If you are submitting a quantitative research proposal for a grant application, it is suggested that you include a named statistician to be part of your research team and ask them to calculate and justify the participant sample size(s). As part of process, the statistician will use formulas, tables, and power function charts, which have been developed to help researchers determine appropriate *sample sizes* for grant applications. If you want to read more about how to calculate a *sample size,* see Kadam and Bhalerao 2010. However, a simpler example of a table to help researchers understand and determine their *sample size* is provided in Table 6.8.

To recap, so far in developing the stages of your sampling process, we have dealt with (i) *Define the population of interest,* (ii) *Specify a set of participants (or items) that are obtainable to investigate,* (iii) *Specify a sampling method for selecting participants from the population,* and (iv) *Determine the sample size.* The next stage in the sampling process is to (v) *Write the sampling plan* (see Table 6.1).

6.4.5 (STAGE 5) WRITE THE SAMPLING PLAN

The *sampling plan* must support recruitment of enough participants from the *population* to gather sufficient data to answer the research question. A sampling plan consists of a series of steps that are captured in a template (see Table 6.9).

Table 6.9 Participant sampling plan template.

(1) Define the population of interest:

(2) Provide participant numbers, justify this choice, and how many from each site:

(3) Outline the setting, and provide names and addresses of the data collection site(s):

(4) Specify participant inclusion and exclusion criteria:

(5) Outline nonresponse processes:

(6) Specify and justify the sampling method:

(7) Outline recruitment processes:

Within your sampling plan, it is important to outline the precise processes that the recruiter should follow. Mentioning this and specifically in relation to point (5) in Table 6.9, first, it is important to clarify what a nonresponse is.

Nonresponse

In attempts to recruit participants, there will be some women who are unwilling to participate in the study. This brings with it the risk of creating a selection bias through simply recruiting women and/or partners who are keen and willing to participate. For example, women who have breastfed may be more willing to take part in a study about infant feeding that a 'bottle feeding' mum. This in itself could bias results, simply because women who 'bottle feed' may show reluctance to participate through belief that the researching midwife may judge them for not breastfeeding. In addition, it is important to be aware that nonresponse rates are ordinarily higher when the researcher attempts to recruit by email. Hence, several invitation resends may be necessary to recruit adequate participant numbers. Nonetheless and in general, there are several ways of attempting to reduce potential participant nonresponse:

- Design an attractive-looking questionnaire that is easy to complete.

- Personalize the communication by naming the participant.

- Sign your signature in colour.

- If posting, use a first-class stamp and include a stamped addressed envelope.

- Send a personalized information sheet about the up-and-coming survey in advance of the questionnaire.

- Prompt nonrespondents by sending repeat reminders.

- Offer vouchers or some form of reward for taking part.

You may decide to write more than one *sampling plan* if you are undertaking a multisite project. One for each recruiter in individual sites (e.g. maternity units). The *sampling plan* should also be accompanied by a *data collection plan*, as the recruiter is likely to also be the data collector.

To conclude stage five of the sampling process (Table 6.1), a midwifery researcher requires to recruit a stated number of women who meet the inclusion criteria for their study, which accounts for dropout and non-full completion of the data collection instruments (e.g. questionnaire(s)). Within the sampling plan, the target population needs to be stated and details provided about participant numbers that complete data must be gathered from. The next step in writing your research proposal involves writing a *data collection plan* for the data collector to follow once they have recruited appropriate participants, which is (STEP 9) of how to write a research proposal (Describe data collection instruments). In summary, so far in developing the stages of your sampling process, we have dealt with (i) *Define the population of interest,* (ii) *Specify a set of participants (or items) that are obtainable to investigate,* (iii) *Specify a sampling method for selecting participants from the population,* (iv) *Determine the sample size,* and (v) *Write the sampling plan.* The next stage in the sampling process is (vi) *Practical sampling and data collection guidance.*

Table 6.10 Data collection plan template (Continued from Table 6.9).

(8)	Name of data collector:
(9)	Data collection dates (e.g. 1 January 2026 – 30 April 2026).
(10)	Summarize procedures involved in providing informed consent:
(11)	Processes of randomization if an RCT.
(12)	Guide to data collection (e.g. appendix survey instruments and interview schedules).
(13)	Data management plan (e.g. where collected data is inputted and stored).
(14)	Participant retention plan (e.g. send reminders at 1 and 3 weeks).
(15)	Guidance for participant about where to seek optional follow-up support post data collection (e.g. leaflet developed for issue).
(16)	Appendices included.

6.4.6 (STAGE 6) PRACTICAL SAMPLING AND DATA COLLECTION GUIDANCE

Actual sampling and recruitment of participants are followed by data collection, which requires the researcher to write a plan about how the data collector is going to in fact gather data from participants. An example of a data collection plan can be viewed in Table 6.10.

The *participant sampling plan* (Table 6.9) and the *data collection plan* (Table 6.10) become part of the protocol for the research study. As such, the study protocol is a predefined procedural plan for actual implementation of the study. Protocols are essential for all research studies, and are particularly important for experimental methods, precisely because they standardize the actual processes involved and make the study replicable by different multisite research team(s). Hence, writing a research protocol is a key task for any researcher, with how to sample and collect the data in just one component. The protocol is a full description of the practicalities of how to conduct the whole research study. To view a protocol template for both quantitative and qualitative research methods, see: https://www.hra.nhs.uk/planning-and-improvingresearch/research-planning/protocol/. There are also research journals that specialize in publishing research protocols (see https://plos.org/protocols/). To view a published protocol, see Activity 6.2.

Activity 6.2

Access and read the following protocol:

Stålberg, V., Krevers, B., Lingetun, L. et al. (2022). Study protocol for a modified antenatal care program for pregnant women with a low risk for adverse outcomes: a stepped wedge cluster non-inferiority randomized trial. *BMC Pregnancy Childbirth* 22: 299. https://doi.org/10.1186/s12884-022-04406-7.

6.5 SUMMARY OF THE SAMPLING PROCESS

Now that you have carried out Stages 1–6 of the sampling process (Table 6.1), you will have clearly defined the population of interest (Stage 1). You will have specified a set of participants (or items) that are obtainable to investigate (Stage 2). You will have specified a sampling method for selecting participants from the population (Stage 3). You will have determined the sample size (Stage 4). You will have written a sampling plan (Stage 5) and finally, you will have written practical sampling and data collection guidance (Stage 6).

6.5.1 CHAPTER CONCLUSION

This chapter has addressed (STEP 8) of how to write a research proposal (recipe), which includes selecting the setting, participants, sampling method, inclusion and exclusion criteria, and method of recruiting participants or items. The next chapter will now address (STEP 9), which involves describing what data collection instruments you plan to use in your research study, which for example may include questionnaires or conducting interviews, etc. Such processes of data collection may involve you using preexisting validated psychometric scales or developing your own purpose-built questionnaires. *Chapter 7* will now look at a variety of data collection instruments, which you could possibly use in your study. Regardless of the type of data collection (e.g. questionnaire, structured interviews, and measurements), your purpose is to gain information that post analysis will answer the research question. Accuracy of data gathered requires that the data collector be trained in important aspects of the data collection process. For example, procedures of making initial participant contact, how to ask predecided questions, probing answers to gain greater depth of understanding, recording, and storing responses, when to terminate the interview, and methods of debriefing post data collection. Also, how to prepare the data for data analysis using computer software. As such, data preparation is a meticulous process, which includes scrutinizing the data for accuracy and ensuring minimal gaps in completeness, precisely because unfinished, ambiguous, and inconsistent responses cannot be included in the data set. Data collection tools should allow for anonymization and coding, which involves attaching numbers and letters to the gathered data. We will now move on to *Chapter 7*, which has been written to help you select and describe the data collection instruments for your research proposal (STEP 9).

6.6 SELF-ASSESSMENT QUESTIONS (SAQs)

6.1 **Simple random sampling is:**

   (a) Is a non-probability sampling method used to select participants who possess similar characteristics.

   (b) Involves a population being divided into nonoverlapping subgroups.

   (c) Is a process of determining sample size.

   (d) Is used to ensure equal probability of participants being selected to receive an intervention.

6.2 **Which of the following is a type of probability sampling?**

   (a) Convenience sampling.

   (b) Simple random sampling.

   (c) Homogeneous sampling.

   (d) Snowball sampling.

6.3 **Snowball sampling is:**

   (a) Is used to gather data for randomization in quantitative studies.

   (b) Is a form of cluster sampling.

   (c) Involves existing participants recruiting further participants with the same characteristics.

   (d) Is a process of accessing participants to take part in studies during the winter.

6.4 **A population includes:**

   (a) People with the characteristics the researcher wants to study.

   (b) A whole town of people with all sorts of characteristics.

   (c) Is a type of sampling method.

   (d) Involves collecting data from abroad.

6.5 **A sampling frame is:**

   (a) The total list of available items from which a sample is taken.

   (b) Used to collect a specimen.

   (c) A statistical test that allows the researcher to make inferences about a population.

   (d) Is a metal cage that blood samples are held in.

ANSWERS TO CHAPTER 6 SAQs

6.1 **d**

6.2 **b**

6.3 **c**

6.4 **a**

6.5 **a**

Data Collection Methods

CHAPTER 7

STEP (9): Outline data collection instruments.

7.1 DIFFERENCES BETWEEN PRIMARY AND SECONDARY DATA

Primary data is new and original data gathered directly by the researcher as part of following a research proposal. As such, primary data is collected firsthand by the researcher through their direct endeavours and for the purpose of answering their specified research question. As such, primary data is raw data gathered via specified methods, which may include collected physical samples, completed surveys, recorded observations, audiotaped interviews or focus groups, or analysed historical records.

In contrast, secondary data is secondhand material gathered from already published research papers, organizational records, reports, websites, meeting minutes, letters, case notes, etc. Often the midwifery researcher will carry out secondary data analysis in the form of a literature review (see Chapter 3). To view a summary of differences between primary and secondary data, see Table 7.1).

We will now move on and discuss types of data collection tools, but first, we will define this term. The phrase 'data collection tools' refers to the instruments the researcher uses to gather data for their study, which may include paper or online questionnaire(s), gathering specimens, interviews, or focus groups.

7.2 DATA COLLECTION METHODS AND TOOLS

Data are a compilation of information, evidence, or facts from which the researcher draws conclusions. In relation to the two research approaches (see Chapter 2), data collected can be quantitative (deductive and numeric in form) or qualitative (inductive and involve individualized discussion with participants to induce many themes). Whatever approach you take, the data collection tools you select are implemented for the purpose of gathering data that will provide evidence to answer the research question(s). Fit for purpose, there are many different data collection methods. To view some of the more common types, see Table 7.2.

There are many approaches to collecting data, which are selected in terms of appropriateness for the research method that has been chosen, and whether it is quantitative (inductive) or qualitative (deductive) in approach. As part of process, it is important to write a guideline as to how the data are to be collected and beforehand pilot the processes involved.

Research Recipes for Midwives, First Edition. Caroline J. Hollins Martin.
© 2024 John Wiley & Sons Ltd. Published 2024 by John Wiley & Sons Ltd.

Table 7.1   Summary of differences between primary and secondary data.

Primary data	Secondary data
First-time original data produced by the researcher	Preexisting data already gathered
Focused on an immediate and present problem or issue	General relationship to the problem or issue
Real-time data	Relates to the past
Detailed and follows a 16-STEP research proposal.	Gathers many sources of data
Process takes time, money, and workforce	Fairly rapid, cheap, and available
Ethical approval necessary	Often obtained through libraries, etc., and so ethical approval more often not required
Data actually collected in the form of, e.g. physical samples, surveys, observations, interviews, focus groups, and historical records	Data gathered secondhand (e.g. research papers, organizational records, reports, websites, meeting minutes, letters, and case notes)
Answers a specified research question	Has a more general relationship to the topic of interest
Researcher can control the quality of data gathered	Researcher has no control over the quality of data, as already archived
Raw data	Derived data

Table 7.2   Examples of quantitative and qualitative data collection tools.

Quantitative data collection tools	Qualitative data collection tools
Questionnaires	**Questionnaires**
Closed-ended Likert scored questionnaires:	Open-ended questionnaires:
• To identify numerically social attitudes, skills, or behaviours	• To explore individual differences and values that underpin social attitudes, skills, or behaviours
Measurement	**Interviews**
Recording of precise quantities (e.g. weight, height, and blood samples)	One-to-one conversation or focus groups used to explore people's values, attitudes, experiences, skills, and/or behaviours
Recording observations	**Investigating observations**
Recording observations (e.g. behaviours)	Exploring observations (e.g. behaviours)
• How often?	• Why happens?
• Frequency?	• Personalized experiences
• Most common?	• Choices?
	• Exploring underpinning values and emotions attached to decisions

7.3 GUIDELINES FOR DATA COLLECTION PROCESSES

Pilot testing helps the researcher prepare their data collection processes, which is called testing the feasibility. As such, a pilot study is a small-scale preliminary investigation conducted to evaluate feasibility, duration, cost, adverse events, and improve processes involved in the study design, prior to conducting the full-scale research project. During process, the data collection tools are tested with a small sample of volunteers before being implemented to gather data in the main study. This prelude *pilot study* will help the researcher determine how to use predeveloped and validated data collection instruments and test whether the questions are comprehensible. Alternatively, if the researcher has developed their own data collection tools (e.g. questionnaires and semi-structured interview schedules), the *pilot study* will allow the researcher to sort out a snag list. In essence, the *pilot study* should pinpoint where improvements can be made to both the data collection instruments and data collection processes. Within the guideline, it is important to formulate a clear calendar for data collection from start to finish and train fellow researchers to gather the required data. Guidance provided should also provide information about how the data will be stored and protected to ensure participant confidentiality (i.e. numerical tagging). In essence, the plan should include precisely where the data are to be collected, how, when, and by whom. We will now move on to study in more detail different types of data collection methods, starting with questionnaires and their design.

7.4 QUESTIONNAIRES

A questionnaire consists of a list of items (questions) with the whole tool used to collect data about, for example, social attitudes (e.g. opinions towards or against something) or experiences (of partaking in an event). Questionnaires gather either quantitative or qualitative information and sometimes both if a comments section is placed beneath each Likert scale scored item. In quantitative research, numeric continuums are marked by responders to score items, which accumulate to generate total subscale scores and total overall scores. In contrast, qualitative questionnaires consist of open-ended questions that reflect differences in responders' attitudes, skills, and/or behaviours. Either way, a questionnaire is a data collection tool designed to gain specific information with appropriate design crucial for a successful study. Dependent upon whether the researcher has elected to take a quantitative or qualitative approach, they will select a response style that involves closed-ended items in a deductive approach and open-ended questions in an inductive approach. It is normal to have some descriptive data at the beginning of a questionnaire, which identifies participants' personal characteristics, which post-completion are anonymized using numerical tagging. Before completing any survey, the participants are asked to read the preprepared information sheet and are given time to answer questions (see Table 7.3) and then sign a consent form (see Table 7.4). At the beginning of any questionnaire, it is important to gather important details and demographic data relevant to the study (see Table 7.5). In addition, it is important to add contact details of how participants can contact you later, should they have any questions:

Principal researcher:
Professional qualifications:
Telephone number:
Email:
Address:

Table 7.3 Example Participant Information Sheet (PIS).

Project title:

Invitation to participate

You are invited to take part in a research study currently being conducted at ...., in collaboration with the University of .... Before you decide whether to complete the questionnaire or not, it is important for you to understand why the research is being carried out and what it will involve. Please take time to read the following information. Please ask the data collector if there is anything that is not clear. If you agree to take part, you will be asked to sign a consent form that will confirm that you have read the preparatory information before you complete the questionnaire. Thank you for your consideration and time.

What is the purpose of the study?
This questionnaire aims to look at your attitudes and feelings about being a birth partner.

Why have I been invited?
You have been chosen because you are considering whether or not you want to be present at the birth of your baby.

Do I have to take part?
It is up to you to decide whether you want to complete the questionnaire. If you decide you want to, you are free to withdraw at any time without giving a reason why. Take a look at the questionnaire and if you have any questions then please ask the researcher who is collecting the data to answer them.

What will I have to do?
There are no costs to you for taking part in this study. You may complete the questionnaire at a time of your convenience and return it to the researcher who issued it to you.

(continued)

Table 7.3 (Continued)

What are the possible disadvantages and risks of taking part?
No harm to either the person who asked you to be their birth partner, yourself, or the baby can result from this study. You may, however, consider participation to be a slight imposition on your personal life. If you wish to complain or have any concerns about any aspect of the way you have been approached or treated, the normal National Health Service complaints mechanisms are available to you.

What are the possible benefits of taking part in the study?
The data collected may ultimately improve the labour experiences of subsequent birth partners and childbearing women.

Will my taking part in this study be kept confidential?
Confidentiality will be respected with information restricted from anyone not directly involved in the study. Anonymity is provided with questionnaires tagged and stored in a locked filing cabinet. Any information about you, which leaves the researcher's realm, will have your name and address removed so that you cannot be recognized from it.

What will happen to the results of the research study?
The results of this research study will facilitate midwives with improving the quality of parenthood education provided to those who decide to be birth partners. What is found may also be of use to pregnant women planning their birth. The aim is to publish the findings without personally naming participants in any of the reports. We are delighted to share the study results with you. If you are interested, you can contact the researcher at the number and address over page and we will forward the publications to you. If you have any concerns, please do not hesitate to contact the researcher.

Who is organizing the research?
This study has been organized by a team of people who are researchers and lecturers in NAME OF INSTITUTION. NAME OF RESEARCHER has had a career in .... Their contact details are as follows.................

Who has reviewed the study?
This study has been scrutinized by the appropriate Research Ethics Committee (NAME OF RESEARCH COMMITTEE). The role of NAME OF RESEARCH COMMITTEE is to ensure that all studies are conducted with integrity and in line with generally accepted ethical principles.

Providing agreement to participate
If you agree to participate in this study, we thank you. Your contribution is appreciated. Please complete the three replicated consent forms over page: one is for yourself, one is for the researcher and one will be kept in your partner's notes.

Table 7.4 Example of a participant consent form.

Participant identification number for this study:

Centre number:

Study number:

Patient identification number for this study:

CONSENT FORM

Title of project:

Name of researcher   Please initial box

1. I confirm that I have read and understood the information sheet for the above study. I have had the opportunity   ☐
    to consider the information, ask questions, and have had these answered satisfactorily.

2. I understand that my participation is voluntary and that I am free to withdraw at any time without giving any   ☐
    reason and without the childbearing woman's care or legal rights being affected.

3. I understand that the data collected during the study may be looked at by individuals from the NAME OF INSTI-   ☐
    TUTION or by regulatory authorities relevant to my taking part in the research. I give permission for these
    individuals to have access to my data.

4. I agree to take part in the above study.   ☐

Participant name	Date	Signature
Name of person taking consent	Date	Signature

1 for participant; 1 for researcher; 1 to be kept in the childbearing woman's medical notes

Table 7.5 Examples of how to gather important details and demographic data.

(a) Name:

(b) Unit number:

(c) Address:

(d) Parity:

(e) Marital status:

(f) Clinic attended:

(g) Midwives name:

(h) What date is your baby due to be born?

(i) In which maternity unit will the birth take place?

(j) Where do you intend to have your baby (i.e. delivery suite, birthing unit, home, and theatre)?

(k) What is your date of birth?

Following on from demographic details, some tips for filling in the questionnaire are necessary (see Table 7.6). We will now look at some examples of questions/item response styles, starting with quantitative approaches (see Table 7.7).

Table 7.6 Tips for filling in the questionnaire.

(a) Find a quiet place where you will be undisturbed.

(b) Read each statement carefully and once you understand what is being asked, respond fairly quickly. Do not ponder too long over each statement.

(c) The statements are structured as follows. Please circle one of the following.

| Strongly | Agree | Neither Agree or Disagree | Disagree | Strongly Disagree |

(d) Please *do not miss* out any of the items and try to be as honest as possible.

Table 7.7 Examples of numeric responses in quantitative research.

Q   How much have you spent on leisure activities this week?

Total £_____

Q   How would you rate the benefits of back massage during labour?
(Please circle answer.)

- Excellent   (4)
- Good   (3)
- Fair   (2)
- Poor   (1)

Q   How would you rate the success of the following therapies in treating postnatal depression (PND)? (*On a scale of 1–10 with 10 maximum and 1 minimum*)

- Cognitive behavioural therapy (CBT) _____
- Gestalt therapy _____
- Psychotherapy _____
- Neuro-linguistic programming (NLP) _____

Item   I would like to give birth to my baby at home.

	Strongly Agree	Agree	Neither Agree or Disagree	Disagree	Strongly Disagree
Scores	5	4	3	2	1

Q   How severe is the level of bullying and harassment in your workplace?
(*Please circle the continuum below with 10 maximum and 1 minimum.*)

1____2____3____4____5____6____7____8____9____10

Activity 7.1

Access and read the following paper:

Hollins-Martin, C.J. and Martin, C. (2014). Development and psychometric properties of the Birth Satisfaction Scale-Revised (BSS-R). *Midwifery* 30: 610–619. https://doi.org/10.1016/j.midw.2013.10.006

Please note that all participant responses in Table 7.7 are numerical, which will permit descriptive and inferential statistics to be calculated (see Chapter 9). It is also important to understand what a valid and reliable psychometric scale is. The validity of a psychometric questionnaire is a concept that relates to gathering quantitative numerical data and measuring the degree to which that test measures accurately what it sets out to measure. Psychometric validation of a questionnaire involves complex statistical testing, which is usually carried out by a statistician or specifically skilled researcher. If you are interested in psychometric testing of your developed scale, tool, or questionnaire, there are books that specialize in this topic alone (e.g. Irwing et al. 2018). To view an example of a questionnaire that has been developed and then validated by the author, see Activity 7.1.

Moving on to inductive approaches towards questionnaire development, we will now look at some examples of question response styles that take a qualitative approach (see Table 7.8).

In summary, use of questionnaire(s) or survey instruments is a process of data collecting that may involve the researcher using prevalidated psychometric scales, such as the *Birth Satisfaction Scale-Revised* (BSS-R) (Hollins-Martin and Martin (2014), see https://www.bss-r.co.uk/) or the Edinburgh Postnatal Depression Scale (EPDS) (Cox et al. 1987). Alternatively, there may not be a prevalidated questionnaire suitable to answer your research question. Hence, you may consider developing a scale of your own and carry out psychometric statistical testing on your newly developed quantitative instrument. If you decide to do this, it is a good idea to speak to a statistician who may recommend an appropriate statistics plan (see Table 7.9).

Researchers carry out statistical tests to ensure that their newly developed quantitative questionnaire is both reliable and valid. At this point though, you may be asking what the terms *reliable* and *valid* mean.

7.4.1 WHAT ARE RELIABILITY AND VALIDITY?

In research, measuring tools require to be both *reliable* and *valid*.

7.4.2 WHAT IS RELIABILITY?

The term *reliability* means that when you use a measuring tool, it provides the same results upon repeated measurements. For example, if you give a test on Monday and repeat data collection on Wednesday, results should be similar or the same. In contrast, *validity* asks whether the tool is measuring what it is supposed to measure. For example, does a person with high wealth correlate with them having high intelligence? This is an invalid question because money can be inherited, won, stolen, or earned. It is important to note that all instruments measure with errors, and it is the job of the researcher to reduce this error to as small an amount as possible. To example the meaning of error, when a person achieves an exam score of 42% and their real ability is 60%, there is an 18% error. So, what could have caused this 18% inaccuracy? Was it: (i) poor instruction, (ii) dodgy marking, or (iii) a badly worded question? Also, please note that it is normal to have a margin of error unless the researcher achieves 100% accuracy upon repeated measurement.

Another source of error is *content sampling*. For example, in a question paper, there is a limit to the amount of questions that a person can be asked, and therefore it is impossible to sample all the knowledge that they have. This person may know 620 facts and not know 200 facts. Out of the 820 total facts, the question paper asks 200 facts that the person does not know. This example demonstrates that there is a degree of luck involved in question sampling. In addition, administration and the environment can cause a margin of error. For example, whilst sitting for the test, a distracting fly on the window is buzzing, there is a cold draft in the examination room, or external noise diverts participant attention from the task at hand. *Reliability* is about test measurement providing a similar result at two separate recordings with data captured by setting up a *test–retest* or *parallel form* scenario.

Table 7.8 Examples of inductive responses in qualitative research.

Q	What type of leisure activities do you carry out in a normal week?
	Comments: _____
	_____

Q	Please describe what types of pain relief methods helped you cope with pain during your labour?
	Comments: _____
	_____

Q	Please describe how successful therapy was at reducing your postnatal depression (PND) symptoms? (Whichever one is applicable)
	• Cognitive behavioural therapy (CBT)
	Comments: _____
	_____
	• Gestalt therapy
	Comments: _____
	_____
	• Psychotherapy
	Comments: _____
	_____
	• Neuro-linguistic programming (NLP)
	Comments: _____
	_____

Q	How do you feel about giving birth to your baby at home?
	Comments: _____
	_____

Q	Please describe your perceptions of types and levels of bullying and harassment in your workplace?
	Comments: _____
	_____

7.4.3 TEST–RETEST

An example of a *test–retest* scenario to measure *reliability* would involve the researcher issuing ($n = 100$) participants the test on Tuesday (Test 1) and reissuing the same test to the same people three-months later (Test 2). For the questionnaire to be reliable there requires to be a high correlation between *Test 1* and *Test 2* scores. It is rare for results to equal 100%, with 70% acceptable due to performance errors, which may include distractions, fatigue, lack of attention, memory, etc. The best way to deal with these sources of error is to place a meaningful gap between *Test 1* and *Test 2*. Of course, this

Table 7.9   Example of a psychometric plan to validate a quantitative survey instrument.

There are number of ways to evaluate the psychometric properties of a newly developed quantitative questionnaire.

Sample size
A minimum sample size is required in order to perform statistical procedures and particularly those that evaluate the measurement model of the scale. Evaluating the measurement model of a scale generally requires the largest minimum sample size. Thus, this would represent a realistic minimum for a full psychometric evaluation involving a number of tests of validity and reliability.

Evaluation of the measurement model
If the scale consists of subscales, the measurement model assumes that domains represented by the subscale items are correlated. For example, evaluation of a tridimensional measurement model is usually undertaken using Confirmatory Factor Analysis (CFA) and the findings are considered against threshold levels on established measures of 'model fit'. In terms of fully completed scales, a minimum sample size for undertaking the CFA is 20 times larger than the number of items on the scale (e.g. 10 questions then participant numbers equal ($n = 200$), which is considered acceptable for publication by most journals.

Internal consistency
The general accepted measure for internal consistency is Cronbach's alpha (Cronbach 1951), which should calculate at 0.70 or above for whole scale, and all subscales (Clark and Watson 1995).

Known-groups discriminant validity
Known-groups discriminant validity (KGDV) is evaluated in a number of ways, with hypotheses related to group difference at a whole scale or subscale level investigated to confirm this validity domain. An example of this is provided in papers that have used unassisted vaginal delivery compared to an intervention delivery to examine group differences (Romero-Gonzalez et al., 2019; Skvirsky et al. 2019), with any hypothesis-driven and evidence-informed group comparison undertaken in the same way. Dependent on the profile of data, statistical evaluation by parametric or nonparametric tests may be used, for example in the case comparison of two groups and data characteristics suitable for a parametric test, the independent *t*-test would be appropriate.

Divergent validity
Divergent validity assumes no relationship between total or subscale scores and a domain that naturally is not assumed to have a relationship with scores. The usual statistical approach to this is to undertake a Pearson's correlation coefficient (or the nonparametric equivalent test) with the expectation that a statistically significant correlation will *not* be found.

Test–retest reliability
Test–retest reliability may be evaluated by readministering the scale to the same group of participants at a second observation point and testing for a statistically significant relationship between observation points using a Pearson's correlation coefficient (or the nonparametric equivalent test). It is noteworthy that test–retest reliability findings reported in research papers more generally have a too short second observation point to evaluate test–retest reliability. Hence, we would suggest a minimum test–retest period of three months, which is consistent with the recommendations of Kline (2000).

The above are some suggestions for psychometric evaluation of a scale. We would recommend further reading to consider the range of statistical approaches that may be undertaken and the characteristics of the study that should be taken into account. A good paper covering a number of these issues is that of Martin and Savage-McGlynn (2013).

organization may bring with it difficulties with reassembling participants, children growing older, dementia worsening, etc. Hence, an alternative approach to testing questionnaire reliability is to carry out a *parallel form* of scale, questionnaire, or tool issue.

7.4.4 PARALLEL FORM

Testing reliability using *parallel form* involves issuing two similar versions of the same questionnaire at the same time to different participant groups. Processes involve the questionnaire developer preparing two questionnaires that tap into the same subject, with questions similar, but not identical (see Table 7.10).

Parallel form method of measuring questionnaire *reliability* can capture margins of error, specifically due to participant differences in interpretation of the questions asked. Hence, another way the researcher can test *reliability* of the test is to undertake a *split half* test.

Table 7.10 Examples of parallel form questions.

To test for a psychotic personality, the researcher could ask:				
Test 1: (a) When I was young, I used to torture spiders.				
Test 2: (b) When I was young, insects used to flee from my magnifying glass.				
Strongly Agree	Agree	Neither Agree or Disagree	Disagree	Strongly Disagree
5	4	3	2	1
		OR		
To test for an extroverted personality trait, the researcher could ask the following:				
Test 1: (a) I like parties.				
Test 2: (b) I like gatherings of people.				
Strongly Agree	Agree	Neither Agree or Disagree	Disagree	Strongly Disagree
5	4	3	2	1

7.4.5 SPLIT HALF

In a *split half* reliability test, the researcher takes a full questionnaire and splits it into two halves. One participant receives all the odd-numbered questions, whilst another participant receives all the even-numbered questions. A *split half* coefficient is applied to both halves, which is a statistical test that provides a *reliability* coefficient. Problems with *split half* method of testing *reliability* is that the questions may not be similar enough or half the questions are not as good as the whole scale.

To conclude, within statistics and psychometrics, *reliability* is the overall consistency of the measuring tool developed. We will now move on to explore the concept of *validity*. Having looked at some aspects of *reliability,* with similarity we will now look at some types of *validity*.

7.4.6 WHAT IS VALIDITY?

Validity is the accuracy with which a measuring tool reflects what the researcher intended. As such, *validity* is the degree to which the question(s) measure what they claim to measure. Some examples of types of *validity* include *face validity*, *content validity*, *criterion validity,* and *concurrent validity*.

7.4.7 FACE VALIDITY

Face validity is the extent to which a test subjectively covers the concept it reports to measure. As such, *face validity* refers to the transparency or relevance of the test as it appears. In other words, a test is said to have *face validity* when it 'looks like' it is going to measure what it is supposed to measure. For instance, if a test is prepared to measure whether students can perform multiplication, and the people who view it all agree that it looks like a good test of multiplication ability, this demonstrates *face validity* of the test. Another facet of *face validity* is about the test looking plausible to the user. That is, does the test look professional? For example, does the questionnaire look like it has been written on boiled sweet wrappers or is covered in coffee stains? As such, to have *face validity*, the test additionally must look professional and well presented.

7.4.8 CONTENT VALIDITY

Content validity is the extent to which a measure represents all facets of a given construct. For example, a depression scale may lack *content validity* when it only assesses the affective dimension of depression (i.e. feelings) and fails to assess the behavioural components of depression (i.e. shouting or crying). An element of subjectivity exists when determining *content validity* of an instrument with disagreements preventing gain of a high level of *content validity*. *Content validity* is also about the test covering the full landscape of potential content. For example, when measuring intelligence, the researcher needs to sample the full range of content of intelligence (i.e. interpretation of meaning, spatial awareness, and mathematical ability). For example, is intelligence about being good with numbers, ability to write text, understanding social situations, spatial skills, and/or having a good sense of humour? When measuring intelligence, sampling of the full range of content has proved difficult because psychologists lack consensus about the constituents of intelligence. To explain this, sense of humour, musical skills, and physical ability are currently not measured by intelligence tests when one could argue that these talents are in fact components of intelligence.

7.4.9 CRITERION VALIDITY

Criterion validity is the degree to which a questionnaire covers the theoretical representation of the construct under question. *Criterion validity* is subdivided into either *concurrent validity*, *predictive validity*, or *measure validity*, which is dependent upon context. To explain this in more detail.

- *Concurrent validity* refers to a comparison made between the measure and a similar outcome test that measures the same time (e.g. comparing two different types of intelligence tests). If this new scale correlates well (>0.7) with the established preexisting validated scale that measures the same thing, then *concurrent validity* has been established. It is however important to note that *concurrent validity* can only be declared when this other criteria or preexisting robust validated measure already exists. As such, *concurrent validity* is demonstrated when a test correlates well with a measure that has previously been validated to measure the same or similar construct.

- *Criterion validity (also known as predictive validity)* is typically assessed through comparing your test against a preexisting gold standard. The overall aim of *criterion validity* is to correlate what is being measured in your new test, against an already established external benchmark. *Predictive validity* is for example, when a person scores high on an intelligence test and they proceed to do well in their job, then the intelligence test has good *predictive validity* of life success. In contrast, if a person scores high on an intelligence test and they do not do well in their job, then the intelligence test has poor *predictive validity*. Another example that has obvious poor *criterion validity* (*predictive validity*) is to assess intelligence by measuring head circumference, simply because head size does not correlate with intelligence. To distinguish *predictive validity* from *concurrent validity*, *concurrent validity* involves gathering evidence to defend the use of a test and its success at measuring a particularized outcome. To view examples of preexisting intelligence tests that you can compare your newly developed scale against, see Table 7.11.

During process of calculating *concurrent validity*, a statistical validity coefficient is calculated to compare scores of the test against the selected external criterion (i.e. other intelligence tests). To provide a midwifery example, a mother

Table 7.11   Common types of validated intelligence tests.

Universal Nonverbal Intelligence
Differential Ability Scales
Stanford–Binet Intelligence Scale
Peabody Individual Achievement Test
Wechsler Adult Intelligence Scale
Wechsler Individual Achievement Test
Woodcock–Johnson III Tests of Cognitive Disabilities

suspected of being depressed is asked to complete the *Edinburgh Postnatal Depression Scale* (EPDS) (Cox et al. 1987) and achieves a high score. Hence and to achieve *concurrent validity*, an external rating is required that corresponds or agrees with the woman's depressed state. In this instance, a mental health nurse assessment is one *external criterion* and if they diagnose that the woman is depressed, then the EPDS result is decreed valid. Alternatively, or in addition, the woman could complete a *Hospital Anxiety and Depression Scale* (HADS) (Zigmond and Snaith 1983), which is an additional *external criterion*. There does not need to be an exact relationship between the findings of the measuring tool and the *external criterion*, although a high correlation coefficient is better (i.e. 0.9 is excellent, 0.7 is the cut-off of acceptability, and 0.5 is unacceptable). In the case of pure quantitative *criterion validity*, we talk about *measure validity,* which involves the researcher comparing their construct of focus against an external criterion. An example follows:

What is being measured	External criterion
Anxiety	Pulse raised
	Sweaty
	Increased blood flow

Alternatively, anxiety state could be *concurrently validated* against scores on the *Spielberger's Anxiety Scale* (Spielberger 1983), thus providing *concurrent validity*.

To conclude this section about validity testing, rigour in a research project is required to produce a quality piece of work. A rigorous quantitative research study requires to use *reliable* and *valid* measuring tools, which produce consistent and repeatable results. An analogy to exemplify this involves using a 6-inch ruler, which consistently measures 6 inches. At the same time and in terms of *validity*, this 6-inch ruler should provide a *valid* measurement of what it says it is measuring. In this case distance and not intelligence. We will now move on to consider the quantitative data collection method called *measurement*.

7.5 MEASUREMENT

Measurement involves the quantitative assessment of a calculable element of an object. For example, its length, height, or weight. Fit for purpose, a valid and reliable measuring tool is calibrated to set standards. Examples of two everyday measuring tools you will know are weighing scales calibrated to measure kilograms, stones, pounds, and ounces and a ruler which is standardized to quantify metres, centimetres, feet, and inches. In research, accurate measurement is crucial in terms of three aspects:

1. The measurement itself.

2. The margin of error.

3. The confidence level, which is the probability that the actual property of the physical object is within the margin of error (e.g. the researcher measures the length of an object as 1.21 m plus or minus 0.01 of a meter, which represents a 95% level of confidence.

Metrology is the scientific study of measurement and includes estimation of a physical quantity (e.g. distance, energy, temperature, weight, or time). A researcher can measure distance, weight, mass, temperature, or volume of a given object, which is measured in miles or kilometers, calories, degrees Celsius, kilograms, pounds, or stones. Whatever object is being measured, the result will be presented in numeric value. To view a research paper that has used measurement as a form of data collection in maternity care, see Activity 7.2.

Activity 7.2

Access and read the following paper that has used measurement as a form of data collection:

Inskip, H., Crozier, S., Baird, J. et al. (2021). Measured weight in early pregnancy is a valid method for estimating pre-pregnancy weight. *Journal of Developmental Origins of Health and Disease* 12: 561–569. https://doi.org/10.1017/S2040174420000926

A further example of measured data is blood testing, which involves analysis of a blood sample that has been extracted from a person's vein. Examples of measurements taken include full blood count (e.g. haemoglobin, white cells, and platelets), blood group (e.g. A, B, O, or AB), and Rhesus status (positive or negative). We will now move on to look at interviews as a qualitative method of data collection.

7.6 INTERVIEWS

Interviews are a qualitative form of data collection, which involves the researcher asking open-ended questions. The purpose of an interview is to permit the researcher to gather individualized participant responses, whilst taking into consideration spoken words, nonverbal body language, and emotional responses. There are three approaches to interviewing, which include (i) *unstructured*, (ii) *semi-structured*, and (iii) *structured*. First, an *unstructured* interview is a non-directed interview, during which the questions asked are not predetermined. Second, a *semi-structured* interview consists of a list of predetermined open-ended questions and a set of prompts. Third, a *structured interview* takes a systematic approach, which involves the interviewer asking the same list of predetermined questions of all participants in the exact same order. Each of these questions is then rated using a calibrated scoring system.

7.6.1 UNSTRUCTURED INTERVIEW

An *unstructured interview* allows the researcher to learn about aspects that they may not have preconceived when preparing for an interview. For example, asking the participant to tell you about themselves. Some example questions follow:

Q Please describe your ideal scenario.
Q Tell me what you value most about your work experience.
Q Explain what you value most highly in life.

The advantage of an open interview approach is that it enables the researcher to ascertain experiences or knowledge that they had not previously thought of. As such, conversations vary considerably between participants.

7.6.2 SEMI-STRUCTURED INTERVIEW

Semi-structured interviews allow the researcher to explore participants' thoughts, beliefs, and emotions about a predetermined topic and delve down deeply into their individualized world of experience. For example, asking the participant to tell you about their birth experience. Some example questions follow:

Q Please describe your ideal birth scenario.
Q Tell me what you value most about your intranatal experience.
Q Explain what yocand birth.

Suggested prompts

- Can you elaborate on that point?
- How was that for you?
- Can you enlarge upon?

Having a rigorous number of questions keeps the interview on track and keeps it focused upon the research question.

7.6.3 STRUCTURED INTERVIEW

A *structured interview* can be designed to take both a qualitative and quantitative approach to ensure reliability through asking precisely the same questions in exactly the same order with each participant. As such, this approach to data collection allows questions to be accumulated and scored on a continuum. This is similar to a quantitative survey approach, which for example scores participant responses out of 10, with the main difference being that the interview is conducted face-to-face or through a virtual computer setup. As such, comparisons may be drawn with confidence between participant groups (e.g. primiparous and multiparous women) and different longitudinal structured survey interview points. For example, asking the participant to tell you about and also rate their birth experience.

Q Please tell us about and rate your last experience of giving birth in terms of pain experienced.

Low pain 1 2 3 4 5 6 7 8 9 10 High pain

Q How supportive was the midwife(s) when you gave birth to your last baby?

Unsupportive 1 2 3 4 5 6 7 8 9 10 Very supportive

Q Explain how much you valued having your partner present during your last labour and delivery?

Not at all 1 2 3 4 5 6 7 8 9 10 Highly

The responses given will be elaborated upon during the structured interview.

In summary, an interview is a systemized discussion during which the researcher asks questions, and the participant provides answers. Within research, the word 'interview' denotes a one-to-one discussion on a specific topic, which is prearranged between the interviewer and a selected interviewee who meets the inclusion criteria for the study. In contrast, when more than one participant takes part in an organized interview, this is called a *focus group*.

7.6.4 FOCUS GROUP INTERVIEWS

A focus group interview is a structured group process used to obtain detailed information about a specific subject. It is particularly useful for exploring attitudes and feelings and to draw out precise issues that may be unknown to the researcher. A focus group is typically composed of two to nine participants who represent a specific population (e.g. diabetics, women with babies in the neonatal unit, and teenage pregnancy). A focus group session normally lasts between one and two hours, with two hours being the absolute maximum beneficial length. During process, a trained facilitator keeps the discussion on track through asking a series of preplanned open-ended questions written on a preplanned interview schedule. This interview schedule is designed to stimulate discussion between individuals in the group, who then promote and stimulate other members' thinking. There are several steps taken by the researcher who is organizing a *focus group*.

7.6.5 STEPS INVOLVED IN RUNNING A FOCUS GROUP

Define the Purpose

The researcher clearly identifies subject matter they would like to know more about, which will relate to the preorganized research aim(s) and question(s). The researcher then formulates specific objectives that relate to the topic under investigation. For example:

Identify pregnant women's experiences of developing gestational diabetes.

OR

Identify what types of contraception women in Malawi use.

OR

Discover what aspects of perinatal bereavement support are helpful for the experiencer.

OR

Discover reasons why breastfeeding women cease to breastfeed.

Prepare the Interview Questions

A set of questions are developed to provide an overall direction for the group discussion. These questions move from the general to the more specific. Questions should be open-ended, straightforward, unbiased, and focused upon the topic of address. The purpose of these developed questions is to stimulate and guide dialogue, although it is important to note that discussion invariably raises further issues for exploration. To view an example of a semi-structured interview schedule, see Table 7.12.

Table 7.12   Example of a semi-structured interview schedule.

DATE, NAMES OF INERVIEWER(S), AND VENUE

- Thank participants for participating in the interview.
- Tell them why you are interviewing them (e.g. Discover what aspects of perinatal bereavement support are helpful for the experiencer).
- Explain that participation is voluntary, and they can leave at any point.
- Reassure the interview will not influence future care given.
- Tell participant how long the interview will last.
- Gain permission to audio-record the interview.
- Explain that the participant can decline to answer a question or ask for clarification about what is being asked at any point during the interview.
- Explain that confidentiality is assured, with data only shared with team members and that it will be coded.
- Ask participants(s) if they have any questions about what has been explained so far.
- Ask if you can turn on the audio recorder.
- Establish a repour through introductions, etc.
- Commence the open-ended question guide.

Example question guide, which is tailored to answer the aim(s) and research question(s)

(Q1) Were you provided with any resources that helped you understand your condition (e.g. pamphlets and leaflets)?
Example prompt: Can you explain how they helped you?

(Q2) Who did you approach for help and/or advice (midwife, family, friend, etc.)?
Example prompt: If so, how useful were they at helping you understand your condition?

(Q3) What were your concerns surrounding your diagnosis (e.g. pain, employment, mental health responses, and ability to have personal relationships)?
Example prompt: Please can you be more specific?

(Q4) Can you explain what sorts of support were offered to you?
Example prompt: Please can you tell me a little bit more about that?

(Q5) How did you find out about additional support on offer?
Example prompt: Can you elaborate?

(Q6) What stands out for you about your support experience?
Example prompt: How did it help or not help you?

(Q7) What aspect of support was most helpful?
Example prompt: In what way did it help?

(Q8) What aspect of support was least helpful?
Example prompt: In what way did it not help?

(Q9) What support aspect would you recommend for others in the same situation as you?
Example prompt: Can you explain why?

(Q10) Is there anything else that you would like to comment on about the support provided to you?

- Thank participant(s) for attending.
- Inform participant(s) that you have turned the audio recorder off.
- Reassure participant(s) about data security.
- Explain how and when results will be reported.
- Provide a follow-up contact number in case upset later or want to ask a question.

Identify and Recruit Participants

When recruiting participants, the researchers' first task is to identify the key population of interest and construct relevant inclusion and exclusion criteria (e.g. primiparous women who have developed gestational diabetes). Specialized participant groups are recruited in relation to the required characteristics (e.g. age, gender, employment status, place of residence, marital status, social class, income, ethnic group, specified disease, or problem). Participants are invited to take part in a *focus group* with the communication stating purpose, who the researchers are, and what the results will be used for. An informed consent form is signed, and a reminder of the time and place of meeting is sent to the participant's home.

Environment

The researcher books a meeting room, which has comfortable chairs, is free from outside distractions, which has refreshments provided, bathroom facilities, and the room set at a comfortable temperature. Participants are invited to sit in a circle so they can view one another from an equal footing. Conducting a *focus group* in a comfortable environment will promote discussion, idea sharing, and debate.

Conducting the Focus Group Interview

An ideal facilitator uses communication skills that allow them to direct group discussion without themselves taking part in the dialogue exchange. During process, the facilitator strives to create a relaxed informal atmosphere in which participants feel free to express their views. At all times, the facilitator must avoid being judgemental about opinions offered. Questions asked should not be time limited with participants encouraged to express uninterrupted viewpoints. Leads in new directions are encouraged when they relate to the research aim(s) and question(s). All group members are equally encouraged to have their say with those dominating the discussion reigned in from doing so. Some researchers ask participants to write down ideas before the discussion, which can work towards cultivating conversation. The session is audio recorded and later transcribed with the facilitator ideally having a fellow researcher on site to take notes. Having discussed *focus group interviews,* we will now move on to discuss observational data collection.

7.7 OBSERVATIONS

Observation allows the researcher to study people in their natural environment for the purpose of understanding perspectives within a living context. As such, observational data collection has its roots in anthropology and is used by ethnographers. Observational studies involve the researcher systematically recording observable phenomena or behaviour within a natural setting. As such, observational data can be quantitative or qualitative in approach. During process, the researcher uses a variety of techniques to gather data, such as recording behaviours, events, or noting physical features. During process, participants may know whether they are being observed (overt data collection) or not (covert data collection) with data gathered in a structured or unstructured way by the researcher. There are ethical issues surrounding data collection, given that data gathering is often covert, with the observer participating in daily life whilst covertly observing processes, listening to conversations, and questioning people over time. Additional observational data may be gathered from records (e.g. diaries, portfolios, letters, minutes, websites, art, and literature). Whilst observing people in their natural settings, there are a variety of roles the researcher can adopt.

7.7.1 ROLES TAKEN DURING OBSERVATIONAL DATA COLLECTION

Nonparticipation

Nonparticipation involves the researcher having no level of involvement with study participants. For example, data are collected via a one-way mirror or by observing interaction in a group. Whilst this form of data collection has advantages, it does not allow in-depth exploration of people's behaviours in their conceptual worlds.

Complete Observer

The *complete observer* is present in the environment but does not interact with participants to any substantial extent. The *complete observer's* role is to listen, observe, and eavesdrop with detachment sometimes detrimental because the researcher does not hear the whole conversation. During process, a *complete observer* cannot ask questions to qualify what is stated, which inhibits them from grasping the full significance of the information exchange. The researcher may also collect data through videotaping, audiotaping, or photographing unsuspecting participants, which also has ethical implications.

Observer-as-Participant

Unlike the covert activity of the *complete observer*, the researcher's identity is known. During process, the *observer-as-participant* should remain research-oriented and not cross into the friendship domain. One advantage for the *observer-as-participant* is that participants may be more willing to talk to a familiar individual who has declared a positive purpose to their presence.

Observational data collection, as the name implies, is a method of gathering data through observing participants in a natural setting in a covert or overt way. This makes observational data collection participatory in nature, simply because the researcher immerses themselves in the scene whilst taking notes or using systematic recording sheets. To view a research paper that has gathered observations as a form of data collection, see Activity 7.3.

Activity 7.3

Access and read the following paper that has gathered observations as a form of data collection:

Hirata, S., Fuwa, K., Sugama, K. et al. (2011). Mechanism of birth in chimpanzees: humans are not unique among primates. *Biology Letters* 23;7(5): 686–688. https://doi.org/10.1098/rsbl.2011.0214

7.8   SUMMARY OF DATA COLLECTION CHAPTER

To conclude, Chapter 7 has looked at a variety of data collection processes, which has included questionnaires, measurement, interviews, and observations. Whatever approach is selected, data collection is the process of gathering and measuring information about specified variables in a predecided environment, which enables the researcher to answer specified research questions and evaluate findings. Regardless of whether the approach is quantitative or qualitative, the aim of all data collection is to capture honest and quality evidence, which is then analysed and reported to provide credible answers to the predetermined research question. We will now move on to Chapter 8, which proceeds to discuss processes of analyzing qualitative data gathered by the researcher.

7.9   SELF-ASSESSMENT QUESTIONS (SAQs)

7.1   The question in the box below is an example of what type of data collection:

(Q) Attending a support group has reduced the amount of alcohol I drink.

	Strongly agree	Agree	Neither agree or disagree	Disagree	Strongly disagree
Scores	1	2	3	4	5

(a) Quantitative survey data collection

(b) Agreement data collection

(c) Interview data collection

(d) Observational data collection

7.2   Reliability is:

(a) When a research tool has been used and proved itself in another research project.

(b) When a pilot study has been carried out to see if the study is feasible.

(c) The consistency of measurement of a research tool across longitudinal timepoints.

(d) Findings agree with what other researchers have found.

7.3   **What is the correct order of steps when using a questionnaire to gather data?**

   (a)   Write the report, design the questions, analyse the data, and collect data.

   (b)   Design the questions, write the report, collect data, and analyse the data.

   (c)   Design the questions, collect data, analyse the data, and write the report.

   (d)   Collect data, analyse the data, design the questions, and write the report.

7.4   **Which data collection approach does not require ethical approval?**

   (a)   Interviewing participants' experiences of a particular treatment.

   (b)   Seeking out research papers for a systematic review.

   (c)   Asking pregnant women to complete a questionnaire.

   (d)   Taking blood samples from participants to send to the laboratory.

7.5   **Which of the following is not a data collection method?**

   (a)   Searching women's historical obstetric case records.

   (b)   Weighing women at the antenatal clinic.

   (c)   Interviewing women about their experiences at the antenatal clinic.

   (d)   Watching television.

7.6   **What is primary data?**

   (a)   A form of longitudinal data collection.

   (b)   Data collected directly from main sources (e.g. interviews, surveys, and experiments)

   (c)   Secondary data collected by someone other than the primary user.

   (d)   Data collected from a primary school.

ANSWERS TO CHAPTER 7 SAQs

7.1   **a**

7.2   **c**

7.3   **c**

7.4   **b**

7.5   **d**

7.6   **b**

STEP (10): Detail intended data processing and analysis.

8.1 INTRODUCTION TO QUALITATIVE DATA ANALYSIS

Qualitative data analysis involves the research midwife investigating descriptive and conceptual findings gathered via, for example, observations, questionnaires, or interviews. Analysis of qualitative data allows the research midwife to explore ideas presented in:

- Interviews

- Focus groups

- Diaries

- Video recordings

- Photographs

- Case studies

- Case notes

- Documents (e.g. meeting minutes, letters, and stories)

- Observations

- Open-ended surveys

- Concept maps

- Portfolios of evidence

Compared with quantitative data, which is based on numbers that are countable and measurable, qualitative data analysis is interpretation based, descriptive, and captured in language. As such, creative thinking is required to interpret findings and construct stories.

Qualitative data comes in a variety of forms, with interview transcripts derived from open-ended, focused, and exploratory questions that the researcher has pre-written on a semi-structured interview schedule. This predecided semi-structured

Research Recipes for Midwives, First Edition. Caroline J. Hollins Martin.
© 2024 John Wiley & Sons Ltd. Published 2024 by John Wiley & Sons Ltd.

interview schedule will be submitted as an appendix to the research proposal. There is no limit to what constitutes qualitative data, with researchers using observations (both video and participatory), focus groups, texts, documents, multimedia products, public domain sources (e.g. library), policy manuals, photographs, or lay autobiographical accounts. In essence, qualitative data refers to anything that is not quantitative or rendered into numerical form. Remember, what distinguishes quantitative data from qualitative data is assumptions, principles, and values about truth and reality. In contrast, quantitative researchers deem that the goal of science is to discover the truths that exist in the world, whilst qualitative researchers defend that relevant reality is subjective human experience embedded in social context and historical time. As such, the qualitative stance is concerned with uncovering knowledge about how people think and feel about an event. Having clarified what qualitative data is or is not, we will now look at processes of qualitative data analysis.

8.2 BASIC PROCESSES OF QUALITATIVE DATA ANALYSIS

Qualitative research midwives take an interest in *finding, creating*, and *analyzing* texts. For example, *finding* texts involves conducting interviews with participants (e.g. women, partners, family members, midwives, and allied healthcare professionals), or gathering data through the study of clinical transactions, management plans, case notes, or personal correspondence. The next step involves *creating* texts of what participants say during an interview and transcribing these recordings. Alternatively, they may gather qualitative data in recording sheets from the study of recorded texts. Either way, during qualitative data analysis, text is labelled and regularities are studied across similar tags to form themes (also known as categories) and subthemes (also known as subcategories). This is pretty much what content *analysis* is about. During process, the researcher studies meaning and looks for similar narratives with similar overtone in attempts to develop an analytical research story. For example, suppose ($n = 30$) postnatal women are asked by the qualitative research midwife to describe their experiences of labour and childbirth. Out of these ($n = 30$) postnatal women's intranatal descriptions, their recorded experiences will contain patterns of how the perceived events unfolded, which will be both similar and different in terms of birth satisfaction and outcome. As the qualitative research midwife analyses individual texts, they will gradually develop a framework of themes (categories) and subthemes (subcategories) and build a framework of their own research story. To view an example of a final qualitative data analysis table, see Table 8.1.

In Table 8.1, you will see that a story has been summarized, with each theme and its associated subthemes analytically discussed in relation to the literature review that forefronts the research paper. To view the organization of themes and subthemes constructed in a research paper, see Activity 8.1.

Activity 8.1

Access and read the following paper that reports qualitative findings in terms of themes and subthemes in a diagrammatic form:

(See Figure 1 in this paper)

Hewitt, L., Dadich, A., Hartz, D.L. et al. (2022). Midwife-centred management: a qualitative study of midwifery group practice management and leadership in Australia. *BMC Health Serv Res* 22, 1203. https://doi.org/10.1186/s12913-022-08532-y

---

Table 8.1 Themes and subthemes identified in the data.

Themes	Subthemes	
(1) Pain experienced	(1a)	Feeling proud to have coped
	(1b)	Pain relief requested
	(1c)	Perception of help from the midwife
(2) Role of the birth partner	(2a)	Concern for their well-being
	(2b)	Made a difference
	(2c)	Well prepared
(3) Birth satisfaction	(3a)	Felt in control
	(3b)	Continuity of care important
	(3c)	Provided with informed choice

It is important to note that people are individuals and perceive situations differently and according to their experience, gender, culture, education, etc. The following endeavour (Activity 8.2) is designed to highlight subjective differences in how people may perceive a similar situation.

Activity 8.2

(a) Place a pair of tights on a table at home and ask two to six members of your family to explain different ways in which this pair of tights could be used.

(b) As each explanation is provided, write them down on a piece of paper.

(c) Organize the findings into themes and subthemes.

Once you have completed Activity 8.2, consider ways in which you could code your data.

8.3 CODING THE DATA

There are difficulties with coding texts and finding patterns. Coding turns qualitative data (texts) into quantitative data (coded data) because the codes attached create numbers. For example, five participants come up with a similar use for the pair of tights, which is clustered into a theme. The researcher interprets all the written comments gathered and focuses upon naming the themes and telling the story as they have interpreted it. They then look at their identified themes and work out how they relate to one another. The researcher will then deconstruct the text, look for hidden subtexts, try to inform the reader of deeper or multiple meanings, and back up these arguments with appropriate references. The text is discussed and labels are produced for the themes identified. At times, these discussions may take the reader away from the text, just as surely as numerical coding does. Remember quantitative analysis involves reducing themes to numbers, whilst and in contrast, qualitative analysis involves making sense of what dialogue represents. As such, the qualitative researcher constructs their perceived meaning of the themes (categories) and subthemes (subcategories) using their own words. Researchers today have at their disposal a tremendous set of tools for collecting, processing, deconstructing, analyzing, and interpreting meaning of data that relates to human thought and behaviour. Intrinsically, coding of qualitative data follows a structured process.

8.3.1 THE CODING PROCESS

Most of the coding effort should emanate from the research question with often unforeseen discoveries encountered in the data. The processes of coding qualitative data follows a distinct set of steps (see Table 8.2).

Table 8.2   Steps involved in coding qualitative data.

1	Prepare the data for analysis and number each section in a systemized way (e.g. transcripts, notes, documents, or other sources).
2	Read through the data and gain a feel for it.
3	Reread data and mark significant points with codes (e.g. participant 1, page 3, line 5) (P1, p3, L5). Go through each line one-by-one of your transcript and code as much data as you can.
4	Sort codes and combine them into themes (categories) that relate to the research question (see Table 8.1) (e.g. Theme 1 is labelled *pain experienced*).
5	Where possible, sort codes placed under a labelled theme (category) into subthemes (subcategories) (see Table 8.1) (e.g. subtheme (1a) is labelled *'feeling proud to have coped'*; (1b) *pain relief requested*; (1c) *'perception of help from the midwife'*).
6	Look at the overall frame of themes (categories) and subthemes (subcategories) and revise to improve sensemaking.
7	Present themes (categories) and subthemes (subcategories) in an interconnected manner (e.g. akin to Table 8.1 or diagram).

8.3.2 DEFINING CODES

As the research midwife 'defines a code', this will refine their thinking as they progress through the qualitative data analysis. Sometimes the coding strategy will focus on the nature of the content being coded (the what), and other times it will focus on the process (the how). To view some examples of coded narratives, see Table 8.3.

Having looked at some examples of coded quotes, it is important to know that there are different ways of approaching the labelling task, with some researchers coding manually and others using computer software. *Computer-assisted qualitative data analysis software* (CAQDAS) embraces technology designed to support qualitative data analysis. Advantages of using CAQDAS include proficient management of data and transparency of processes. Disadvantages of using CAQDAS include overemphasis on coding qualitative data, which may distract from analytical procedures and time spent in learning the software program (Vignato et al. 2022). Different systems and research methods guide coding of qualitative data. For example, automated coding, generative or open coding, axial coding, selective coding, factual or descriptive coding, interpretive coding, pattern analysis, and content analysis.

Automated Coding

Automating coding applies *string and pattern searches* to locate keywords in documents, which essentially requires the use of a software program. One problem with using keywords is that more abstract concepts cannot be characterized by a single word or phrase. Consequently, the researcher should not totally rely on automated keyword searches to provide the foundation for their data analysis, with it was important for them to also immerse themselves in their transcript data.

Table 8.3 Themes and subthemes.

	Codes	Examples of coded narratives extracted from interview transcripts
Themes (1, 2, or 3) and subthemes (a, b, or c) identified	Participant = P	(*n* = 20) participants in total
	page = p	Please note there would be several quotes for each theme and subtheme.
	Line = L	
(1) Pain experienced	P7, p3, L16	'The pain was excruciating, and I was not prepared for that'.
(1a) Feeling proud to have coped	P3, p1, L17	'I handled my labour pain well. . . . . . .I think, but I had rehearsed and rehearsed in preparation. . .yeah'.
(1b) Pain relief requested	P18, p5, L28	'I said to the midwife, I did. Give me everything (referring to pain relief). . . .yeah everything you've got. OK and thanks'.
(1c) Perception of help from the midwife	P9, p6, L26	'The midwives were great, yes, they were. They made me laugh, and I chanted through the pain. It was sore though. Yes, really painful'.
(2) Role of the birth partner	P1, p4, L4	'Alex. He's my partner. . .came to classes with me and joined in. They worked, and he felt confident to support me, and he was with me all. . .or most of the way'.
(2a) Concern for their well-being	P20, p2, L23	'I worried about him all the time. He was not happy, no not happy at all. He told me afterwards he was scared, which was hard for him as he is a man's man'.
(2b) Made a difference	P3, p6, L15	'Having him there. . . .Dave my husband was great. After all, it's our baby. I don't think; I would have done so well. Yeah, he made it different, better'.
(2c) Well prepared	P7, p7, L17	'I was ready, really ready, to have my baby. I went to classes and everything. Read books, listened to podcasts. It all helped'. It did!
(3) Birth satisfaction	P19, p3, L23	'My birth experience was great, really great. It was sore, but it was all good in the end. I made it and will go again'.
(3a) Felt in control	P2, p4, L32	'I felt in control most. . .yeah most of the time. But at the end it was hard. I think I may have lost it. I was shouting at the top of my voice'.
(3b) Continuity of care important	P16, p5, L24	'Having a midwife, I knew was good. I met her four times at the clinic. Yeah. The one in Alloway. She was really kind and I felt she knew me too. That helped, and I thought she cared'.
(3c) Provided with informed choice	P8, p4, L2	'The midwife explained most things to me. . .at times, I did not understand, but she repeated and answered questions, etc. I got to write a plan for my birth, and she asked me what I wanted'.

Generative or Open Coding

Generative or *open* coding is used in *grounded theory research method* and involves development of themes (categories) and subthemes (subcategories) from concepts that emerge within the data. It is an open process, given that exploration of the data is carried out without the researcher making any prior assumptions about what they might discover.

Axial Coding

Axial coding is also used in *grounded theory research method* and involves building connections within and between themes (categories) and subthemes (subcategories) for purpose of deepening the theoretical framework that underpins the data analysis. Axial coding involves connecting or linking data together to reveal codes, themes (categories), and subthemes (subcategories) grounded within participants' voices.

Selective Coding

Selective coding is also used in *grounded theory research method* and builds relationships between themes (categories) and subthemes (subcategories), which becomes the configuration of the theoretical analysis. Selective coding involves the qualitative researcher selecting a core theme (category) and systematically relating it to other themes (categories). During process, the qualitative researcher should maintain an open mind about the codes they create.

Factual or Descriptive Coding

Factual or *descriptive coding* represents ideas that are more concrete, which may include actions, definitions, events, properties, settings, conditions, or processes. *Factual* or *descriptive coding* aims to capture extracts from the data through the use of a single word that encases the overall concept retrieved from the data. Words used will characteristically describe the data in a highly concentrated way that allows the researcher to quickly label the content.

Interpretive Coding

Interpretive coding is used to select and reorganize data to identify themes (categories) and subthemes (subcategories), with observations interpreted through the eyes of the participant and embedded within the social context. Interpretation involves viewing or experiencing the phenomenon from the subjective perspectives of the participant. *Interpretive coding* is informed by the philosophical traditions of hermeneutics, phenomenology, pragmatism, symbolic interaction, and critical theory.

Pattern Analysis

Pattern analysis focuses on conceptual relationships, chronologies, taxonomies, language analysis, and/or repetitions. It does not involve counting instances of a phenomenon, which is more characteristic of *content analysis*.

Content Analysis

Content analysis has its roots in the quantitative paradigm since numbers of participant reports of a similar concept are counted. Hence, *content analysis* is quantitative and focused on counting and measuring. Once the code words have been developed and the associated quotes counted, the researcher analyses the results.

Different methods of analyzing and coding qualitative data lead to different answers, insights, conclusions, and response actions. Essentially, coding methods are aids to sorting and organizing sets of qualitative data, followed by intellectual processing to transform data into findings. In relation to the different qualitative research methods, we will now look at specific analytical strategies that qualitative researchers can use.

8.4 SPECIFIC ANALYTIC STRATEGIES

An appreciation of the more common analytic approaches can be helpful towards understanding what a researcher states about how their data was sorted, organized, conceptualized, refined, and interpreted. There are a variety of ways that qualitative data may be analysed. For example, phenomenological analysis, constant comparative analysis, ethnographic analysis, and narrative and discourse analysis. When deciding which specific analytic strategy, you intend to use to analyse your qualitative data, make sure it matches the whole qualitative research method (recipe). If you are planning a research proposal to take forward for master or doctorate study, ensure you select an expert in your chosen method to be one of your supervisors and approach them for advice. Some examples of specific qualitative analytic strategies follow.

8.4.1 INTERPRETATIVE PHENOMENOLOGICAL ANALYSIS (IPA)

IPA is a qualitative method of data analysis, which provides deep and detailed investigations of individualized participants' lived experiences that relate to the research question. IPA generates accounts of lived experiences from the storyteller's perspective as opposed to detailing preexisting theoretical preconceptions. As such, IPA is an interpretive form of analysis, which endeavours to make sense of each person's human situation in turn as interviews are conducted, before producing generalized research findings. This makes IPA the perfect method for investigating complex topics, which are emotionally loaded and ambiguous. Experiences of labour and childbirth are a good example of this because individual experiences of pain, interactions with midwives, expectations, and rollout of events are complex to explain. Hence, IPA data analysis is committed to examining how participants make sense of their major life experiences.

When analyzing qualitative data as a tradition, IPA encourages researchers to 'bracket' their preconceptions to prevent them from influencing their interpretation of the 'lived experiences' of each participant (Creswell 2013). As such, the researcher first describes their own experiences of the topic in question, records these as preconceptions, and attempts to avoid letting their views interrupt the participant's account and analysis of their data. Some argue that bracketing of own preconceptions is an impossible task to ask of a researcher, which is a question that is open to debate. In attempts to bracket preconceptions and according to Creswell (2013), the researcher develops a list of significant statements and forms a foundation from which they attempt to understand the phenomenon. These statements may emerge from the interviews themself and/or from other relevant research sources that have explored the topic of interest. Post developing these statements, the researcher then groups them into larger units of information, called 'meaning units' or themes (categories). The next step involves the researcher writing a description of 'what' the participants experienced in relation to the phenomenon of interest. Creswell (2013) calls this 'textural description' of participants' experiences, which must be accompanied by participants' verbatim examples. Next, the researcher writes a description of 'how' the experience happened, which is called a 'structural description'. Finally, the researcher writes a composite description of the phenomenon, which incorporates both the 'textural description' and the 'structural description' (Creswell 2013). With IPA, each interview transcript is transcribed verbatim and printed off as a hard copy. Each interview, in turn, is then analysed with significant parts marked using color-coded pens according to common identified themes. As such, IPA according to Smith et al. (2009) permits the researcher to deeply explore the 'lived experiences' of each individual participant to gain understanding of the phenomenological significance and how it impacted them. The last step of IPA analysis involves the researcher writing a long paragraph and mini statement, which informs the reader 'what' the participant experienced and 'how' within a contextual format.

8.4.2 GROUNDED THEORY CONSTANT COMPARATIVE ANALYSIS

In qualitative *grounded theory research method*, there is a continual interplay between data collection and data analysis, with the researcher using *constant comparative analysis*. During the process of *constant comparative analysis*, similar coded data points are gathered to form themes (categories), which are then coded and compared across already identified themes (categories), with patterns identified and refined as new data being obtained from subsequent participants. *Constant comparative analysis* permits the analyst to use preexisting or emergent theory against which new pieces of data are compared. As such, *constant comparative analysis* involves the researcher taking one piece of data (one interview, one statement, or one theme) and comparing it with all others that may be similar to develop conceptualizations of relationships between the pieces of data. For example, by comparing the accounts of two different people who have had a similar experience, a researcher might pose analytical questions. An example of this is, how is this text or theme (category) different from that, and how are these two texts or themes related. The aim of the researcher is to generate knowledge about common patterns and themes within human experience. This process continues until all data sets have been compared with each other. *Constant comparative analysis* is well suited to grounded theory, which is because the method explains fundamental social processes involved in human behaviour and experience. For example, the stages of grieving and processes of recovery involved. *Constant comparative analysis* creates knowledge that is generally descriptive or interpretive to develop ways of understanding human phenomena within the context experienced.

8.4.3 ETHNOGRAPHIC ANALYSIS

Ethnographic analysis is derived from anthropology's tradition of interpreting the processes and products of cultural behaviour. Ethnographers document aspects of human experience, such as beliefs, kinship patterns, and ways of living. Healthcare professionals use ethnographic analysis to uncover and record variations in how different social and cultural groups understand and enact health and illness. When a researcher uses an ethnographic method, they have learned about a culture or group through their own immersion and engagement in fieldwork or participant observation and then proceed to portray that culture in written text. *Ethnographic analysis* uses an iterative process in which cultural ideas that arise during active involvement 'in the field' are transformed, translated, or represented in a written document. *Ethnographic analysis* involves sifting and sorting through pieces of data to detect and interpret thematic categorizations, whilst searching for inconsistencies and contradictions, and at end of process generating conclusions about what is happening and why.

8.4.4 NARRATIVE AND DISCOURSE ANALYSIS

Many qualitative researchers have discovered the extent to which human experience is shaped, transformed, and understood through linguistic representation. The subjective characterizations of life experiences take on meaning when attempts are made to articulate them in communication. Putting experience into words, whether we do this verbally, in writing, or in thought, the aim is to transform the actual event into a communicable representation. Thus, speech forms are not the experiences themselves. Instead, speech forms are socially and culturally constructed devices for creating shared understandings. *Narrative analysis* is a strategy that recognizes the extent to which stories provide insight into lived experiences. Through analytic processes, the main narrative themes accounted for by participants facilitate discovery and understanding of how individuals make sense of their lives. In contrast, *discourse analysis* recognizes that speech is not a direct representation of human experience. Instead, *discourse analysis* is a linguistic tool shaped by numerous social or ideological influences. *Discourse analysis* draws upon theories developed in sociolinguistics and cognitive psychology to aid understanding of what is represented. A critical inquiry of the language used by a participant is conducted to uncover societal influences that underlie human thoughts and behaviours. Although both *narrative analysis* and *discourse analysis* rely heavily on speech as the most relevant data form, the reasons given for analyzing language between the two differ. In essence, *narrative and discourse analysis* are methods of analyzing the structure of text and utterances of participants, which considers the content and sociolinguistic context.

To summarize this section, each specific analytic strategy turns raw data into new knowledge. During each analytical process, the qualitative researcher engages in active and demanding systematic methodical processes, which involve reading, understanding, theming text, and interpreting data. The language of analysis is sometimes confusing, and it can be challenging to interpret and understand how the findings have evolved from the data. For example, when describing processes that are involved in data analysis, some researchers may use unusual language, such as claiming that conceptual categories have *emerged* from the data. Such research language will gradually be accumulated, with researchers continuing to learn across their career spectrum.

8.5 COGNITIVE PROCESSES INVOLVED IN QUALITATIVE DATA ANALYSIS

The term qualitative research encompasses a wide range of philosophical positions, methodological strategies, and analytical procedures. The cognitive processes involved in qualitative research work to facilitate better understanding of how the researcher's cognitive processes interact with qualitative data to bring about findings and generate new knowledge. As such, qualitative analysis involves:

- *Comprehending* the occurrence under study.

- *Synthesizing* a portrait of the occurrence that accounts for relations and linkages within its aspects.

- *Theorizing* about how and why these relations appear as they do.

- *Recontextualizing* new knowledge about occurrences into context of how others have articulated it.

These steps depict a series of intellectual processes by which raw data are considered, examined, and reformulated to become a research product. During qualitative data analysis, the researcher requires to:

- Prompt themself constantly that the goal is to explore individual and situational perspectives.

- Keep reminding themself of what the research question is. They can introduce secondary ideas but must stay focused on the question asked.

- Be the intellectual intermediary between what has been said and how it relates to the research question.

- Identify from a range of interview transcripts, topics that accurately answer the research question. For example, in response to the question: why do students drop out of university? Excerpts may reflect opinions, such as financial problems, pregnancy, failing course work, high workload, or a difficult course. In this instance, five themes have been identified and each should be critically discussed.

- Decide whether to work with paper transcripts or use a software program to code their data.

Unquestionably, qualitative data analysis is a complex and enigmatic phase of any qualitative research method. For novice midwifery researchers, the data collection processes involved in a qualitative research method may feel more comfortable than undertaking the statistical analysis involved in a quantitative research method. This may be because midwives base their clinical proficiency upon learning about women, partners, and families. During processes of caring, midwives identify commonalities and variations among and between women, babies, and families to provide individualized person-centred care. Nonetheless, simply creating a database is not enough when conducting a qualitative research method. To generate findings that transform raw data into innovative knowledge, the qualitative researcher must engage in vigorous and challenging analytic processes throughout the data analysis phase of the method. To enable themselves to undertake this task, they will be required to read, understand, and interpret the data gathered. To have a go at considering how you could organize some data into themes and subthemes, gather together some research-interested family and friends and have a go at Activity 8.3 and Activity 8.4.

Activity 8.3

Meet with a group of peers (three to five people) and together formulate their responses to the following:

(1) Write all the things a *brick* could be used for.
(2) Assort these lists into core themes (categories).
(3) Subdivide each theme into subthemes (subcategories).
(4) Present a table of the core themes (categories) and subthemes (subcategories).

Activity 8.4

Undertake a database search and find a qualitative research paper that relates to the work of a midwife. Answer the following questions.

(1) How was the data collected?
(2) How was the data analysed?
(3) How many themes (or categories) were identified?
(4) What were these themes (or categories) called?
(5) What were the key conclusions of this paper?

Now that you have a bit more experience at learning how to induce themes (categories) and subthemes (subcategories) from qualitative data, have a go at *Activity 8.5*.

Activity 8.5

The research question is: What situational aspects of a maternity unit promote obedient behaviour from junior midwives?

Themes:

(a) *An obligation to follow hospital policies.*
(b) *Hierarchical control.*
(c) *Fear of consequences from challenging a senior person.*

Assort the following quotes into the above themes:

(1) *Participant 39: Its positional power isn't it and how they use that power. . .There's a difference in power balance, definitely.*
(2) *Participant 21: I would, I would in this case because thinking ahead of the possibilities of, ummm, problems ahead.*
(3) *Participant 19: I'd have to if she's under his care 'cos you know, I've got my own professional practice, but I am employed, and I'm under the auspices of the hospital policies.*
(4) *Participant 60: I wouldn't refuse to do it because again I just think that someone higher up asked you to do it.*
(5) *Participant 36: I would be thinking if I don't do it and if anything goes wrong then I would never forgive myself.*
(6) *Participant 38: I used to know this consultant who went to bezerk when they had more than one (birth partner present during labour).*
(7) *Participant 29: It's like I'm defeated, if you know what I mean. I would have to follow them (guidelines).*
(8) *Participant 15: In the eyes of the court if I don't do it and something happens, then he's going to say "I didn't follow his instructions" or whatever.*
(9) *Participant 44: The costs of being direct with some of these individuals is one that they tend to go a shade of puce and they and you know that they are going to make your life a misery for the next goodness knows how long.*
(10) *Participant 41: I think there is a definite power struggle that goes on. . .I don't just mean between professionals, but between women, professionals, and the doctors themselves.*
(11) *Participant 60: Ummm, I feel quite strongly, and I think that for litigation reasons. . ...that's in your best interests.*
(12) *Participant 35: Well it depends, but on that particular personality here, it probably would because I know what she would be like if I didn't agree.*
(13) *Participant 44: I would say that I disagree. It is sort of one of those situations where I would feel a bit narked that I would be having to do this, but it's there, and it is in black and white. That is the issue, you have to work within these guidelines.*
(14) *Participant 43: But again if he has made the decision (the doctor). You have got to; you have got to follow.*
(15) *Participant 10: I would challenge, but it can often be quite intimidating to do so. I do though remember the feelings of helplessness, anger, and frustration I felt.*
(16) *Participant 49: I would probably say, if that's the policy, you know. Yeah, you are not making that decision for that person, you are making that decision for the senior person's breathing down your neck and saying this is the policy and I am not happy with this. I would in reality of the situation; I would go along with the system.*
(17) *Participant 15: So, I suppose you are more likely; I am more likely to do what a consultant requests than I am probably a registrar.*
(18) *Participant 57: Well, I think I would probably have found it difficult, but I mean I might be lying there actually. It's difficult, isn't it? I think I might well be obliged to follow the guidelines if I was junior.*
(19) *Participant 8: It's difficult in that it is the consultant. If it is a more junior doctor or a sister you could say, "I don't think that is needed." When it is a consultant, it is difficult.*

8.6 SUMMARY OF ANALYZING QUALITATIVE DATA CHAPTER

Within this chapter, we have discussed general processes involved in qualitative (inductive) data analysis (STEP 10) of the 16-step guide to writing a research proposal. During process, the key purpose of the researcher is to dig deep into what is occurring within the data to identify and make sense of themes (categories) generated for purpose of answering the research question. A summary of the processes involved include:

- Reading transcripts several times to identify themes (categories) and sub themes (subcategories).

- Developing a coding frame to mark transcripts.

- Acknowledging emerging new narratives and using decided coding method to label similar segments of interview text. This rigorous and methodical coding of transcripts will allow relevant themes (categories) and subthemes (subcategories) to be clustered by similarity and labelled.

- Relabelling of emerging themes (categories) through repeatedly studying the transcripts and reconsidering possible meanings and how these fit into the other newly developed themes (categories) and subthemes (subcategories).

- Condensing raw data into a brief summarized format.

- Establishing comprehensive relationships between the study objectives along with debating similarities and differences across subgroups of participants.

- Ensuring that links made are transparent and defensible.

- Developing a theoretical model (i.e. diagram) to explain the themes (categories) and subthemes (subcategories) identified.

- Acknowledging when no relevant new themes (categories) or subthemes (subcategories) can be identified.

- Writing a critical discussion of coded quotes and what the themes (categories) and subthemes (subcategories) mean, and relate these to the overall study objectives, aim(s), research question(s), and subquestion(s) (STEP 6).

- Publishing a peer-reviewed research paper to explain the research method (STEPS 1–16), which in addition to the 16-step model includes *findings*, *discussion*, *study limitations*, and *recommendations for midwifery practice and future research*.

Now that we have summarized processes involved in qualitative data analysis, we will proceed to *Chapter 9*, which discusses processes involved in analyzing quantitative data (STEP 10).

8.7 SELF-ASSESSMENT QUESTIONS (SAQs)

8.1 The purpose of qualitative data analysis is to:

(a) Establish cause-and-effect relationships.

(b) Manipulate the data.

(c) Triangulate the data.

(d) Structure themes to make sense of the data.

8.2 Which of the following is not a characteristic of qualitative data?

(a) Rich descriptions.

(b) Taking a constructivist approach towards building themes.

(c) Describing relationships between variables.

(d) Interpretation of the data.

8.3 Which of the following are features of qualitative data analysis?

(a) Data is analysed during and after collection.

(b) There is no one way to understand the phenomenon of interest.

(c) Reality is described in language that may have different meanings for different people.

(d) All of the above.

8.4 **The logic of qualitative data analysis is described as:**

(a) Subjective.

(b) Deductive.

(c) Designed to support a hypothesis.

(d) Objective.

8.5 **The first step in qualitative data analysis involves:**

(a) Manipulating the data.

(b) Transcribing the data.

(c) Interpreting data.

(d) Coding the data.

8.6 **The purpose of qualitative data analysis is to:**

(a) Establish a cause-and-effect relationship.

(b) Manipulate the data.

(c) Structure themes to make sense of the data.

(d) Triangulate the data.

ANSWERS TO CHAPTER 8 SAQs

8.1 **d**

8.2 **c**

8.3 **d**

8.4 **a**

8.5 **b**

8.6 **c**

Analyzing Quantitative Research

STEP (10): Detail intended data processing and analysis.

9.1 INTRODUCTION TO QUANTITATIVE DATA ANALYSIS

The purpose of quantitative data analysis is to discover patterns and relationships between defined variables the research midwife has observed. Compared with qualitative data analysis (*which is interpretation-based, descriptive and captured in language*), quantitative data analysis is based upon numbers (*which are countable, measurable and rendered in numerical form*). Statistics is the currency of quantitative data analysis, and involves organizing collected data in appropriate ways, analyzing it, interpreting findings, and presenting the results in comprehensible ways. Before applying statistics to answer a midwifery, neonatal, or organizational problem, first a statistical plan is written and agreed with a qualified statistician. Within each quantitative research proposal, this statistical plan is presented immediately after the data collection section, which describes data collection instruments (STEP 9). Before we move on to describe and explain some statistical methods of quantitative data analysis, it would first seem reasonable to ask what the term statistics means.

9.2 WHAT THE TERM STATISTICS MEANS?

Statistics is a mathematical body of science, which involves collecting, analyzing, interpreting, and presenting data in numerical form. As such, statistics includes extracting and summarizing information from gatherings of numerical facts, which may be collected in a variety of ways. For example, every four years the government in the United Kingdom (UK) accumulates data about its residents on a specified date. This exercise is called a *census*, which is conducted to find out global and local facts about specified groups of people within the UK population. For example, data may be collected to calculate the birth rate, number of children under five years of age, quantity of women aged between 20 and 40, or numbers of people who have developed a specified disease. As part of process, data collection includes many methods of selecting samples of participants from clearly defined populations, with typically the data analysed used to inference conclusions about the total matching population. The statistical tests selected ensure that conclusions drawn are *reliable*, and from these *reliable* results, *statistical inferences* are drawn. *Statistical inferencing* is the process of conducting calculations on numerical data to deduce properties of a distribution of probability.

Research Recipes for Midwives, First Edition. Caroline J. Hollins Martin.
© 2024 John Wiley & Sons Ltd. Published 2024 by John Wiley & Sons Ltd.

As such, *statistical inferencing* infers properties about the population of interest, through evaluating a related hypothesis and deriving estimated findings. During the process of quantitative data analysis, two types of *statistical inferences* are used, which include *statistical estimation* and *hypothesis testing*. Since samples are selected from specified populations using a random approach, the mathematical theory of probability underlies *statistical inference*. In general, statistical methods are applied to analyse data obtained from quantitative research methods, such as a *randomized controlled trials* (RCT) and other experimental designs. Statistical analysis is applied to the data collected, which is organized, examined, interpreted, and presented in the final thesis or paper published to answer the specified research question. When writing a research proposal, the researcher must be clear about what they want from their data, so they are equipped and able to answer their specified research question. Consequently, templates of the intended *descriptive statistics* and *inferential statistics* are listed in a plan (STEP 10). Ordinarily, the research midwife should ask a statistician to advise them and check that what they have proposed will achieve their project goals. In many instances (*such as working on a funded project*), it is prerequisite that a statistician prescribes the analysis, creates the appropriate spreadsheets for the researcher to enter their numerical findings in, analyses the data, and writes up the results section of the research report.

When applying statistics to answer a specified research question, it is first necessary to specify the *population* under exploration. Populations can be large (e.g. *all women of childbearing age living in a particular city*), and so appropriate representative sampling is used to ensure that inferences and conclusions can be safely extended from the sample population to the whole population of women of childbearing age in the specified city. Experimental research involves recording measurements of the variables under study, applying an intervention, and then repeating these measurements to determine if the manipulation has modified the values in question. For example, a population of postnatal women has been diagnosed with depression using the *Edinburgh postnatal depression scale* (EPDS). As a treatment, these depressed postnatal women receive a specified schedule (intervention) of *cognitive behavioral therapy* (CBT), and postdelivery the EPDS is again used to measure their depressive symptoms.

In contrast to this example, an observational study instead involves watching the behaviour of people in a population and does not involve an experimental manipulation of an intervention. The two main statistical approaches used in quantitative data analysis include *descriptive statistics* and *inferential statistics*. *Descriptive statistics* are used to summarize data gathered from a sample of the population for purpose of calculating *modes, medians, means,* and other *measures of dispersion* (i.e. *range, interquartile range,* and *standard deviations*). In contrast, *inferential statistics* operates on the principle of *probability theory*.

Organizing a statistical plan involves first developing the *hypotheses* and *null hypotheses* (STEP 6), which the calculations will accept or reject. Disproving the *null hypothesis* is a central task in any experimental research method, with the statistical goal being to calculate a probability (*p*-value) that rejects the *null hypothesis* and supports the *hypothesis*. It is important to note that producing statistical data may encounter errors, such as systematic (bias), reporting incorrect numbers, missing data, or producing biased estimates, with specific statistical techniques developed to address such inaccuracies. *Confidence intervals* allow the researcher to express how closely the sample estimate matches the true value of the whole population (i.e. a whole city). For example, a 95% *confidence interval* is a range provided when sampling and analysis are repeated under the same conditions to produce two different datasets. In response, the results found from these sample populations may be extrapolated (inferred) to the whole population in 95% of all possible cases. Relationships between two sets of data can also be *correlated*. In this event, two variables that may or may not be the cause of one another are *correlated*, or otherwise caused by a third phenomenon (variable), which is called the *confounding variable*. We will now elaborate on some of these statistical concepts.

9.3 WHAT ARE DESCRIPTIVE STATISTICS?

Descriptive statistics are used to describe the main features of a collection of numbers gathered during data collection in a research study. *Descriptive statistics* are different from *inferential statistics,* given that they aim to make summaries about the collection of numbers that have been gathered. In other words, *descriptive statistics* create sum-ups about a sample, as opposed to making inferences about the *population* being examined. *Descriptive statistics* are not about probability theory (creating *p*-values) but instead produce illustrating summaries about what the researcher has found. Examples of different types of *descriptive statistics* include calculating *measures of central tendency (mode, median and, mean), measures of dispersion (range, Inter Quartile Range [IQR] and standard deviation)*.

9.3.1 MEASURES OF CENTRAL TENDENCY

Measures of central tendency describe the data according to the following three measures: *mode*, *median*, and *mean*

- *Mode:*
  The *mode* is the value that occurs with the greatest frequency. In other words, the 'most popular' value. For instance, a range of integers 3, 1, 8, 2, 6, 5, 2 is calculated. To analyse the *mode*, place these numbers in order as follows 1, **2, 2**, 3, 5, 6, 8. The *mode* is the number that occurs most frequently, which in this case is the number 2.

- *Median:*
  The *median* is the middle value in a set of numbers. For instance, a range of integers 3, 1, 8, 2, 6, 5, 2 is calculated. To analyse the median, place these numbers in order as follows 1, 2, 2, **3**, 5, 6, 8. The median is the middle number, which in this case is the number 3. Please note that when there is an even number of scores, the middle two scores are averaged (i.e. 1, 2, 2, **3, 4**, 5, 6, 8), with the median calculated to be 3.5.

- *Mean:*
  The *mean* is the average number and represents the sum of all the observations divided by the number of observations. The *mean* is also known as the arithmetic mean or average number, and is represented as follows:

$$\text{Mean} = \frac{\text{Sum of all observations}}{\text{Total number of observations}}$$

$$\text{Mean} = \frac{3+1+8+2+6+5+2 = 27}{27 \text{ divided by } 7 = 3.8}$$

Now attempt to calculate the *mean*, *median*, and *mode* of the data in Activity 9.1.

Activity 9.1

Ten students are asked 'how many cups of coffee they consumed during the previous week?'

Student number	Cups of coffee drunk
1	3
2	12
3	5
4	0
5	7
6	12
7	18
8	12
9	0
10	8

Q Calculate the *mean*, *median* and *mode* of this data

9.3.2 MEASURES OF DISPERSION

The *mode, median,* and *mean* give no indication of the spread of the data (i.e. numerical values measured). For example, are all the number values close to the centre or are they spread out more evenly? Such *measures of dispersion* describe how closely the data cluster around the *measure of central tendency*. On the whole, three main measures are calculated, which include the *range, inter quartile range* (IQR), and *standard deviation*.

- *Range:*
  The *range* represents the distance between the highest and lowest numerical value and is based only upon these two numbers. That is, no account is made of the distribution of scores between the lowest and highest values. As such, the *range* is greatly effected by outliers. That is, values that are a large distance away from the main body of data.

- *Inter Quartile range (IQR):*
  The IQR is used alongside the *median* and describes the middle 50% of the data. Hence, the IQR represents 25–75% of the data (percentiles divide the data into 100 equal parts). The IQR measures the spread of the middle half of the data, and as such it is the range of the middle 50% of the sample. The IQR is used to assess variability of where most of the values lie, with larger values indicating that this central portion of data expands out further.

- *Standard deviation:*
  The *standard deviation* is used alongside the *mean* and measures how much the observations vary from the mean (average) number. The researcher starts by calculating the difference between each observation and the *mean* and uses these differences to work out the *standard deviation*. A *standard deviation* is calculated according to the following equation:

$$SD = \sqrt{\frac{\text{sum of squared distances from the mean of all abservations}}{\text{total number of observations}^{-1}}}$$

Returning to the coffee cup story in Activity 9.1, view the calculated *range, IQR,* and the *standard deviation* (see Box 9.1).

The good news for budding midwifery researchers is that statistical packages will calculate these figures for you, with many types of software packages available on the market. For example, the *statistical package for the social sciences* (SPSS) (IBM Corp. 2020) is a common software used to analyse data. We will now move on to look at *distribution of data*.

9.4 DISTRIBUTION OF DATA

The shape of a histogram gives a rough idea of the *distribution of the data* gathered by a researcher. The statistical function of a *data distribution* is to specify all possible values of a *variable,* and also quantify the relative frequency that particular data points occur. This could also be interpreted as the probability of how often a plotted *variable* occurs. All populations can have their scatterings of data presented as a distribution, with the main purpose being to help the researcher decide upon the correct test for analyzing the data. For example, say a midwife researcher collects 400 data points (e.g. total scores from 400 fully completed EPDS scales), the meaning for future management of postnatal women has no value unless the researcher categorizes it in a purposeful way. In essence, methods of distributing data aim to organize the raw data collected in graphical representations (e.g. block plots, charts, or histograms), which when viewed can provide really useful information. As such, *distribution of data* presented on a plotted graph could present as a *normal distribution,* or alternatively, a *positive skew* or *negative skew*. An example of data that presents as a *normal distribution* follows.

BOX 9.1	HOW TO CALCULATE THE *RANGE*, *IQR*, AND THE *STANDARD DEVIATION* FOR THE EXAMPLE OF DATA PRESENTED IN ACTIVITY 9.1

Student number	Cups of coffee drunk
1	3
2	12
3	5
4	0
5	7
6	12
7	18
8	12
9	0
10	8

Range = highest to lowest = $18 - 0 =$ **18**

Inter-quartile Range (IQR) $= 0, 0, 3, 5, 7, 8, 12, 12, 12, 18$

75th percentile (12) − 25th percentile (2.25) = **10**

$$Standard\,deviation = \frac{\sqrt{\left(7.7^2 + 7.7^2 + 4.7^2 + 2.7^2 + 0.7^2 + 0.3^2 + 4.3^2 + 4.3^2 + 4.3^2 + 10.3^2\right)/9}}{\sqrt{\left(59.29 + 59.29 + 22.09 + 7.29 + 0.49 + 0.09 + 18.49 + 18.49 + 18.49 + 106.09\right)/9}}$$

Standard Deviation = **5.87** (mean was 7.7)

9.4.1 THE NORMAL DISTRIBUTION

One shape of particular importance in statistics is a *normal distribution* (see Figure 9.1).

When data is *normally distributed*, the outline of the curve is symmetrical and bell-shaped. Many *variables* of interest may present as a *normal distribution*, with possible examples including childbearing women weight, height, or blood pressure. Statistical tests that are based on a *normal distribution* are known as *parametric tests*.

9.4.2 PARAMETRIC TESTS

Parametric tests are statistical tests, which assume that the data follows a pattern of *normal distribution* when plotted on a graph. Hence, it is appropriate to plot data points before deciding what statistical *parametric test* to use. *Parametric tests* often focus upon statistically analyzing data and comparing one mean against another mean collected from a different group of participants. Before doing this, the parameters of both groups have to be clearly defined and fixed. As such, parametric tests compare the *mean* of variance of plotted data. Some examples of parametric tests include:

- T-test when ($n < 30$) participants, which is classed into *Sample One* and *Sample Two*.
- An *analysis of variance* (ANOVA), which may be a *One-way ANOVA* or *Two-way ANOVA*.
- Pearson's Correlation Coefficient (r).
- Z-test for larger samples of participants ($n > 30$).

These *parametric tests* are hypotheses testing statistical investigations provide generalizations about the *mean* of a population. As such, a T-test works on the assumption of *normally distributed* data underpinning the variable of interest.

Now returning to *standard deviations*, let us look at its relationship to *normally distributed* data (see Figure 9.2).

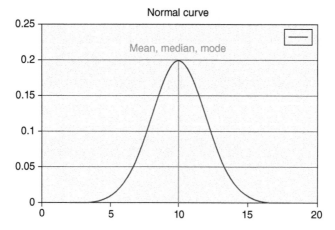

FIGURE 9.1 Graph of plotted data that presents as a normal distribution.

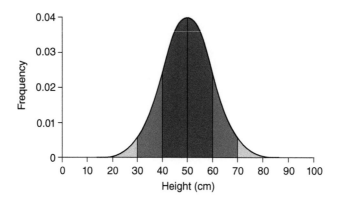

FIGURE 9.2 Standard deviations within normally distributed data.

In Figure 9.2, the *mean* on the height axis is 50 cm. The *standard deviation* lies on both the right and left side of this mean, with each standard deviation covering 10 cm of the dark blue area. Hence, the *mean* of 50 cm is reported as plus or minus one *standard deviation*, which covers between 40 and 60 cm of the data and contains 68% of the measured data. If we include the mid-blue area, we call these 2 standard deviations from the *mean* (i.e. 30–70 cm), which contains 95% of all the recorded measurements. With a standard deviation for a *normally distributed* variable:

- 68% of observations are between +1 and −1 *standard deviation* from the *mean*

- 95% of observations are between +2 and −2 *standard deviations* from the *mean*

- 99.8% of observations are between +3 and −3 *standard deviations* from the *mean*

From these plotted measures, we can view the spread of the data (see Figures 9.2 and 9.3).
What follows is a summary of the key points made so far.

Summary of Key Points

- Measures of *central tendency* consist of the *mode, median,* and *mean.*
- Measures of *dispersion* consist of the *range, inter quartile range* (ITQ), and *standard deviation.*
- Many variables are *normally distributed.*
- With a *normal distribution,* we know that ranges of observations fall within fixed percentages.

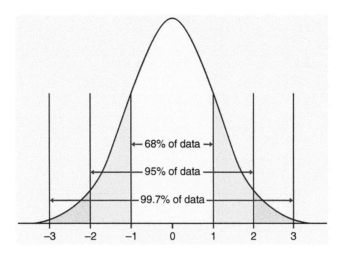

FIGURE 9.3   Percentages of data within normal distributed data.

Noting that most data sets rise towards the centre, and as data plotted moves out from the midpoint progressively fewer cases occur. Sometimes *data distribution* is described as being *skewed*. Some key points that relate to *skewness* follow.

- *Skewness* refers to the symmetry of the distribution curve.

- Distributions that are asymmetric are described as being *skewed*.

- With a *skewed* distribution, some values are outlying from the others.

- Direction of *skew* refers to the direction of the longer tail, and not where most of the values are located

    To view a *negatively skewed distribution of data* (see Figure 9.4).
    In contrast, to view a *positively skewed distribution of data*, see Figure 9.5.

9.4.3 SKEWNESS AND ITS RELATIONSHIP TO CENTRAL TENDENCY

The *median* is the preferred measure to use when dispersion of numerical data is not symmetrical (i.e. *skewed*). In contrast, the mean is the preferred measure to use when dispersion is symmetrical (i.e. normally distributed). Statisticians recommend that it is best to use statistical *non-parametric tests* when data is *skewed* and not *normally distributed*. So what are *non-parametric tests*?

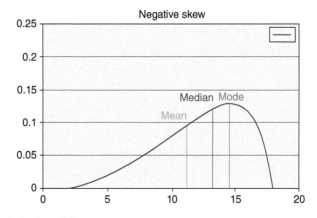

FIGURE 9.4   Illustration of negatively skewed data.

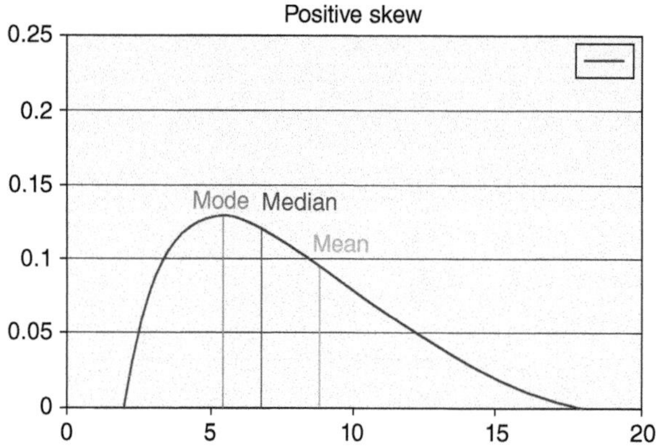

FIGURE 9.5 Illustration of positively skewed data.

9.4.4 NON-PARAMETRIC TESTS

Non-parametric tests do not require data to be *normally distributed.* As such, a *non-parametric test* is defined as a test of the hypothesis that is based upon having no underlying assumptions about the *data distribution* (e.g. *skewness*), and hence is a distribution-free test. A *non-parametric test* assumes that the variable of interest is measured at a *nominal* or *ordinal* level. Differences between *nominal, ordinal, interval,* and *ratio* data are discussed further in this chapter. First, we will discuss the differences between *parametric* and *non-parametric tests* (see Table 9.1).

In essence, *descriptive statistics* present statistical summaries to describe the data. Processes involved summarize a sample, as opposed to inferring results in terms of the population under scrutiny. As such, descriptive statistics are not developed to analyse *probability theory*. In a research proposal, the midwifery researcher will state that they will present a table of descriptive statistics, which will present results in terms of the overall sample size, subgroup sample sizes (intervention groups and control), numbers of participants in differing intervention (treatment) groups, and demographic information (e.g. age range and mean age, and sex). Hence, *descriptive statistics* ordinarily involve summaries about the sample and observations that have been made in the research study. *Descriptive statistics* are presented in tables as quantitative summaries of the statistical findings, and/or in visually easy-to-understand graphs. For example, the number of postnatal women who breastfed in a particular named city is a descriptive statistic, along with how long they elected to do so. Midwives may proceed to use such percentages to measure the effectiveness of an educational intervention designed to socially influence women to breastfeed in the first place and for a longer window of time. In summary, *descriptive statistics* provide useful summaries of the data. We will now move on to discuss some aspects of *inferential statistics*.

Table 9.1 Main differences between parametric and non-parametric tests.

Parametric tests	Non-parametric tests
A statistical test based on normally distributed data.	A statistical test based upon skewed or arbitrarily distributed data
Interval/Ratio	Nominal/Ordinal
Mean used	Median used
Population known	Population unknown
e.g. Pearson correlation coefficient	e.g. Spearman
Paired T-test	Mann–Whitney test
ANOVA	Kruskal Wallis test

9.5 WHAT ARE INFERENTIAL STATISTICS?

Through use of *inferential statistics*, midwifery researchers attempt to draw conclusions that extend beyond the immediate descriptive data set of numerical values gathered. Put simply, *inferential statistics* are used to infer the results from the sample of data gathered and extrapolate findings to the outside population with same characteristics. Using the pre-mentioned breastfeeding example, the researcher may have collected data from a small sample of postnatal women ($n = 100$), which have been sampled from the whole population of breastfeeding women in the same named city. When making these extrapolations, researchers make judgements about the probability that an observed difference between groups in their sample population represents the entire same population. Hence, they need to know whether their success (i.e. the effectiveness of an educational intervention to increase the number of women who breastfeed in the city) happened by chance or accident. When conducting an experiment, the researcher compares one or more treatments (*variables*) issued to *intervention group(s),* with probability calculations measured against results from a *control group* who do not receive the intervention (treatment). Probability calculations that compare *mean* differences in scores between the *intervention group* and the *control group,* declare whether the positive treatment effect happened by chance or accident.

When writing a research proposal, the research midwife develops a *research protocol* to guide study delivery processes, which will keep the method consistent throughout. As such, this protocol is a recipe that ensures that all the researchers involved in the study are clear about the steps involved in data collection, analysis, and reporting of results. When carrying out an experimental research method (recipe), the commonest inferential test used is *probability testing*, which is undertaken to compare mean performance between two groups to identify if the intervention (or variable) has made a difference to the treatment receiving group. For example, the researcher may want to know whether students from diverse healthcare disciplines differ in test scores, or whether the aforementioned breastfeeding intervention group differ in success rates compared against the control group who did not receive the educational package. When a researcher wants to compare the average performance between two groups, they use a statistical *T-test,* which calculates a ratio that quantifies how significant the difference is between the two groups means, at the same time as taking the distribution of data into account.

Inferential statistics are derived from a family of statistical models known as the *general linear model*, which includes the *T-test, analysis of variance (ANOVA), analysis of covariance (ANCOVA), regression analysis*, and many of the *multivariate methods* like *factor analysis, multidimensional scaling, cluster analysis, discriminant function analysis*, and so on. Program outcome evaluations compare the program who receives an intervention against a non-program group (control), with the research method (recipe) used being an experimental research method (recipe) (e.g. *randomized controlled trials* [RCT]). A two-group RCT is ordinarily analysed with a *T-test* or *one-way ANOVA*, whilst multi-group experiments are analysed using an *analysis of variance (ANOVA)*. In contrast to RCT's, quasi-experimental analysis does not use random assignment of participants to specialized groups. This lack of random assignment complicates analysis considerably, because the researcher has to adjust the pre-test scores for measurement error, which is called *reliability corrected model of covariance*. At this point, statistics can become confusing, and it is recommended that the research midwife speak to a statistician for advice about their specific study design.

In contrast and observational studies, the researcher's goal is to investigate causality and draw conclusions about the effect(s) of *independent variable(s)* upon *dependent variables*. An experimental research study (e.g. RCT) involves taking measurements before the variable is delivered to the intervention group to manipulate the change, and then repeating these measurements postdelivery to find out if the intervention (or variable) has altered post-intervention scores. In contrast, an observational study does not involve experimental manipulation. Instead, data is gathered and *correlations* calculated between *variables*, with the calculated *correlation coefficient* indicating the extent by which two variables fluctuate together. Hence *correlations* describe the relationship between variables, which may be weak or strong and in a positive or negative direction. As such, *correlations* cannot declare the cause and effect of results, and instead only an association between the two variables of interest (see Chapter 5; Section 5.5 to view graphs). We will now look at types of data produced from quantitative studies.

9.6 TYPES OF QUANTITATIVE DATA PRODUCED

There are several types of data that may be produced from quantitative research methods (recipes). For example, data gathered may be *nominal, ordinal, interval, or ratio* in measurement, instead of being *numerical*. These distinctions influence choice of statistical tests that the researcher applies to the data.

9.6.1 NOMINAL DATA

Nominal scales are used for labelling variables, which have no quantitative value. These scales consist of categorical responses or labels. For example, what is your gender (male or female), or what is your hair color (brown, black, blonde, gray, or other), which is non-numeric in identity. As such, a *nominal* group is a gathering based upon same characteristics.

9.6.2 ORDINAL DATA

Ordinal scales rank variables in hierarchical order. For example, in response to a question asking a participant how they feel today, the respondents may rank responses in the following order (very happy, happy, neither happy nor unhappy, unhappy, and very unhappy). As such, ordinal data is non-numeric and clusters group variables into descriptive categories, which are then ordered on a hierarchical scale from high to low.

9.6.3 INTERVAL DATA

Interval data is numeric data measured along a scale, in which each point is equal in distance from each other. Hence, interval data is always numeric in form, standardized, and equal. A classic example of an interval scale is temperature, straightforwardly because differences between values are all the same. For example, the difference between 70° and 60° is a measurable 10°, and the difference between 80° and 70° is also 10°. Time is a further example of an *interval* scale in which the increments are known, consistent, and measurable. *Interval* scales are useful because statistical analysis on the data sets opens up to producing values of *central tendency*, such as *mode, median, mean*, and *standard deviation*. The *T-test* is the most used method of evaluating differences in mean scores between two groups. For example, the *T-test* can be used to test for a difference in test scores between a group of labouring women who were given a drug and a control group who received a placebo.

9.6.4 RATIO DATA

Ratio data is quantitative in nature and has the same properties as numerical interval data. The difference being that it has equal ratios between each data point and the absolute of zero, which means there are no negative numerical values or values below zero (0). An example of ratio data includes a childbearing woman weighing in at 80 kg, which is double the value of 40 kg. There can be no negative values, because a childbearing woman cannot have a negative value of weight. As such, years of age and weight are good examples of *ratio* data. In terms of probability calculations, we are now going to return to and enlarge the story of calculating probability.

9.7 CALCULATING PROBABILITY

Calculating *probability* is the process of determining the chance of an event occurring. Reiterating the point and to build the story, the *T-test* is the most common statistical test used when a researcher wants to know if any differences between mean scores between groups happened by chance, or in other words were brought about by the *intervention* (independent variable) (e.g. a drug or treatment). This is called *probability*, which means the relative likelihood that an event will or will not occur. For example, how likely is it that when the sky is cloudy, will it rain? If everything were predictable, there would be no need for probability. Probability is:

- Based on previous experience.
- The probability of a given outcome is the number of times that outcome occurs divided by the total number of trials.
- If the outcome is certain, it has a probability of 1
- If an outcome cannot occur, it has a probability of 0
- It is often presented as a percentage (%)

For example, if the calculated *probability* is ($p = 0.01$) for an event, the chance of the occurrence happening by chance or accident equals 1 in 100. Declaring the opposite, a calculated probability value of ($p = 0.99$) supports that the occurrence is likely to happen, operating at a chance of 99 in 100. The equation of probability calculation is represented as:

$$p(A) = \frac{\text{Number of occurrences of } A}{\text{Total number of possible chances}}$$

To clarify, *probability* is called the '*p-value*, which represents the *probability* value. The smaller the '*p*'-value is, the more likely the *hypothesis* will be supported and the *null hypothesis* rejected. The minimal accepted "*p*'-value is ($p = 0.05$), which means there is a 1 in 20 chance that the change in effect due to the experimental intervention happened by chance (accident). To develop your understanding of *calculating probability*, undertake Activity 9.2.

Activity 9.2

To predict the probability of achieving a *Head (H)* when tossing a coin, spin a coin 20 times and measure how many *Heads (H)* you achieve and how many *Tails (T)*.

$$p(H) = \frac{\text{Number of occurrences of } H}{\text{Total number of possible chances}}$$

Your answer should be similar to 0.5, 50%, or half of the number of tosses:

$$\frac{H}{H+T} = \frac{1}{2} = 0.5$$

Alternatively, if a person buys a lottery ticket and there are 100 000 tickets for sale, the probability of winning first prize is:

$$p(\text{first prize}) = \frac{1}{100\,000} = 0.00001$$

In other words, there is a 1 in 100 000 chance that the purchaser will win the lottery prize draw money. With similarity, when carrying out a quantitative research study, it is important to estimate the *probability* of an outcome or event occurring. Returning to the *normal distribution* curve. Flip a coin 20 times and count the number of *Heads (H)*, and then repeat this process 10 000 times. The distribution of *Heads (H)* on a graph will look akin to Figure 9.6.

9.7.1 THE RELATIONSHIP OF PROBABILITY TO SAMPLES AND POPULATIONS

Statistical *probability* analysis is based on acquiring data from a sample of participants with similar features (Intervention Group versus Control Group) and using the mean data between groups to calculate a '*p*'-value, which if:

- The result is ($p < 0.05$), this equals a 1 in 20 chance that the result happened by accident.

- The result is ($p < 0.01$), this equals a 1 in 100 chance the result happened by accident.

- The result is ($p < 001$), this equals a 1 in 1000 chance the result happened by accident.

- The result is ($p < 0001$), this equals a 1 in 10 000 chance the result happened by accident.

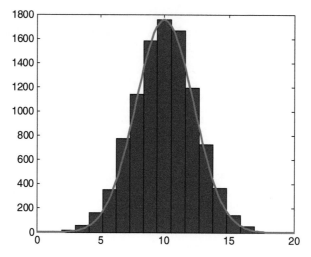

FIGURE 9.6 The distribution of *Heads (H)* on a graph.

From the calculated '*p*'-value (*p* <0001 being the best value), the researcher can make inferences about the success of the named intervention (variable), and its potential effects on the whole population that presents with the same inclusion criteria.

This *inference* to the whole population, is why this form of statistics is known as *inferential statistics*, as opposed to *descriptive statistics*. The relationship between the sample population of participants selected and the whole similar population is not certain, with probability used to estimate this uncertainty. Now to develop greater understanding of relationships between population and sample statistics.

9.7.2 RELATIONSHIP BETWEEN POPULATION AND SAMPLE STATISTICS

If a researcher collects repeated samples of the same size from a population, it is unlikely that the estimates of the population parameters (e.g. the population mean) would be the same in each sample. Each sample taken is likely to result in a different mean. To view an example, see Box 9.2.

Hence, if the researcher takes repeated samples (e.g. 20) of height measurements of the same size ($n = 100$) from the whole population of Scottish women (TOTAL = 20000), it is doubtful that the estimates of mean for each sample would be the same in all 20 samples. By quantifying how much estimates vary between all of the sample means, the researcher can work out how precise their estimates are likely to be. This is known as the *sampling error* or the *standard error of the mean*. In reality, we often only take one sample from the population, and use our knowledge of the *normal distribution* to draw inferences about the population as a whole. Now we will move on and discuss a bit more about the term variables.

BOX 9.2	**EXAMPLE OF A RELATIONSHIP BETWEEN A SAMPLE MEAN AND THE WHOLE POPULATION**

We are interested in knowing if the average height of Scottish females has increased since 1950. In 1950, we know the average height was 154 cm. If we were to take repeated samples of ($n = 100$) females from a population of ($n = 10000$) women, we would arrive at a different mean from each sample taken. As the researcher is only capturing one sample, how will they know how much it varies from the true population mean?

9.8 RESEARCH VARIABLES

Within a quantitative research study, a *variable* straightforwardly denotes an event the midwifery researcher is trying to measure. For example, length of first stage of labour or fundal height. Alternatively, this event may be a person (e.g. primigravids, multiparous, or neonates). A *variable* can also be physical, social, or demographic (e.g. religion, socioeconomic group, and language spoken). Many variables are crystal clear (e.g. gender and blood group), whilst others may be vague (e.g. food and lifestyle). Whatever the researcher is attempting to explore, in a quantitative experiment they will manipulate a *variable* to test cause-and-effect relationships (e.g. the effects of cognitive behavioural therapy [CBT] on post natal depression [PND] scores). In this example, the *independent variable* is the cause (i.e. the CBT therapy), and the *dependent variable* is the effect (e.g. *Edinburgh postnatal depression scale* [EPDS] scores), which is being used to measure changes in participants depression scores. As such, the CBT is being used to manipulate changes in postnatal women's PND scores. To further explain *dependent* and *independent variables*.

Dependent variables are also known as response or outcome variables, which change (or respond) depending upon the values of other variables (e.g. blood pressure or depression rating [e.g. as measured by the EPDS]).

Independent variables are stand-alone events that cannot be changed by other variables in the study (e.g. a childbearing woman's age, which cannot be changed because there is nothing you can do to change it). As such, a woman's age is independent of all else. Hence, an *independent variable* stands alone and remains unchanged by other *variables* the researcher is trying to measure (e.g. what drugs the woman takes or counselling [e.g. CBT] she receives will not change her age). Other examples of *independent variables* include gender identity, culture, and level of education reached, all of which remain unchanged through delivering CBT. We will now return to discuss the *standard error of the mean*.

Standard error of the mean is the *standard error* of a statistic, which informs the researcher how much that statistic is likely to vary from one sample to another within the population of interest. In other words, the *standard error of the mean* is a calculated measure of how confident the researcher is about having attained the *true population mean*. So how does the researcher use this *standard error*.

9.8.1 USING THE STANDARD ERROR

If the researcher takes enough samples from the population and calculates the mean for each sample, they can then plot all these mean values on a graph (see Figure 9.7).

As a reminder, *normal distribution* is the probability that the distribution is symmetrical about the mean, which shows that the data plotted near the mean is more frequent in occurrence than data plotted further away from the mean. In figurative form, a normal distribution presents as a 'bell curve', as is illustrated in Figure 9.7 in which the *normal distribution* presents as 95% of the mean values lying +2 and −2 *standard errors* from the mean of all the samples (i.e. within the red and green areas). And so, what exactly is a *confidence interval*?

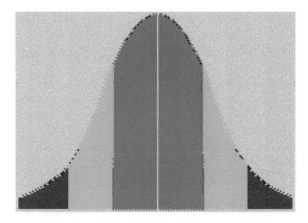

FIGURE 9.7 Means of gathered samples from the whole population to illustrate standard errors.

9.8.2 CONFIDENCE INTERVALS

A *confidence interval* is the mean in the researcher's approximation, plus and minus the variation in the approximation. As such, the *confidence interval* is the range of values the researcher expects their estimate to fall within if they were to repeat the study, and they would state this ascertain within a certain level of confidence. Hence, within a 95% confidence interval, the researcher has a 5% chance of being wrong (1 in 20). In contrast, within a 90% confidence interval, the researcher has a 10% chance of being wrong (1 in 10). Hence, a *confidence interval* is:

- The *range of values* between which the true value for the population is likely to lie.

- Is based on the *observed sample mean* and the *standard error of the mean*.

In practice, a researcher ordinarily would only take one sample from the population, and use what is known to construct a *range* around the *sample mean* within which they can be 95% sure the population mean will lie, and from a *normal distribution* of data they will know that approximately 95% of the sample means lie between two *standard errors* above or below the population mean (i.e. within the red and green areas within Figure 9.7). When this happens, they can be 95% certain that the true population mean lies between −2 and +2 *standard errors* from the mean. And so, how does calculating a confidence interval relate to *hypothesis testing*.

9.9 HYPOTHESIS TESTING

Hypotheses testing involves statistical analysis in which the midwifery researcher explores their assumptions about the population parametres, which is then used to estimate the relationship between two measured variables. Examples of midwifery *hypotheses* can be viewed in Table 9.2.

A *null hypothesis* is typically an equality statement of the *hypothesis*, which proposes no difference between variables being measured in the sample population. As such, the *null hypothesis* proposes that there is no difference between the particularized characteristics or variables of interest in the clearly defined population. Examples of *null hypotheses* that match the *alternative hypotheses* displayed in Table 9.2 can be viewed in Table 9.3.

In essence, a *null hypothesis* is a supposition, which propositions that there is no relationship between two measured variables (or characteristics) of quantitative data gathered from the sample taken from the clearly defined population of interest. In contrast, the *hypothesis* predicts a link between the variables of interest.

The midwifery researcher tests their *hypothesis* on a data set to statistically evidence plausibleness of the proposed *null hypothesis*. As such, the statistical analysis is carried out on the ideally randomized sample of measurements gathered from the sample of consenting participants that have been extracted from the population of interest. During process, two *hypotheses* are tested, which include the proposed (i) *hypothesis* and the (ii) *null hypothesis*, with

Table 9.2 Examples of hypotheses that relate to midwifery practice.

1	Childbearing women who have been diagnosed with anorexia nervosa deliver infants of lower birth weight than mothers who have uncomplicated pregnancies.
2	There is a relationship between higher levels of maternal/infant skin-to-skin contact and reduced crying in babies between 1 and 28 days old.
3	Women who attend parenthood education classes experience reduced levels of pain during labour compared with non-attending mothers.

Table 9.3 Examples of null hypotheses that match the alternative hypotheses in Table 9.2.

1	Childbearing women who have been diagnosed with anorexia nervosa deliver infants of similar birth weight as mothers who have uncomplicated pregnancies.
2	There is no relationship between levels of maternal/infant skin-to-skin contact and crying in babies between 1 and 28 days old.
3	Women who attend parenthood education classes experience similar levels of pain during labour as non-attending mothers.

essentially the *null hypothesis* representing a counter position to the *hypothesis* (compare Tables 9.2 and 9.3). As you can see, both are mutually exclusive to each other and only one can be supported as being statistically correct. In other words, only one out of these two possibilities (*hypothesis* or *null hypothesis*) can be supported by the statistical outcome, with the *null hypothesis* stating an assumption that the event (*hypothesis*) will not occur. Hence, a rejection of the *null hypothesis* assumes acceptance of the *hypothesis*. H0 (pronounced *H-naught*) is the statistical symbol for a rejected *null hypothesis*, and Ha (or sometimes H1) is the statistical symbol for a supported *hypothesis*. To appropriately test your hypothesis, sampling, and data collection must be representative of the population of interest to produce accurate results.

Once the collected data has been entered into computer spreadsheets, the next step is to select an appropriate statistical test to conduct the analysis. Some statistical tests compare within-group variance, which is about how the data spreads inside the group (e.g. of primigravids). In contrast, other statistical tests compare between-groups variance, which is about how different categories differ from each other (e.g. primigravids versus multigravidas). In the between-groups example, when the variation is large enough and there is little or no intersection, the statistical test will calculate a low or smaller *p*-value (e.g. $p = 0.001$) (smaller is better), which means that the difference between groups (e.g. primigravids versus multigravidas) is 1 in 1000 times possibility that the result happened by chance (i.e. accident). In contrast, when the result is $p = 0.01$ there is a 1 in 100 times probability that the result happened by chance (i.e. 1%), or $p = 0.05$ where there is a 1 in 20 times probability that the result happened by chance (i.e. 5%). All of these *p*-values produce a *significant difference* between groups or variables. Please note that these percentages reduce the possibility of the researcher wrongly rejecting the *null hypothesis*.

The next step is to determine whether the *null hypothesis* should be rejected, which if so, assumes acceptance of the *hypothesis*. As part of this process, the *p*-value is a metric that expresses the likelihood that an observed difference could have happened by chance (i.e. accident). If the *p*-value is small enough (i.e. less than or equal to $p = 0.05$), the researcher rejects the *null hypothesis* with $p = 0.05$ the largest acceptable probability value. Better values include smaller ones (i.e. $p = 0.01$ and even better $p = 0.001$).

In summary, producing a *significant difference* does not provide a simple 'yes' or 'no' answer to the research question. Interpretation comes down to the level of statistical significance applied to the numbers and refers to the probability of a value that rejects the *null hypothesis*. Henceforth, the standard approach is to test the *null hypothesis* against the *hypothesis*. While in principle the acceptable level of statistical difference is a subject for debate, the smaller the *p*-value, the lower the probability of the result happening due to an error or chance. We will now introduce some statistical tests, which represent the beginnings of statistical understanding.

9.9.1 TYPES OF STATISTICAL TESTS THAT TEST THE HYPOTHESIS

a. *Z-Test*

To establish whether the relationship between groups (e.g. primigravids versus multigravidas) and the variable (e.g. treatment) is statistically significant, a *z-test* is used. Per se, the *z-test* checks whether the two-group means are the same (e.g. Group 1: primigravids and Group 2: multigravidas). Criteria for using a *z-test*, first involves knowing what the standard deviation is, and second having a sample size that includes 30 data points or above. Another statistical test that the researcher can apply to establish whether the relationship between groups and the variables is statistically significant, is a *t-test*.

b. *T-Test*

A *t-test* is a statistical test that is carried out to compare the means between two groups (e.g. primigravids versus multigravidas) to establish whether or not the group means differ in relation to each other, or the variable under test (e.g. treatment).

To elaborate, *t-tests* can be used to test for a difference in test scores between a group of childbearing women who were given a drug and a control group who received a placebo. The researcher wants to know if any differences found happened by chance or were brought about by the drug. In summary, the probability value ('*p*'-value) indicates whether the difference in results between two groups happened by chance (accident) and are presented as numerical quantities.

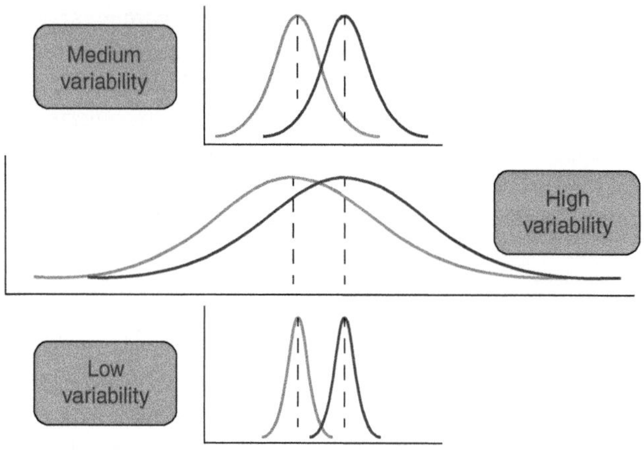

FIGURE 9.8   Illustration of widths of variability.

p-value	probability of result happening by chance
0.05	5 in 100
0.01	1 in 100
0.001	1 in 1000

When selecting a *t-test*, there are certain assumptions that should be made about the data. These assumptions include:

1. A minimal number of ($n = 30$) participants in each group.

2. *Numeric data* involves allocation of numbers that can be used in calculation.

3. *Normal distribution* of data.

4. Variation of scores in groups is not reliably different (see Figure 9.8).

When these conditions are not met, the researcher evaluates differences in means between groups using a *nonparametric* alternative (e.g. *Cohen's kappa* or *Mann–Whitney* tests). *Nonparametric* methods are *distribution-free* methods since they do not rely on the aforementioned assumptions about the data. The next reasonable question to ask, is which statistical test is the most appropriate to test for significant difference in mean scores between the groups and variables use in my experimental study?

9.10 HOW TO SELECT THE APPROPRIATE STATISTICAL TEST

What follows are some examples of well-known statistical tests, which have been embedded into a decision grid. Which test to select is dependent upon three factors:

1. Whether the data is *nominal, ordinal,* or *numerical.*

2. Whether the data is *non-normally distributed* or *normally distributed.*

3. How many groups are involved in the study.

To view a decision grid, which can help you select the most appropriate statistical test for use in your quantitative study (see Figure 9.9).

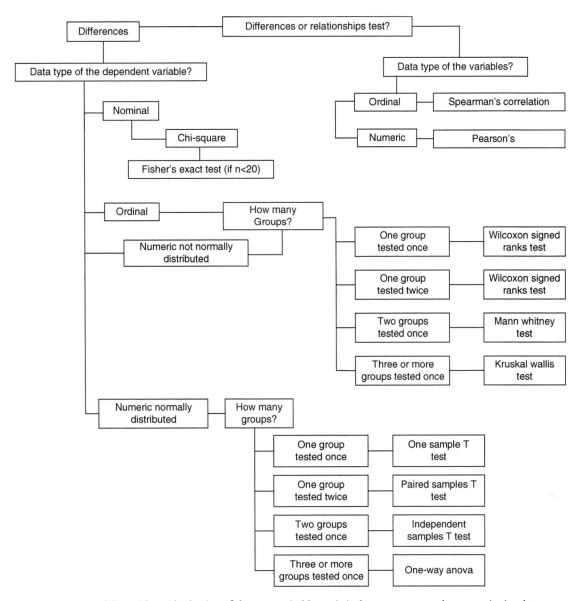

FIGURE 9.9 Decision grid to aid selection of the most suitable statistical test to use to analyse quantitative data.

9.10.1 SIGNIFICANT DIFFERENCE BETWEEN GROUPS

All the statistical tests in Figure 9.9 compare means between study groups, to test the hypothesis and determine whether the variable has had an effect upon the sample population under study. In other words, these statistical tests compare group means and evaluate whether there is a significant difference between group values. Returning to calculating statistical probability, which is based upon acquiring data from a sample of participants with analogous characteristics, an example follows:

Group 1 = Intervention Group of ($n = 100$) participants who received the treatment (e.g. antidepressants for PND).

Group 2 = Control Group who receive a placebo (e.g. sugar pill).

($p \leq 0.05$): When the calculated mean values of *Group 1* and *Group 2* are compared and if the result is ($p < 0.05$), then there is a 1 in 20 chance that the effectiveness of the antidepressant improved mean values in *Group 1* (intervention group). This means the antidepressant improved PND scores as measured by a robust psychometric scale (e.g. Edinburgh postnatal depression scale [EPDS]), and there is a 19 out of 20 chance that the improvement was due to the antidepressant. Alternatively this could be phrased as, there is a 1 in 20 chance the improvement in EPDS scores happened by accident.

$(p \leq 0.01)$: When the calculated mean values of *Group 1* and *Group 2* are compared and if the result is $(p < 0.01)$, then there is a 1 in 100 chance that the effectiveness of the antidepressant improved mean values in *Group 1* (intervention group). This means the antidepressant improved PND scores as measured by a robust psychometric scale (e.g. EPDS), and there is a 99 out of 100 chance that the improvement was due to the antidepressant. Alternatively this could be phrased as, there is a 1 in 100 chance the improvement in EPDS scores happened by chance (accident).

$(p \leq 0.001)$: When the calculated mean values of *Group 1* and *Group 2* are compared and if the result is $(p < 0.001)$, then there is a 1 in 1000 chance that the effectiveness of the antidepressant improved mean values in *Group 1* (intervention group). This means the antidepressant improved PND scores as measured by a robust psychometric scale (e.g. EPDS), and there is a 999 out of 1000 chance that the improvement was due to the antidepressant. Alternatively this could be phrased as, there is a 1 in 1000 chance the improvement in EPDS scores happened by accident.

To conclude, the smaller the *p*-value, then the better the result (e.g. $p = 0001$ is better than $p = 001$), which is better than $(p = 0.05)$, with anything bigger than $p = 0.05$ (e.g. $p = 0.06$) an insignificant value. If the *p*-value is significant, then this *inference* can be made to the whole population (e.g. women with the same matched characteristics experiencing PND). In relation to Figure 9.9 and selecting appropriate tests to identify significant differences between groups and variables, examples of studies that use a *one sample t-test* (Box 9.3), *paired samples t-test* (Box 9.4), *independent samples t-test* (Box 9.5), *analysis of variance (ANOVA)* (Box 9.6), and *Chi-square test* (Box 9.7) follow.

BOX 9.3   EXAMPLE STUDY THAT HAS USED A *ONE SAMPLE T-TEST*

The *one sample t-test* is a statistical hypothesis test used to establish whether the mean calculated from the sample data gathered from a single group is different from an assigned value specified by the researcher. The *One Sample t-Test* is carried out when there is only one population from which a sample of data has been gathered (Group 1). An example of a *One Sample t-test* follows:

Example of a *one sample t-test*
The *one sample t-test* is used to compare the mean score of a sample of third year student midwives $(n = 113)$ who complete the *Rosenberg self-esteem scale* (Rosenberg 1965). In this study, the mean scores of data gathered from this group of students calculated at 4.04, which the researcher compared against their other stated value of 3.9. Results are reported as follows:

Data collected	Participant numbers	Mean	Standard deviation
Rosenburg self-esteem scale	$(n = 113)$	4.04	0.65
Reported as		Mean = 4.04 ± 0.65	

The calculated group mean for this sample is 4.04, which is significantly higher than the other stated population mean of 3.9. The results of this *one sample t-test* are as follows:

Data collected	Significant difference	Mean difference	95% confidence interval
Rosenburg self- esteem scale	$p = 0.024$	0.14	0.65
Reported as	$p = 0.02$		

The significant difference between the Group 1 mean of 4.04 and the other stated population mean of 3.9 calculated as $(p = 0.02)$, which means there is a 1 in 50 probability that the result happened by chance, which represents a significant difference. Hence, the *hypothesis* is supported, and *null hypothesis* is rejected:

Hypothesis
There is a significant difference between the sample mean and other stated population mean.

Null hypothesis
There is no significant difference between the sample mean and other stated population mean.

BOX 9.4	EXAMPLE STUDY THAT HAS USED A *PAIRED SAMPLES T-TEST*

A *paired samples t-test* compares the means of two measurements gathered from the same individual (participant) or object (e.g. haemoglobin). Such paired measurements can denote scored data gathered at two separate times (e.g. pre-test and post-test scores), with an intervention delivered between these two longitudinal time points. As such, a *paired samples t-test* compares the difference between two variables, and tests if the mean discrepancy is significantly different (i.e. between X and Y). An example of a *paired samples t-test* follows:

Example of a paired samples t-test
The *paired samples t-test* compares participants' mean test scores prior to (Test 1) and post completion (Test 2) of an education program (intervention). The aim is to find out whether this education program improved scores on the data collection instrument. Results are reported as follows:

Data collected	Participant numbers	Mean	Standard deviation
Pre-test scores	(n = 30)	2.43	0.26
Post-test scores	(n = 30)	2.53	0.28

The difference between the mean pre-test and post-test scores, in this case, calculated at $2.53 - 2.43 = 0.10$, with the researcher wanting to know if 0.10 is a significant result. The results of this paired samples t-test are as follows:

Data collected	Significant difference	Mean difference
Pre-test mean scores and Post-test mean scores	$p = 0.53$	0.10

When the significance value is equal to or less than $p = 0.05$, there is a significant difference between the two data collection points. However, if the significance value is greater than $p = 0.05$, this means there is no significant difference. In this instance, $p = 0.53$ is larger than $p = 0.05$, which signifies that the education program (intervention) was unsuccessful at improving participant learning. Hence the *null hypothesis* is supported, and the *hypothesis* rejected:

Hypothesis
There is a significant difference between the means of the two variables (pre-test and post-test).

Null hypothesis
There is no significant difference between the means of the two variables (pre-test and post-test).

Instead, the researcher may elect to look at correlations between the two variables, which involves plotting pre-test and post-test scores on a graph.

Data collected	Participant numbers	Correlation	Significant difference
Pre-test mean scores and Post-test mean scores	(n = 30)		
(n = 30)		0.829	$p = 0.001$

This significant difference of $p = 0.001$ calculated represents a strong *positive correlation*.

9.11 CORRELATIONS

A *correlation* describes the relationship between different variables (e.g. X and Y), and this can be described as weak or strong. However, it is important to note that a *correlation* does not indicate cause of an effect. An example of a perfect *positive correlation* can be viewed in Figure 9.10.

A *correlation* is a statistical measure that demonstrates the extent to which two variables (e.g. X and Y) relate to each other. *Correlations* are linearly related and a common method of describing the relationship between variables without commenting on what the cause and effect of any change is. In other words, a *correlation* is a statistical measure that

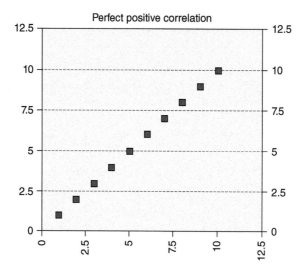

FIGURE 9.10 Illustration of a perfect positive correlation.

indicates the extent to which two or more variables fluctuate in relation to each other. A good example of a *positive correlation* is the number of calories a student midwife burns working on a maternity ward, and the increase in number of calories burnt. A calculated *positive correlation* is situated at:

- 1 demonstrates a perfect linear relationship.
- 0.8 indicates a fairly strong relationship.
- 0.6 indicates a moderate positive relationship.
- 0.5–0.7 indicates variables that correlate moderately.
- 0.3–0.5 indicates variables that have a low correlation.
- 0 is a correlation coefficient that indicates no relationship between variables.

In contrast, a *negative correlation* represents the relationship between two *variables*, which involves one *variable* increasing, whilst the other *variable* decreases.

An example of a perfect *negative correlation* can be viewed in Figure 9.11.

When a *negative correlation* has been calculated the *correlation coefficients* range from +1 to −1, with values below zero expressing a relationship between the two *variables* which is inverse. A strong *negative correlation* indicates a meaningful connection, which illustrates that as one *variable* goes up, the other one comes down. For example, a researcher might find that there is a *negative correlation* between student midwives' performance in assessments and the amount of time they are absent from the university. A calculated *negative correlation* is situated at:

- −1 demonstrates a perfect negative relationship.
- −0.8 indicates a fairly strong negative relationship.
- −0.6 indicates a moderate negative relationship.
- −0.5–0.7 indicates variables that have a moderate *negative correlation*.
- −0.3–0.5 indicates variables that have a low *negative correlation*.
- 0 is a *correlation coefficient* that indicates no relationship between *variables*.

In relation to *Figure* 9.9 and the number of groups, examples of a study that is designed to use an *independent samples t-test* can be viewed in (Box 9.5).

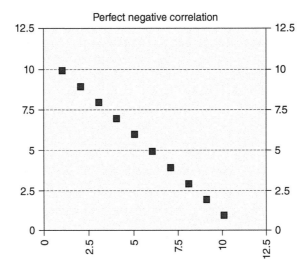

FIGURE 9.11 Illustration of a perfect negative correlation.

BOX 9.5	EXAMPLE STUDY THAT HAS USED AN *INDEPENDENT SAMPLES T-TEST*

The *independent samples t-test* is a statistical test that compares the means of two independent groups to establish whether the associated population means are significantly different. It is a parametric test, which assumes that the data is normally distributed. An example of an *independent samples t-test* follows:

Example of an *independent samples t-test*
The *independent samples t-test* is used to compare mean scores between two groups on a given variable. For example, comparing the mean blood pressure of a group of pregnant women who have received drug treatment for hypertension (e.g. an anti-hypertensive drug) versus the control group who receive a placebo (a sugar pill). In this study, the mean scores of data gathered from the intervention group of pregnant women calculated at 3.35, which the researcher compared against the control group value of 2.23. Results are reported as follows:

Data collected	Participant numbers	Mean	Standard deviation
Placebo group (Control group)	(n = 200)	3.35	5.477
Anti-hypertensive group	(n = 200)	2.23	5.134

The calculated group mean for the control group is 3.35, which is significantly higher than the anti-hypertensive group mean of 2.23, which inform us that the women who received the placebo on average had higher blood pressure than those who took the anti-hypertensive drug. The results of the *independent samples t-test* are as follows:

Data collected	Significant difference	Mean difference
Placebo group (Control) and Anti-hypertensive group	p = 0.004	1.12

The significant difference between the control group mean of 3.35 and the anti-hypertensive group mean of 2.23 is calculated at (p = 0.004), which indicates that there is a 4 in 1000 probability that the result happened by chance, which represents a significant difference. Hence the *hypothesis* is supported, and *null hypothesis* is rejected:

Hypothesis
The means of the two groups are significantly different (anti-hypertensive group versus control group).

Null hypothesis
The means of the two groups are not significantly different (anti-hypertensive group versus control group).

9.11.1 ANALYSIS OF VARIANCE (ANOVA)

Returning to Figure 9.9, an *ANOVA* is a statistical test that is used to compare variance between (2+) group means. In other words, an *ANOVA* is used to determine the statistical differences between the means of several diverse groups. For example, an *ANOVA* will determine if there are significant differences in blood sugar levels before, during, and after treatment between different groups of women with diabetes. The sample population is a set of pregnant women, which are then subdivided into multiple groups based upon characteristics (e.g. age group, parity, and maternal weight), with each group receiving a particular treatment for a specified trial period. At the end of this trial period, every participant's blood sugar is measured and charted in the same way. The means are then calculated for each group, with an *ANOVA* used to compare group and variable means to identify whether there are statistical differences within and between them all. Before conducting an *ANOVA*, three assumptions are made about the data:

Assumptions

1. The populations must be approximately normally distributed.

2. The samples must be independent.

3. The variances of the populations must be equal.

The consequence of an *ANOVA* calculation produces an 'F statistic', which identifies differences between the within-group variance and the between-group variance.

The result of the ANOVA allows the researcher to support or reject the *null hypothesis*. When there is a significant difference between the groups, then the *null hypothesis* is not supported, and the F ratio will be bigger. In relation to Figure 9.9, examples of studies designed to use different types of *ANOVA*'s can be viewed in (Box 9.6).

BOX 9.6	EXAMPLE STUDIES THAT USE *ANALYSIS OF VARIANCE (ANOVA)*

An *ANOVA* is used to test for statistical differences between two or more groups to find out if there is any significant difference between the means of these groups. An example of an *ANOVA* follows:

Example of an ANOVA
In this example, the *ANOVA* is used to compare mean scores in a clinical trial designed to test if there are significant differences between different groups of diabetic pregnant women, types of treatment (diet, Metformin medication, and insulin) and resulting mean *blood sugar* levels before and after treatment. With an *ANOVA*, the statistical mean comparisons are being made to calculate *p*-values between three groups and two observation points.

Depending on the number of groups and variables, the *ANOVA* is defined in different ways (e.g. 3×3, 2×2, 3×2). Some examples of *ANOVA*'s follow:

Example of a 3 × 3 ANOVA			
Groups of participants (*n* = 300)	Mean blood sugar before Variable 1	Mean blood sugar during Variable 2	Mean blood sugar after Variable 3
(1) Diet (*n* = 100)	15	10	8
(2) Metformin medication (*n* = 100)	15.5	8	6
(3) Insulin (*n* = 100)	16	7	5

Example of a 2 × 2 ANOVA		
Groups of participants (*n* = 200)	Mean blood sugar before Variable 1	Mean blood sugar after Variable 2
(1) Metformin medication (*n* = 100)	15.5	6
(2) Insulin (*n* = 100)	16	5

BOX 9.6   (CONTINUED)

Example of a 3 × 2 ANOVA		
Groups of participants (*n* = 300)	Mean blood sugar before Variable 1	Mean blood sugar after Variable 2
(1) Diet (*n* = 100)	15	8
(2) Metformin medication (*n* = 100)	15.5	6
(3) Insulin (*n* = 100)	16	5

An example study that has used and reported use of *ANOVA* analysis can be viewed in (Activity 9.3).

Activity 9.3

Access and Read the Following Paper That Reports the Results of a One-Way ANOVA Analysis (See Table 3)

Baranowska, B., Pawlicka, P., Kiersnowska, I., et al. (2021). Woman's needs and satisfaction regarding the communication with doctors and midwives during labour, delivery and early postpartum. *Healthcare*. 9, 382. https://doi.org/10.3390/healthcare9040382

9.11.2 CHI-SQUARE TEST

Returning to Figure 9.9, a chi-square statistical test is used to examine differences between variables that are categorical and gathered from a random sample for purpose of judging fit goodness between expected and observed results. The following assumptions are made about a *Chi-square test*.

1. It is a quantitative test used to determine whether a relationship exists between two *categorical variables (non-numeric)*.

2. Each variable can have two or more categories.

3. It is used when you want to know whether there is an association between two or more variables (i.e. X and Y)

4. Data is not *normally distributed* (it is skewed).

To view examples of graphed data that is negatively skewed, normally distributed, and positively skewed (see Figures 9.12–9.14).

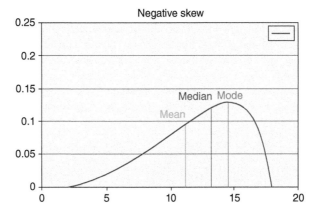

FIGURE 9.12   Negatively skewed data.

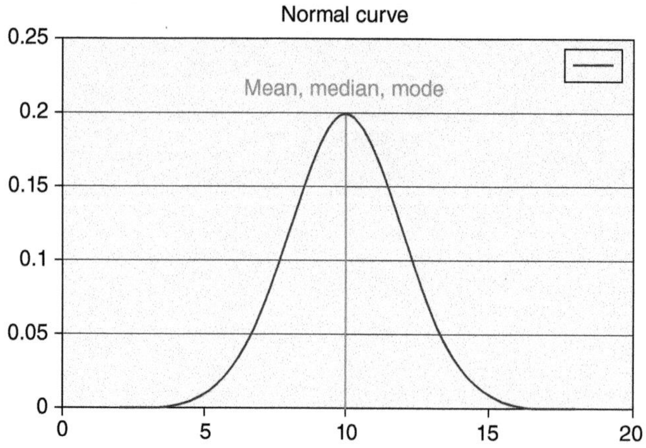

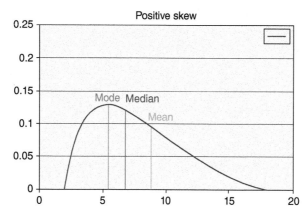

FIGURE 9.13   Normally distributed data.

FIGURE 9.14   Positively skewed data.

In relation to Figure 9.9 and an example of a study designed to use a *Chi-square test* (see Box 9.7).

BOX 9.7   EXAMPLE STUDY THAT WILL USE A *CHI-SQUARE TEST*

The *Chi-square test* is a statistical test that examines the differences between variables that are categorical and gathered from a random sample for purpose of judging fit goodness between expected and observed results. As such, it is a non-parametric test or distribution-free test, which tests a stated hypothesis and is based upon rankings or distribution into categories, which have qualitative labels. The cells of the table are made up of counts (frequencies) of the individuals with the characteristic of interest (in this case morning sickness). For each cell of the table, the expected counts are calculated assuming that the *null hypothesis* is true. The row and column totals for the table are needed to calculate expected values. An example follows:

Parity	Morning sickness present	Morning sickness absent	Total
First-trimester primigravids	12(14)	17(15)	29
First-trimester multiparas	14(12)	11(13)	25
Total	26	28	54

BOX 9.7   (CONTINUED)

Twenty-nine out of 54 participants are *first-trimester primigravids*, which equals 54%. If there is no relationship between parity and morning sickness, one *expects* each column of first row to have the same proportion (e.g. 54% of 26 = 14). Likewise, for *first trimester multiparas'*, the proportion is 25 out of 54, which equals 46% and again *expect* each column of the second row to have the same proportion. Compare the *observed* counts (frequencies) of table cells with the *expected* counts. Once *expected* frequencies are calculated, the *Chi square* is worked out. If the p-value associated is small ($p < 0.05$), there is evidence to reject the *null hypothesis* in favour of the *hypothesis*.

Hypothesis
First-trimester multiparas are more likely to suffer from morning sickness than first-trimester primigravids.

Null hypothesis
There is no association between parity and morning sickness.

9.11.3 FISHER'S EXACT TEST

Fisher's exact test is used in the analysis of categorical data (nominal data) when *sample* sizes are small (less than <20). It is used to examine the significance of the association between two variables in a 2×2 contingency table. The *p*-value from the test is computed.

9.11.4 SPEARMAN'S CORRELATION

Spearman's correlation is a *non-parametric* measure of *correlation*. It is used to assess the relationship between two variables, without making any assumptions about the *frequency distribution* of the *variables*.

9.11.5 PEARSON'S CORRELATION

Pearson's correlation calculates a correlation between −1 and +1 that measures the degree of association between two variables (X and Y). A positive value for the correlation implies a positive association. A negative value for the correlation implies a negative or inverse association.

What has been embraced in this chapter is simply a taster of knowledge regarding statistical tests and analysis. There are so many statistical tests that are beyond the capacity and scope of this chapter, with it advised that the midwife seek advice from a statistician when designing their research study.

9.12 SUMMARY OF ANALYZING QUANTITATIVE DATA

This chapter has been designed to further midwives' knowledge about some statistical tests available to analyse quantitative data gathered. Please note that there is a lot that has not been addressed, with a recommendation made that any statistics plan be tailor-made to match each individual project designed. Within each written research proposal (recipe), the researcher is required to list their quantitative data analysis intentions. To illustrate this, an example is provided in Box 9.8, which addresses *STEP (10): Detail intended data processing and analysis.*

It is usual to seek the advice of a statistician for confirmation that the data analysis intentions are best fit to test the hypotheses and provide appropriate answers to the research question(s). Statisticians have studied statistics to degree level and beyond, and therefore are qualified to comment on the design of proposed quantitative data analysis. Statisticians can advise, propose analysis in context, look for patterns in the data, help make decisions, advise on findings, and often write the end report. Also, if a grant is being applied for, the data analysis plan should be presented as an appendix at the back of the final submitted research proposal. If the research proposal is being written with a view to commencing a PhD or other

BOX 9.8	EXAMPLE OF INTENDED DATA ANALYSIS (STEP 10)

This study consists of two groups and 4 data collection points.

- Group 1: Women 20–30 years of age

- Group 2: Women 30–40 years of age

- 4 data collection points (a, b, c, d)

   (Please note that the details of data collection and instruments used will be clearly outlined in STEP 9 of the research proposal).

Proposed data analysis.
Demographic data will be analysed, and a table produced which will describe population characteristics (i.e. age, ethnicity, marital status, income, education, and employment). *(A purpose-built survey instrument will outline processes of collecting demographic data in STEP 9 of the proposal).* The data collected will be submitted to significance tests, with the p-value calculated to support or reject the null hypothesis for each instrument used. Multivariate ANOVA's will be calculated, with tables and graphs of results produced.

(1) Data collection instrument 1:
Groups 2×4 (a, b, c, d) ANOVA will produce 'p'- values between groups.

(2) Data collection instrument 2:
Groups 2×4 (a, b, c, d) ANOVA will produce 'p'-values between groups.

(3) Data collection instrument 3:
Groups 2×4 (a, b, c, d) ANOVA will produce 'p'-values between groups.

(4) Data collection instrument 4:
Groups 2×4 (a, b, c, d) ANOVA will produce 'p'-values between groups.

   Advice of a statistician will be sought to advise on contents of the statistical plan, and check data analysed and what is reported. *(Naming this statistician and time they would spend would be expected if your research proposal is part of a grant application).*

type of doctorate, the midwife will be expected to collect the data, enter the results into spreadsheets, conduct the analysis, and write the report. Of course, this will be under the vigilance of the research supervisory team and possibly an advising statistician. Beyond this preliminary Chapter 9 has been dedicated to a basic introduction of how to analyse quantitative data (STEP 10), it is recommended that the reader seek further knowledge from a book that is devoted to the topic of statistics (e.g. Scott and Mazhindu 2014). There is also the option of attending study days and/or completing modules that are committed to the topic of statistics, before describing the data collection tools (STEP 9), detailing intended data processing and analysis (STEP 10), and in preparation for the actual task of exploring the data. Now that we have summarized a few processes involved in analyzing quantitative data, Chapter 10 proceeds to discuss the role and procedures involved in gaining ethical approval for the research study you propose (STEP 11).

9.13 SELF-ASSESSMENT QUESTIONS (SAQs)

9.1   **The intervention in the following quantitative study is:**

   (a)   Attending 10-weekly parenthood education classes.

   (b)   Having self-efficacy measured before and after the intervention.

   (c)   Triangulating the data.

   (d)   Doing nothing to educate oneself.

9.2   **Which one of the following variables is not categorical?**

   (a)   Asking the participant to declare their gender (e.g. female, lesbian, and bisexual).

   (b)   Age of the participating childbearing women.

   (c)   Answering true or false to a questionnaire item.

   (d)   Marital status of a person (e.g. single, partnered, married, and divorced).

9.3   **Women's pulse rates equal 69, 62, 82, 74, 94. The medium for this list is:**

(a)   94.

(b)   62.

(c)   69.

(d)   74.

9.4   **When testing the null hypothesis and the level of significance (*p-value*) is smaller, the likelihood that the result happened by chance is:**

(a)   irrelevant.

(b)   Reduced.

(c)   Remains the same.

(d)   Increased.

9.5   **What statistical test is used to assess differences or relationships when the data type of the variables is ordinal (see Figure 9.9)?**

(a)   Spearman's correlation

(b)   One-way ANOVA

(c)   Wilcoxon signed ranks test

(d)   One sample T-test

9.6   **What statistical test is used to test differences when the data type of the dependent variable is nominal (see Figure 9.9)?**

(a)   Paired samples T-test

(b)   Mann–Whitney test

(c)   Chi-Square if $(N > 20)$ or Fisher exact test if $(N < 20)$.

(d)   Pearson's

9.7   **What statistical test is used to test differences when the data type of the dependent variable is ordinal numeric not normally distributed, and one group tested twice (see Figure 9.9)?**

(a)   Kruskal Wallis test

(b)   Chi-Square

(c)   Paired samples T-test

(d)   Wilcoxon signed ranks test

9.8   **What statistical test is used to test differences when the data type of the dependent variable is ordinal numeric not normally distributed, and two groups tested once (see Figure 9.9)?**

(a)   Paired samples T-test

(b)   Fisher exact test

(c)   Spearman's correlation

(d)   Mann–Witney test

9.9   **What statistical test is used to test differences when the data type of the dependent variable is numeric normally distributed, and three or more groups tested once (see Figure 9.9)?**

(a)   Chi-Square

(b)   One-way ANOVA

(c)   Wilcoxon signed ranks test

(d)   Paired samples T-test

ANSWERS TO CHAPTER 9 SAQs

9.1 **a**

9.2 **b**

9.3 **d**

9.4 **d**

9.5 **a**

9.6 **c**

9.7 **d**

9.8 **d**

9.9 **b**

The Role and Procedures Involved in Gaining Ethical Approval

(STEP 11) Declare any ethical considerations and outline data protection procedures.

10.1 ETHICAL ISSUES THAT RELATE TO IMPLEMENTATION OF RESEARCH

Since World War ll, there has been a gradual developing consensus about key ethical principles that should underpin a research project. Three notable events stimulated this interest (see Table 10.1).

Occurrences of the like influenced reconsideration of ethical standards and consensus that human participants require protection from risky scientific researchers.

10.1.1 EXAMPLES OF WHY ETHICS COMMITTEES HAVE EVOLVED

1. *Nazi human experimentation*
   The Nazi human experiments involved a series of medical procedures carried out on prison participants during World War ll and the Holocaust. During process, German Nazi physicians forced prisoners to participate in experiments that more often resulted in their death, and which caused trauma, disfigurement, and permanent disability. For example, in Auschwitz (Poland) and other camps, selected inmates were subjected to hazardous experiments designed to develop new weapons and aid recovery of injured military personnel. In addition, Dr Josef Mengele performed unnecessary experiments on identical twins. Post war, the perpetrators of these crimes were tried in court (called the Doctors' trials), which led to development of the Nuremberg Code of medical ethics (Burrows 2019).

2. *Alder Hey organs scandal*
   The Alder Hey organs scandal involved unauthorized removal, retention, and disposal of human tissue and organs between 1988 and 1995. During process, organs were retained in more than 2000 pots, which contained body parts of over 850 infants. These pots were uncovered at Alder Hey Children's Hospital in Liverpool, with the scandal leading to development of the 2004 Human Tissue Act, which overhauled legislation surrounding handling of human tissue in the United Kingdom. (Bauchner and Vinci 2001).

Research Recipes for Midwives, First Edition. Caroline J. Hollins Martin.
© 2024 John Wiley & Sons Ltd. Published 2024 by John Wiley & Sons Ltd.

Table 10.1 Notable events that influenced development of ethical principles to underpin research.

---

(1) *The Nuremberg War Crimes Trial following World War II brought to public awareness that German scientists had used captive humans as participants in macabre experiments* (Burrows 2019).

(2) *The Alder Hey organs scandal* (Bauchner and Vinci 2001).

(3) *In the 1960s, the Tuskegee Syphilis Study involved withholding of effective treatment for syphilis from infected African American participants* (Wanamaker 2018).

---

3. *Tuskegee study of untreated syphilis in African American Males*

The Tuskegee study was an experiment (clinical trial) carried out between 1932 and 1972 by the *US Public Health Service* (Wanamaker 2018). The aim was to observe the natural history of untreated syphilis. During process, the African American male participants were only told that they were receiving free health care from the Federal government of the United States. The *US Public Health Service* conducted the trial in collaboration with Tuskegee University, which is historically a black college in Alabama. A total of ($n = 600$) impoverished unaware African American men took part in the trial. Out of these ($n = 399$) with latent syphilis entered the intervention group, and ($n = 201$) without syphilis the control group. As an incentive to participate, these men were promised free medical care, and in process were given placebos, ineffective treatments, and diagnostic procedures. Participants with syphilis were not informed of their diagnosis, even though they could infect others, develop blindness, deafness, mental illness, heart disease, bone deterioration, collapse of the central nervous system, and experience early death. Instead, these men were told they were being treated for 'bad blood' and that the study would last 6 months, with the project extending to 40 years. None of the infected men were treated with penicillin, which in 1947 became the standard treatment for syphilis. This 40-year study breached ethical standards, given that the researchers knowingly failed to treat participants appropriately after penicillin was found to be an effective treatment for syphilis. Also, participants remained ignorant of the study purpose, which was to observe the natural course of untreated syphilis. Victims included participants who developed complications and died of syphilis, 40 wives who contracted the disease, and 19 children who were born with congenital syphilis. The Tuskegee Syphilis Study led to writing of the 1979 Belmont Report and establishment of the *Office for Human Research Protections (OHRP)*. On the 16th May 1997, President Bill Clinton apologized on behalf of the United States to victims of the study (Wanamaker 2018).

10.1.2 WHAT DOES RESEARCH ETHICS MEAN?

Research ethics involves the application of fundamental ethical principles when undertaking scientific research. Such principles include caution as regard human experimentation, animal experimentation, various aspects of academic scandal, including scientific misconduct (e.g. fraud, fabrication of data, and plagiarism), whistleblowing, and regulation of research. The World Health Organization (WHO) has written standards and operational guidance for ethics review of health-related research with human participants (WHO 2011). This WHO document was developed to provide guidance to researchers and *Research Ethics Committees* (RECs) overseeing the ethical aspects of health-related studies involving human participants. A researcher's adherence to these guidelines helps promote ethical conduct of their study and protects the rights and well-being of participants (WHO 2011). In response, a fundamental component of all contemporary research ethics guidance is that research proposals must be subject to prior ethical review by a registered REC. Such ethical review is intended to ensure that the ethical principles and practices put forward in the WHO (2011) guidelines will be followed during the study.

10.1.3 MORAL OR ETHICAL CONSIDERATION

Moral or ethical consideration is not an option. It is central to the development of a research proposal. When most people think of morals, they think of rules for distinguishing between right and wrong, such as 'do unto others as you would have them do unto you'. Ethics are norms that distinguish between acceptable and unacceptable behaviour. Most people learn ethical norms at home, school, and through religion. There are also many ethical disputes about what is right or wrong. To resolve these conflicts societies, formulate laws to enforce widely accepted standards of behaviour. In addition, many different disciplines, institutions, and professions have norms for behaviour that suit the aims and goals of their own organization.

10.2 ETHICAL TERMS

There are a number of expressions used to portray ethical issues. These have evolved to guard civil rights of research participants:

a. <u>Voluntary participation</u> is a principle that requires that the person is not pressurized into participating in a research study. This is especially applicable when researchers have 'captive audiences', such as prisoners, the unconscious, and children.

b. <u>Informed consent</u> requires that the participant be fully informed about events and hazards that may be implicated during the study. Consequently, the participant must provide written evidence that they have read the information sheet, have been given opportunity to ask questions, and that they consent to the procedures involved.

c. <u>Risk of harm</u> includes both physical and psychological elements. There are two standards that are applied to protect the privacy of research participants.

   i. <u>Confidentiality</u> assures that identifying information is not made available to anyone who is not directly involved in the study.

   ii. <u>Anonymity</u> requires that the participant remains anonymous in terms of data storage, publication, and occasionally to the researcher(s). In a *randomized controlled trial* (RCT) blinding is carried to create anonymity to reduce researcher bias (Monaghan et al. 2021). One example of this is blinding in clinical trials. One method of blinding is to use outwardly identical medications, e.g. randomly assorting participants into two groups using computer-generated randomization. Group 1 receive the functioning pill, and Group 2 (control) receive a placebo pill. Both pills issued are physically identical, making it impossible for participants and researchers to discern which one is active. There are three types of blinding:

   Single-blinded trial: Only the researcher undertaking the study knows what treatment or intervention is being administered to the participant.

   Double-blinded trial: Neither the researchers nor the childbearing women or neonates know what treatment (intervention) they are getting.

   Triple-blinded trial: The treatment (intervention) is unknown to (a) the participant, (b) the individual(s) who issue the intervention, and (c) the researchers who assess outcomes.

d. <u>Right to service</u> requires that a no-treatment control group (a group of participants who do not receive the treatment) is implemented as part of an RCT design.

e. <u>Institutional Review Board (IRB)</u> is a panel of people who review grant proposals with respect to ethical implications and decide whether further action is required to assure the safety and rights of participants. Their aim is to protect both the researcher and institution from potential legal problems that may arise from neglect of relevant ethical issues.

10.3 PREVENTING HARM

Ethicists are concerned with possible negative effects that may result to participants and researchers during the study. Harm is considered to involve any injury to the rights, safety, or welfare of the participant. Examples include physical, psychological, social, financial, or economic factors. It is the responsibility of the researcher to avoid, prevent, and minimize risk of harm to participants and researchers. To view some potential cause(s) of harm, see Table 10.2.

Table 10.2 Potential cause(s) of harm during a research study may include:

(a) *Physical*: Actions that may result in injury or death.

(b) *Psychological:* Deception or mishandling of information that may result in emotional trauma to the participant.

(c) *Social*: Gathering information that may be hazardous to the social position of a participant or their community.

(d) *Financial/Economic*: Exposure may result in loss of benefits, insurance, or employment.

(e) *Participants' Rights*: Failure to gain informed consent or respect participants' autonomy.

The principle of minimizing harm requires that the study involve the fewest number of participants as is possible to achieve acceptable results. Also, to carry out the least number of tests to gain data to answer the research question(s).

10.3.1 RISK

The study should involve a minimal set of risk(s). For example, the probability of anticipated harm from participating in the study is no greater than that which would be experienced in everyday life. When more than minimal risks are involved, any predictable possibility must be explained to the participant before and during provision of informed consent. To explore further aspects of risk (see Activity 10.1).

Activity 10.1

- Consider an area of midwifery practice that you think merits research attention.
- Can you think of a situation where a treatment (intervention) may place the childbearing women or neonate at risk of physical or emotional harm?

   In relation to the research proposal you are writing, you will need to add a section titled **Ethics** (STEP 11), which will involve you declaring any ethical considerations and outlining data protection procedures.

10.3.2 DECEPTION

Aspects of deception, concealment, or covert observation require consideration by the ethics committee, since voluntary and informed consent cannot be obtained when the real research question is being hidden or participants are being observed out with their awareness. An example of this is observing participants' behaviour through a one-way mirror in a natural situation, such as during labour, at a clinic, or in the postnatal ward. In some fields of research, for example, psychology, exceptional circumstances may arise when the study of human behaviour requires deception, concealment, or covert observation. The ethics committee may consider such circumstances acceptable when:

a. The study would be jeopardized by participants knowing the true purpose of the study.

b. The research question cannot be answered any other way.

c. Participants do not experience increased risk due to the activities undertaken.

d. Disclosure to participants is maximized.

e. Participants are provided with de-briefing post participation.

f. Participants are allowed to withdraw from the research study at any time.

   It is up to the ethics committee to decide whether the study is worth, or merits being carried out. What follows is a very famous example of an experiment that was considered to be deceptive.

10.3.3 THE MILGRAM (1963) EXPERIMENT

Where deception is unavoidable, debriefing of participants is obligatory post data collection. Post event, the researcher should explain the real purpose of the study. What follows is an example of an experiment where debriefing post experiment was considered necessary (Milgram 1963, 1974). The example offered has been selected because it is an interesting keystone experiment that effected ethical changes in social psychology (see Table 10.3).

10.3.4 PRIVACY

A fundamental requirement is that information disclosed during the research study is kept confidential. There is a duty not to release information to people who are not involved in the study unless the participant agrees. It is usual for any quotes to be tagged with a participant number. An infringement of privacy may be justified if a childbearing woman or infant is at

Table 10.3 The Milgram (1963) experiment.

Stanley Milgram (1963) wanted to discover how far people would be prepared to go to carry out the requests of an authority figure. He designed a bogus experiment on the pretext that the purpose was to study the effect of punishment on memory. Milgram carried out 19 variations of his experiment and compared results with those of a baseline voice feedback condition. In Milgram's baseline voice feedback condition, the participant was introduced to another man who was alleged to be another participant, but in fact was a confederate of the experimenter. The confederate had been specially trained to respond in a particular way during the experiment. The experimenter (dressed in a white coat) told the two participants that they would be assigned a role as either teacher or learner and that the teacher would then proceed to teach the learner to remember a list of word pairs. The two men drew lots to decide who was to take each role, but in fact, this was rigged so that the genuine participant always became the teacher. The participant then viewed the learner being strapped into a chair and electrodes attached to him (electrical connections), which were linked up to a shock generator. The learner at this point mentioned that he had heart trouble but the experimenter assured him that, 'although the shocks can be extremely painful, they cause no permanent tissue damage'. The participant was then shown to a separate room where the shock generator was placed on a table. The participant was told that each time the learner made a mistake in recall of the list of word pairs, he was to administer a shock by pressing one of the thirty switches on the shock generator. The first switch was labelled '15 V-mild shock' the next '30 V' and so on up to '450 V' and the participant was told to press the 15-V switch first and then move one switch up the scale each time the learner made a mistake. When all the instructions were clear, the session began. Milgram wanted to know how far up the scale of shocks the participants would go when told to continue by the experimenter. This was despite the sound of cries and pounds on the wall from the learner (an actor faking) asking the participant to stop giving the shocks and, later, the learner's complete silence. The results were unexpected and dramatic with 65% of the men in the baseline condition proceeding up to the 450-V level. At the end of the session, (when the participant had reached 450-V or had refused to continue) the true purpose of the experiment was revealed, and the participant was told that no shocks had in fact been delivered to the learner. The results of Milgram's experiments provided overwhelming evidence that the majority of people are unable to defy orders of authority and will proceed to administer painful electric shocks when commanded to do so.

(see: https://www.youtube.com/watch?v=fCVII-_4GZQ)

Table 10.4 Extract from the NMC Code (NMC 2015), which justifies when a midwife can breach participant confidentiality.

(17)	Raise concerns immediately if you believe a person is vulnerable or at risk and needs extra support and protection. To achieve this, you must:
(17.1)	Take all reasonable steps to protect people who are vulnerable or at risk from harm, neglect, or abuse.
(17.2)	Share information if you believe someone may be at risk of harm, in line with the laws relating to the disclosure of information.
(17.3)	Have knowledge of and keep to the relevant laws and policies about protecting and caring for vulnerable people.

risk of abuse. For example, in the *nursing and midwifery council* (NMC), professional standards of practice and behaviour for nurses, midwives, and nursing associates (NMC 2015), under the section called 'preserve safety', it informs the midwife of situations that it is acceptable to breach participant confidentiality (see Table 10.4).

10.3.5 CONFIDENTIALITY

It is the duty of the researcher to protect the confidentiality agreed in the informed consent process. Anonymity must be protected as regards personal information and record keeping. Personal information may be classified into one of three types of data:

1. *Identified data*
   Refers to data collected which has identifiers attached, which if found or published will reveal precisely who the participant is or was. To view examples, see *Table 10.5*.

2. *Potentially identifiable data*
   Identified data must be removed and tagged in accordance with a coding system, which is replaced by a symbol, a series of significant numbers and letters that are declared and mean something, or an alternative pseudo-name. Such coding or tagging make the anonymizing process reversible, which may be necessary if the researcher needs to reidentify participants again at a later date. In qualitative research, recordings of interviews or focus groups are considered identifiable data, even when the recordings have no recognizable markings on them, precisely because voices may be

Table 10.5   Identifiers that should be removed from data and tagged in accordance with a coding system.

Name: (full name and title)

Address: (city, county, and postal code)

Dates directly related to a person: (date of birth, admission, discharge, etc.)

Contact details: (telephone, email address, account numbers)

Other identifiers: certificate/license numbers, car registration plates, finger/voice prints, photographs, etc.

distinguishable. Hence, participants' recordings are stored under a double lock and key. Transcriptions of interview tapes are also potentially identifiable data, and therefore also must be coded.

3. *De-identified data*
   Refers to information that is anonymous and not re-identifiable. That is, the data has never been identified or the identifiers have been permanently removed. As such, de-identification becomes an irreversible process.

The processes involved in how researchers will address assuring participant anonymity must be clearly outlined in a 'data protection plan', which is an appendix to the research proposal. Together, these are sent to the appropriate ethics committees for review. The *European University Institute* has written a helpful guide on good data protection practice in research (EUI 2022).

10.4   WHAT IS ETHICAL APPROVAL?

The basic ethical question is whether risks to the participant can be justified compared against potential contribution of study findings to the overall body of knowledge. All *Ethics Committees* issue guidelines as to what studies require ethical approval and how the process is carried out, with advisors available to guide researchers through the process. Ethical consideration for human studies is based on the Helsinki Declaration (1975) (World Medical Association 2013), which has been adopted globally as the yardstick for clinical research trials. It is best to err on the side of caution and submit to the ethics committee any study that involves patients, human volunteers, or human material for ethical approval. Animal experimentation and embryological and genetic research are also subject to strict control by the Home Office in the United Kingdom.

10.5   WHY IS ETHICAL APPROVAL NECESSARY?

The Second World War crimes trials led to the Nuremberg Code (1947) (Czech et al. 2018). The Nuremberg Trials were a series of court cases most notable for the prosecution of prominent members of political, military, and economic leadership of Nazi Germany post defeat in World War ll. The trials were held in the Palace of Justice in the city of Nuremberg (Germany) between 1945 and 1946. The Doctors' Trial was the first of 12 trials for war crimes. Twenty of the 23 defendants were medical doctors, with all accused of having been involved in Nazi human experimentation. The defendants were faced with charges of performing medical experiments without participants' consent, afflicting brutalities, and torturing concentration camp prisoners. They were also accused of performing mass murder of hostages by gas and lethal injection, and stigmatizing civilians as old, insane, incurably ill, and deformed. As a consequence of the Nuremberg Trials, seven doctors were acquitted, nine were imprisoned for life, and seven were hanged. The behavior of these doctors provoked the formulation of ethics principles (see Table 10.6).

10.5.1   THE DECLARATION OF HELSINKI

The Declaration of Helsinki is regarded as one of the most authoritative set of principles in research. The Helsinki Declaration (1975) (World Medical Association, 2013) is widely regarded as the cornerstone document of human research ethics.

Table 10.6 As a consequence of the Nuremberg Trials, the following principles were embedded into generic international ethics protocols.

(1) Voluntary consent from participants is essential.

(2) Experiments conducted must be for the good of society.

(3) Anticipated results should justify the experiment.

(4) Researchers must avoid causing unnecessary suffering.

(5) There must be no risk to the participant of death or disability.

(6) Risks should not outweigh benefits.

(7) Participants should be protected by proper facilities.

(8) The research should only be conducted by scientifically qualified persons.

(9) Participants should be free to withdraw from a study at any time.

(10) The experiment must be terminated if risks develop of possible injury or death.

Although it is not a legally binding instrument in international law, it draws its authority from the degree to which it has influenced national legislation, regulations, and guidelines (World Medical Association 2013), which impact upon research practice in both symbolic and instrumental roles. In response, all research carried out within midwifery practice should be conducted with integrity and in line with generally accepted ethical principles. Hence, it is a mandatory requirement of the universities and health and social care institutions that research with human participants is conducted in line with an approved research ethics application. Researchers who have designed studies that involve human participants and have not sought approval from the ethics committee have breached the rules.

10.6 MONITORING OF RESEARCH PROJECTS

All research projects require to be scrutinized to ensure that they are and remain within ethical guidelines. Universities are committed to ensuring that all research with human participants is conducted according to accepted ethical principles. Research committees are established to enable researchers to obtain approval for their work as efficiently as possible and to protect *principal investigators* (PIs) by ensuring that all aspects of their research studies comply with the regulations. A component of protecting researchers within legislation is to ensure that applications are approved in good time before the preferred start date of a project. It is a legal offence to undertake a study without approval from the appropriate committees.

10.6.1 CODES AND POLICIES FOR RESEARCH ETHICS

Given the importance of considering ethics when conducting research, it should come as no surprise that many different professional organizations, government agencies, and universities have adopted specific codes, rules, and policies that coordinate and monitor research activity. When undertaking a research project, researchers are required to complete and submit the applicable forms to the appropriate ethics committees.

10.7 OBTAINING ETHICS COMMITTEE APPROVAL

When undertaking a research project that involves participants who are being recruited through the *national health service* (NHS) (United Kingdom), researchers are required to complete and submit two sets of forms to the appropriate ethics committees. Applications for ethical approval must be made to:

1. The appropriate university ethics committee

2. The *integrated research application system* (IRAS) for an NHS application.

10.7.1 WHAT DOES THE INTEGRATED RESEARCH APPLICATION SYSTEM (IRAS) DO?

When undertaking research that involves childbearing women, partners, neonates, and/or maternity care staff, in the United Kingdom, the researcher submits their application for ethical approval to NHS IRAS. To access an (IRAS) application form follow the link:

> https://www.hra.nhs.uk/approvals-amendments/what-approvals-do-i-need/research-ethics-committee-review/applying-research-ethics-committee

A few weeks later the applicant may be called to a meeting with a multi-disciplinary IRAS committee in the locality that they wish to conduct their study.

10.7.2 WHAT DOES THE IRAS COMMITTEE DO?

Your research proposal will be reviewed by a multi-disciplinary committee, which typically consists of doctors, midwives, Allied Health Care Professionals, academics, and lay members. The committee is ordinarily composed of around 15 members (10 professionals and 5 laypeople). The 10 professionals represent different relevant disciplines, e.g. an anesthetist, hematologist, nurse, social worker, occupational therapist, physiotherapist, radiographer, and physiotherapist. The purpose of the meeting is to gain clarification about specific aspects of the proposed research study. The bulk of applications are accepted subject to minor changes. Ensure that along with the NHS IRAS application form, other relevant documentation is provided, e.g. the researchers' curriculum vitae, relevant protocols, questionnaires, focus group directions, sample diaries (or guidance notes), and a demonstration of data collection. If feasible, the student's research supervisor should be present. Aluwihare-Samaranayake (2012) examines some of the ethical dilemmas that may be experienced, which demonstrate that both the participant and researcher equally contribute to the transparency of the ethical process. As such, guidelines and principles are designed to minimize harm, increase the sum of good, guarantee trust, ensure research integrity, satisfy professional standards, and cope with challenging problems that occur across the study period (Aluwihare-Samaranayake 2012).

What follows is a general summary of some of the principles that ethics committees scrutinize.

Honesty

Honesty in relation to the study design, with no fabrication, falsification, or misrepresentation of study content or data. No deception of professional colleagues or participants. Also, absence of conflicts of interest and honest representation of public involvement. Conflicts of interest may involve the researcher experiencing financial gain, career advancement, or having an invested bias towards a wanted study outcome. Effective means of identifying and managing conflicts of interest typically focus upon researcher disclosure, which may cause substantial internal cognitive dissonance (Romain 2015).

Integrity

Bias in the research method (recipe) in situations where objectivity may be in question. For example, pharmaceutical companies' financial interests, where the fruits of the study include valuable products that will advance maternity care. At the same time, such products will fuel growth in pharmaceutical, biotechnology, and appliance industries that create medications, devices, and saleable products that earn enormous sums of money for investors (Romain 2015). Tensions between these opposing forces have increased interest in medical ethics and research integrity.

Carefulness

Good documentation practice in clinical research is essential, with no irresponsible errors, negligence, and good record keeping (Bargaje 2011). A researcher should keep meticulous records of research activities and be open to criticism and new ideas. They should honour patents, copyright, and other forms of *intellectual property* (IP), and not use results without permission. Also, credit must be ascribed where due.

Confidentiality

Protection of personal communications, such as recordings, transcripts, data, personal information, and consent sheets is essential. Whilst conducting a study, the researcher must inform participants of the precautions they will undertake to protect their confidentiality. As such, childbearing women should know who will or may have access to their information (Divall and Spiby 2019, Petrova et al. 2016).

Responsible Publication

Publishing research papers in academic journals is ordinarily the final stage of the project. During writing, the authors must ensure that their study is presented in an honest, accurate, and balanced way. Researchers should present results clearly, honestly, and without fabrication, falsification, or inappropriate data manipulation. The research method (recipe) is clearly and unambiguously written, and in enough detail to make the study repeatable in a changed population by a different researcher. The team should adhere to journal requirements, with authors taking collective responsibility for the final paper submitted. In addition, the authorship should accurately reflect individuals' contributions to the work, funding sources, and relevant conflicts of interest (Wagner and Kleinert 2014).

Responsible Participant Informed Consent

Obtaining informed consent from a childbearing woman requires open and honest communication between the researcher and the study participant (Gov, UK Service Manual 2022). Requirements include ensuring participants know what they are agreeing to, and that they understand that the project is ethical and complies with data protection laws. Consent is required from all research participants, regardless of whether you know them. For consent to be fully informed, participants must be told:

- Who is undertaking the study?
- The purpose of the study.
- Type of data being collected.
- Procedures involving their participation.
- How findings will be used.
- Who will be allowed to view the raw data.
- That participation is voluntary and that they can withdraw from the study at any point with no personal repercussions.
- How long data will be kept.
- Their rights and where they can make a complaint.
- Whether data collection is being observed and by whom.
- Whether and if the session is being recorded.
- Which organization is responsible for holding their data and how to contact them if they wish their data to be withdrawn.
- Other service providers, e.g. transcribers.

You need to explain these factors in a *participant information sheet* (PIS). In addition, an assurance of continued support and access to post interview counselling should be offered.

Respect for Participants

To maintain participant trust and confidence during a research study, participants are treated with respect. This includes the need to provide a valid consent process and provide protection for women who have had their capacity for informed consent compromised. It is also important to promote dignity and consider potential effects the research can have on communities and culture. The above are factors that the *research ethics committee* (REC) members will consider when viewing a research proposal (Pieper and Thomson 2014). Part of showing respect involves providing information about the study and gaining participant consent to take part in the study. This requires that a *participant information sheet* (PIS) is written, and a *consent form* is signed. Save two duplicates of the consent form:

- One paper copy for the participant
- One copy for the research data file

To view an example of a PIS, see Table 10.7 and consent form (see Table 10.8).

Table 10.7   Example of a PARTICIPANT INFORMATION SHEET (PIS).

TITLE: Ensure the title is consistent throughout all documentation.

INVITATION PARAGRAH
- Invite potential participants to take part in the study about. . .
- Reassurance that participation is entirely voluntary.

WHAT IS THE PURPOSE OF THE STUDY?
- Write a brief outline in layman's language.

WHY HAVE YOU BEEN INVITED TO TAKE PART
- Explain the specifics about why they are candidate for participating in the study.
- Inform how many participants you will be recruiting.

DO I HAVE TO TAKE PART?
- Inform the potential participant that their participation is entirely voluntary.
- Inform the potential participant that they can withdraw from the study at any time without providing a reason, and that withdrawal will not affect their future maternity care provision.

WHAT WILL HAPPEN IF THEY DECIDE TO TAKE PART IN THE STUDY
- Explain what will be required of them.
- If this is a longitudinal study, explain each data collection session independently.
- If the study is collecting data about one part of maternity provision, be specific that the rest of their care will be as usual during their visit(s), e.g. provide a table of events to illustrate.
- If randomization is part of process, explain how it will be carried out.
- Outline any plans for long-term monitoring or follow-up.

WHAT SHOULD I CONSIDER?
- Explain what the inclusion and exclusion criteria are.

ARE THERE DISADVANTAGES FROM TAKING PART?
- Provide a fair and honest evaluation of the possible consequences of key procedures.

WHAT ARE THE BENEFITS OF TAKING PART?
- Explain any direct benefits of taking part. If there are no benefits, make this explicit.
- Explain long-term benefits to the wider community of the study, e.g. to childbearing women.
- Explain why you are conducting the study.

WILL MY GENERAL PRACTITIONER BE INFORMED?
- Answer this question and if the answer is 'yes', how their GP will be notified, e.g. by letter.

WILL MY PARTICIPATION IN THE STUDY BE KEPT CONFIDENTIAL?
- Explain how confidentiality will be ensured.
- Outline clearly who will be able to access their data.
- Explain that research auditors maybe given access to ensure the study is complying with data protection regulations.
- That any publications will not declare participants' names and contributions.

WILL I BE REIMBURSED FOR PARTICIPATING
- Make it clear if the participant will be reimbursed for their time, and in what way.
- Are others who accompany reimbursed in terms of travel, meals, and childcare.
- At minimum, their travel should be reimbursed.

WHAT IF THERE IS A PROBLEM?
- If the participant wants to complain, whom should they contact (provide contact point).

HOW HAVE THE PUBLIC BEEN INVOLVED IN THIS STUDY?
- Service users helped design this study and what their contribution will be ongoing.

WHO HAS FUNDED THE STUDY?
- Name the organization or person.

WHO HAS REVIEWED THE STUDY?
- Provide details of the research ethics committees which has approved the study.

Table 10.7 (Continued)

WHAT WILL HAPPEN TO THE DATA I PROVIDE?
- General data protection regulations (GDPR) require you to mention who the data controller is (e.g. NHS Foundation Trust or a Named University).
- Outline how data will be stored in the short and longer term.

WHO CAN I CONTACT FOR FUTHER INFORMATION?
- Thank the participants for reading this PIS, whether they elect to participate or otherwise.
- Provide contact details.

ADD A VERSION NUMBER AND DATE
- To keep track of most contemporary version.

Table 10.8 Example of a research participant CONSENT FORM.

Insert name of study, LOGO of university or NHS trust, and a version number and date		
Please tick appropriate boxes	**Yes**	**No**
Taking part in the project		
I have read the *participant information sheet* (PIS) dated DD/MM/YYYY	☐	☐
I have been provided with the opportunity to ask questions about the study.	☐	☐
I agree to take part in the study and understand that participation will include………	☐	☐
Add in what the participant will be doing, i.e. completing a questionnaire, being interviewed and audio or video recorded, and participating in a focus group, with separate tick boxes for each.		
I understand that my participation in this study is voluntary and that I can withdraw at any time before (provide DATE), without providing a reason why. I also understand that there will be no adverse consequences for my future maternity care provision if I were to withdraw.	☐	☐
How my information will be used during and after the project		
I understand that my personal details, e.g. name, telephone number, address, and/or email addresses will not be available to researchers or people outside this study.	☐	☐
I understand that my words may be quoted in publications, reports, websites, and other related research outputs and that I will not be named unless I provide specific consent.	☐	☐
I understand that other authorized researchers will have access to my data and that they agree to preserve confidentiality in relation to the information I provide.	☐	☐
I understand that other authorized researchers may use my data in publications, reports, websites, and other research outputs and that they agree to preserve confidentiality in relation to the information I provide.	☐	☐
I give permission for the data I provide (specify what data) to be deposited in (name data repository) so it can be used for future research and/or learning.	☐	☐
I assign the copyright of materials generated from my participation to the (named university, etc.).	☐	☐
Name of participant (printed) Signature Date		
Name of researcher (printed) Signature Date		

The importance of data protection   In the United Kingdom, the data protection act (2018) regulates the rules surrounding how personal data is used by organizations, businesses, and/or the government (Gov.uk 2022). The data protection act (2018) patrols implementation of *general data protection regulation* (GDPR). In response, everybody who uses personal data must follow rigorous rules called 'data protection principles' that ensure information is:

- Used fairly, lawfully, and transparently.
- Used for specified and explicit purpose(s).
- Used in adequate, relevant, and limited ways.
- Accurate and kept up to date.
- Kept for no longer than is essential.
- Handled in an appropriate and secure way, which includes protection against unlawful/unauthorized processing, access, loss, destruction, and/or damage.

The data protection act (2018) ensures that people:

- Are informed about how their data is being used.
- Have access to their personal data.
- Have incorrect or out-of-date data corrected.
- Have data erased.
- Can stop or inhibit processing of their data.
- Have a say in how their data is reused by different services.
- Can object to how their data is processed in particular circumstances.

The *data protection act* (DPA 2018) aims to prevent people or organizations from holding and using inaccurate information about people, which applies to personal and private or business-based information. The DPA (2018) outlines the framework for appropriate data protection law in the United Kingdom. It is adjacent to the GDPR, and tailors how the GDPR applies within the United Kingdom. A data breach is a security incident that affects confidentiality, integrity, and/or availability of personal data, such as accidentally losing, destroying, corrupting, or disclosing personal information about a participant. Such breaches may involve:

- Providing access to an unauthorized third-party
- Sending personal data to an incorrect recipient
- Stolen computers containing lost personal data
- Tampering with personal data without authorization
- Loss of availability of personal data.

Within every research proposal, it is important to append a data protection plan. To view an example, see Table 10.9.

Social Responsibility

It is also important that midwifery researchers strive to prevent social harm when conducting a research study. Each midwifery researcher is responsible for any impacts from decisions and/or activities on childbearing women, infants, and their partners. There are four principles of research ethics for midwives, which are the same as for any researcher who collects data from human beings. The four principles include:

- Respect for autonomy
- Beneficence
- Non-maleficence
- Justice

Table 10.9 Example of a data protection plan (DPP).

Title of Project:

(a) *Existing data*

The research objectives require that qualitative data be gathered that currently is not available from other sources.

(b) *Information about data collected*: This project involves primary data collection. We intend to conduct face-to-face interviews with childbearing women ($n = 16$), in line with the data protection policy. Data will be collected and stored using digital audio recording (e.g. MP3), with soundtracks typed up according to agreed formats and standards. The principal investigator (PI) (CJHM) will undertake the interviews, carry out consented recordings, and write the transcriptions. These will be written in Microsoft Word, with methods of note-taking, recording, transcribing, and anonymizing semi-structured interview data developed and agreed with the supervisory team. Interview transcripts will be coded in NVivo.

(c) *Quality assurance*: The PI will be responsible for overall quality assurance. Detailed protocols for extracting data will be developed, piloted, refined, and agreed with the supervisory team. Quality will be assured through routine monitoring and periodic cross-checks against written protocols. Systems for notetaking, recording, transcribing, and data storage will be clearly outlined. The supervisory team will check through transcripts for consistency with agreed standards.

(d) *Backup and security*: Data will be backed up regularly, which will include regular email sharing with the supervisory team. Up-to-date versions will be coded and stored on the university server (allocated X drive), which is secure and backed up regularly as per the university research data management (RDM) policy. Additional protection will be afforded through use of passwords and backup hardware.

(e) *Ethical issues*: A letter explaining purpose, approach, and dissemination strategy for the study and an accompanying consent form have been prepared (e.g. see Appendices 1–4). A clear verbal explanation will also be provided to each participant prior to interview. Confidentiality will be maintained by ensuring recordings are not shared, those transcripts are anonymized, and details that will identify participants are removed from transcripts and write-ups. Where there is risk of identification, participants will be shown sections of transcript to ensure they are satisfied that no unnecessary risks are being taken with their interview data. Some interviewees may be more comfortable if some sections of their interview are not recorded or made public, and when stated such requests will be respected. In such circumstances, recording will be paused, or sections of text removed from transcripts.

(f) *Expected difficulties with data sharing:* Transcripts will be recorded and transcribed in English, which will limit accessibility of the data to alternative-speaking cultures.

(g) *Copyright and intellectual property right*: The institutional partners (named maternity unit and named university) will jointly own the data generated. Online and archival sources will be cited and clearly acknowledged in the database and research outputs. Permission will be sought to share research findings on public websites (e.g. named charity).

(h) *Responsibilities*: The PI will be responsible for collecting, transcribing, input, back-up, quote extraction, sharing, and archiving data, under guidance of the supervisory team.

(i) *Preparation for data sharing and archiving:* Data sharing will be through publications and online institutional websites. The project will have a dedicated space on the university/maternity unit website to facilitate this.

Applying realism, any research that involves humans can rarely achieve 'zero risk', simply because by nature humans are sensitive and each has variation in what is perceived as threatening. Nonetheless, we must always attempt to follow these four stated principles of social responsibility.

Non-discrimination

It is important that midwifery researchers attempt not to discriminate against colleagues or students based on sex, race, or ethnicity. Being treated with equality is a deep-seated value, regardless of a person's age, race, colour, sex, nationality, language, religion, ethnical, or social origin. Discrimination may be direct or indirect. Direct discrimination is providing differential treatment of one person compared with another in the same situation based upon their characteristics (age, race, colour, sex, nationality, language, religion, ethnical, or social origin). In contrast, indirect discrimination involves treating people all the same, when a treatment has altered outcomes for a different group of people. For example, there isare significant foetal growth differences between Asian, Black, Hispanic, and white pregnancies. Hence, applying different ethnic-specific growth charts is important when assessing foetal growth antenatally (Kiserud et al. 2017).

Legality

Ethical competence in research is a cornerstone of professional midwifery practice (Clarke 2015). Hence, all studies must obey relevant laws and institutional and government policies. Midwifery researchers are answerable for being aware of the regulatory frameworks, which have over the years escalated in complexity. Hence, it is important for both the university and each individual midwifery researcher to comply with the relevant legislation. For example, general data protection regulation (GDPR).

Human Participants' Protection

It is the midwifery researcher's ethical and legal responsibility to demonstrate that their study will not cause undue harm to women, partners, and participating neonates. Also, in the event that if harm is caused, this must be justified through outlining balanced societal benefits from the study results. Overall, the study design must minimize risk or harm, and maximize benefits for participants. During process, respect for human dignity, privacy, and autonomy must be considered, with special precautions taken in the case of vulnerable populations (i.e. children, people with dementia, or learning disability). During project design, the researcher must demonstrate that they have considered protection of potential participants' rights and welfare, with competent, informed, conscientious, compassionate, and responsible approaches taken.

10.8 GENERAL QUESTIONS ASKED FOR ON AN ETHICS APPLICATION?

Please seek advice from the appropriate ascribed ethics committee advisor at the university. In some universities, the ethical website is referred to under the name 'research integrity'. There will also be a site on the university intranet that provides guidance and forms to complete when applying for ethical approval for your proposed research study. The universities policies and procedures that govern the research process and are appropriate to you will be on such a site. An example of an ethics statement that will represent (STEP 11) of the research proposal can be viewed in (Table 10.10).

Table 10.10   Example of an ethics statement (STEP 11).

This research proposal will be carried out in full compliance with research ethics principles. The *principal investigator* (PI) will take full responsibility for explaining suitable details to participating childbearing women. Each research participant will be issued with a one-page *participant information sheet* (PIS), which outlines the study purpose, who the researchers are, who has funded the study and why, and how the findings will be disseminated and used (e.g. see Appendix 1). This PIS also includes contact information, should the participant request further information, wish to withdraw participation, or want their data removed from the study without consequences for future care. An assurance of anonymity and confidentiality is also afforded. Where needed, the PIS will be translated, although it is expected that English will be the main language spoken by participants. Taking part in this study will be voluntary, with informed consent discussed individually with each potential participant. As this study is using face-to-face survey research method, it is anticipated that spoken consent will additionally be recorded. The survey instrument, data collection sheet, and consent form can be viewed in (e.g. Appendices 2–4).

   The first phase of data collection involves gathering survey data from women who attend an antenatal clinic, with personal identifiers removed and anonymity of participants secured through use of unit codes and pseudonyms. Raw data from each survey will be saved in a password-protected computer, with access restricted to the PI (e.g. CJHM) and one research assistant (RA) (e.g. GN). The data will subsequently be systematized and stored in a password-protected external storage drive, which will be placed in the secure office of the PI (e.g. CJHM). The data protection plan can be viewed in (e.g. Appendix 5).

   The second phase of data collection includes carrying out two focus groups that aim to understand participants' concepts of maternity care they have received. We will meet with the antenatal clinic midwives to develop an appropriate workshop forum, and review our approaches to participation, confidentiality, and dissemination of information and results. Feedback on focus group findings will be offered to midwives and associations through a summary research report.

   The PI will submit this research proposal, along with relevant appendices to the university *school of health and social care* (SHSC) ethics committee and subsequently to the NHS ethics committee and maternity unit *research and development* (R&D) team.

10.8.1 CHAPTER CONCLUSION

Chapter 10 has addressed the concept of providing an environment that recognizes and supports research excellence through following ethical principles. Research should be carried out to the highest possible level of integrity, which involves writing a research method (recipe) that ensures that findings are robust and defensible. Before designing (STEP 11) of your research proposal, you should first familiarize yourself with the *university ethics policies* and maternity unit *research integrity* intranet, which are designed to govern processes of applying for ethics approval. There will also be a designated advisor who can provide advice. Now that STEP 11 (*Declare any ethical considerations and outline data protection procedures*) has been written, it is important to address the remaining stages of the 16-step model, with examples presented in Chapter 1:

STEP (12): Produce a timetable and consider potential problems that may occur.

STEP (13): Estimate resources that may be required.

STEP (14): Detail a public engagement plan.

STEP (15): Append a reference list.

STEP (16): Appendix relevant additional material.

Chapter 11 now provides a template for writing a 16-step research proposal.

10.9 SELF-ASSESSMENT QUESTIONS (SAQs)

10.1 **Which of the following is an ethical issue in research?**

  (a) Probability

  (b) Confidentiality

  (c) Consensus

  (d) Confidence

10.2 **Which of the following is the most important aim of a 'consent form'?**

  (a) To gain participants' consent to take part in the research project.

  (b) To inform participants about how much time they will require to give when taking part in the study.

  (c) To inform participants about the procedures involved in the study.

  (d) To help the participants understand what will happen to them during the study.

10.3 **Which of the following is not appropriate to include in a research participants' informed consent form?**

  (a) Information about how the research data will be used.

  (b) The name and contact details of the researcher.

  (c) The aims of the study.

  (d) The names and contact details of other people participating in the study.

10.4 **Which of the following is not an ethical practice?**

  (a) Obtaining someone's informed consent to participate in the research study prior to commencement.

  (b) Sharing data with other organizations which have a legitimate interest in the findings.

  (c) Using pseudonyms to protect participants from identification.

  (d) Keeping data under lock and key.

10.5 What is the overriding principle governing ethical research behavior?

    (a) To preserve the anonymity of participants.

    (b) To avoid dealing with sensitive topics.

    (c) To obtain the informed consent of the participants.

    (d) To protect research participants and their communities from harm.

10.6 When publishing research, which of the following may present ethical problems?

    (a) Upsetting participants by appearing to misrepresent their views.

    (b) Damage to participants when the media represents a lack of understanding of the principles.

    (c) Damage to the participants due to insufficient anonymity.

    (d) All of the above.

ANSWERS TO CHAPTER 10 SAQs

10.1   **b**

10.2   **a**

10.3   **d**

10.4   **b**

10.5   **d**

10.6   **c**

An Empty Template for Designing a 16-STEP Research Proposal

11.1 RECAP ON HOW TO DESIGN A RESEARCH PROPOSAL

By the time you have read this book, you will be equipped with enough skills to start developing your own research project. Ordinarily, the task of writing a research proposal is carried out in conjunction with a research supervisor who is experienced in the art of doing so. Chapters 1–10 are structured to equip the reader with essential skills to begin populating the 16-STEPS involved in writing a research proposal (see Table 11.1).

Your research proposal is intended to provide logic and structure to the envisioned study, which should follow sequential steps that spell out the recipe. Before commencing your journey, the following activities must be decided:

- Identify a problem in your area of professional midwifery practice.

- Decide which research method is appropriate to address the identified problem. Review the related literature and highlight a gap that could become the rationale for conducting this study. If required, substantiate this rationale with any documents that have expressed need for this investigation (e.g. government policy directives).

- Outline any areas of your proposed study that could raise ethical concern and discuss these with your supervisory team.

- Present a clear overarching research question.

- Provide justification for the selected research method, and its suitability to answer your stated research question.

- Follow the 16-STEP model (Table 11.1) and address each section with an underscored subheading. The chapters of this book provide sequential guidance on how to address each of the 16-STEPS.

A template follows, which the midwifery researcher can adhere to as they progress through development of their research proposal.

11.2 AN EMPTY 16-STEP RESEARCH TEMPLATE

11.2.1 STEP (1): GIVE THE RESEARCH PROPOSAL A TITLE

The title of the proposal should reflect the scope of the envisioned piece of research. The writer needs to present a consistent title throughout all of the relevant documents, which will include the proposal itself, ethics application, appendices, forms, questionnaires, etc. Ordinarily, the title will reflect the research question and research method selected. As a guide, take a look at titles of peer-reviewed published papers. An empty box is now presented for you to write your considered study title:

STEP (1): Give the research proposal a title

Research Recipes for Midwives, First Edition. Caroline J. Hollins Martin.
© 2024 John Wiley & Sons Ltd. Published 2024 by John Wiley & Sons Ltd.

Table 11.1   The 16-steps involved in writing a research proposal.

STEP (1)	Give the research proposal a title.
STEP (2)	Provide relevant personal and professional details.
STEP (3)	Provide a short abstract or summary of around 300 words.
STEP (4)	Supply six keywords to describe the research proposal.
STEP (5)	Construct an introduction that contains a relevant literature review and rationale.
STEP (6)	State the objectives, aim(s), research question(s), sub-question(s), Hypotheses, and null hypotheses of the proposed research study.
STEP (7)	Outline the research method.
STEP (8)	Select setting, participants, sampling method, inclusion and exclusion criteria and method of recruitment.
STEP (9)	Describe data collection instruments.
STEP (10)	Detail intended data processing and analysis.
STEP (11)	Declare any ethical considerations and outline data protection procedures.
STEP (12)	Produce a timetable and consider potential problems that may occur.
STEP (13)	Estimate resources that may be required.
STEP (14)	Detail a public engagement plan.
STEP (15)	Append a reference list.
STEP (16)	Appendix relevant additional material.

11.2.2 STEP (2): PROVIDE RELEVANT PERSONAL AND PROFESSIONAL DETAILS

On the front page of the research proposal, state the names and titles of the *Principal Investigator* (PI), *Supervisor(s)*, *Co-Applicants*, and their professional qualifications. In addition, each stated member of the research team must provide a short up-to-date *curriculum vitae* (CV), which contains a list of their peer-reviewed publications. These CV's will be the first appendices attached to the research proposal. Also, when you attach this CV at the back of your research proposal, remember to direct the reader to it by referencing it as Appendix 1 or 2 or 3 etc. in the main body of your proposal at the end of where it has been discussed. If the research proposal is for a university assessment, it is usual that appendices do not count in the word count, but please check this with the module leader. A box is now presented for you to add your personal details and those of your research colleagues.

STEP (2): Provide relevant personal and professional details

Name and title of principle investigator (PI):

Professional qualifications:
   Telephone number:
   Email number:
   Role(s) in study:
   (CV Appendix 1)

Name of Co-applicant (C1):
   Professional qualifications:
   Telephone number:
   Email number:
   Role(s) in study:
   (CV Appendix 2)

Name of Co-applicant (C2):
   Professional qualifications:
   Telephone number:
   Email number:
   Role(s) in study:
   (CV Appendix 3)

11.2.3 STEP (3): PROVIDE A SHORT ABSTRACT OR SUMMARY (AROUND 300–400 WORDS)

This abstract should present a clear outline of the proposed research study. It is usual to write the abstract after you have developed the research proposal, which will be once you have thought the whole study through. A well-written abstract will contain appropriate and sequential subheadings:

a. A sentence about the context of the proposed study **(Background)**.

b. The goal of the research study **(Aim)**.

c. The chosen research method (recipe) **(Method)**.

d. Intended participants, sampling method, numbers (e.g. $n = 50$) **(Participants)**.

e. Where the research will be conducted (e.g. named maternity unit) **(Setting)**.

f. List tools that will be used to collect data (e.g. questionnaire(s), semi-structured interview schedule(s) etc. **(Proposed data collection)**.

g. State proposed descriptive and inferential statistics if quantitative data OR thematic/content analysis of qualitative data, etc. **(Proposed data analysis)**.

h. Describe how results will be reported (e.g. using descriptive graphs and 'p'- values if quantitative data OR themes and subthemes if qualitative data) **(Proposed reporting of results).**

i. Describe in a sentence what the relevance of the results are (e.g. potential benefit(s) for the maternity unit, midwives, OR neonatal unit) **(Potential relevance of conclusions)**.

j. Describe in a sentence what could come out of this study (e.g. results will inform a guideline, protocol, teaching aid, subsequent study, and leaflet) **(Potential recommendations for practice).**

A box is now presented for you to write your abstract, which in essence is a short outline summary of your proposed research study.

STEP (3): Provide a short abstract or summary of around 300 words

Background:
Aim:
Method:
Participants:
Setting:
Proposed data collection:
Proposed data analysis:
Proposed reporting of results:
Potential relevance of conclusions:
Potential recommendations for practice:

11.2.4 STEP (4): SUPPLY SIX KEYWORDS TO DESCRIBE THE RESEARCH PROPOSAL

Keywords are supplied to facilitate librarians, search engines, and yourself to identify relevant research papers within the databases. As such (STEP 4) provides research papers for the literature review (STEP 5). Once the study is completed and a paper is being submitted to a peer-reviewed journal for potential publication (e.g. *Midwifery*, *Women and Birth*, and *Journal of Reproductive and Infant Psychology*), these keywords will be requested. Appropriate keywords will aid identification of the published paper and increase its chance of being referenced in the future by others. Please note, that the number of paper citations will work towards increasing each of the author(s) h-index. If in future you become a jobbing academic, your personal h-index is the metric that measures the citation impact of your published papers. A box is now presented for you to write six appropriate keywords that characterize and capture the content of your proposed research study.

STEP (4): Supply six keywords to describe the research proposal

1

2

3

4

5

6

11.2.5 STEP (5): CONSTRUCT AN INTRODUCTION THAT CONTAINS A RELEVANT LITERATURE REVIEW AND RATIONALE

Chapter 3 presents a synopsis of how to search the literature and critique published research papers. The purpose of carrying out a literature review is to summarize and critically appraise prior research that has been carried out in your selected field of interest. Once you have done this task, it is important to consider where the research gaps are in current knowledge and produce a rationale for why you think your proposed research study will be of value to future midwifery practice. Chapter 3 outlines different types of literature review methods, and from these, you need to select the most appropriate one to preface your study. If your research proposal is for a dissertation, you may be asked to carry out a full literature search, which will be accommodated within a prescribed word limit. Alternatively, there may already be a published literature review that already proposes a gap. Alternatively, you may plan a literature review as PHASE 1 of 3 study PHASES, within your research proposal. Whatever you choose, ensure you look at the assessment guidelines and marking grid carefully before you commence, and check any plans made with your supervisor(s).

Many universities have a designated specialist librarian who teaches students how to carry out a literature review. If so, you can speak to this designated person if problems arise. Remember there are different types of literature reviews. For example, if it is a quantitative study you are proposing, a *systematic review* method may be the most fitting. Alternatively, if it is a qualitative research method you have selected, a *narrative systematic review* or *scoping review* may be more appropriate. The type of literature review you intend to conduct is a discussion you require to have with your research supervisor. During process and at the end of your PRISMA diagram, you may only have a few papers that directly relate to your chosen topic. You need to carefully critique each of these papers and describe relevance of findings to the body of knowledge in your literature review (see Chapter 3). Per se, each paper's findings are summarized and discussed in relationship to the aim of your proposed research study. Where appropriate, it is important to recognize strengths and weaknesses of these research papers in terms of participant numbers, rigour and/or appropriateness of choice of selected research method. In a *systematic review*, the papers are graded for rigour, and if a *narrative review* the findings are discussed in relation to the state of knowledge on the chosen topic. Previously published literature reviews can provide a useful summary of what is already known about a particular topic, such as identifying a problem, a gap in knowledge, or unresolved controversy for which they are proposing a tentative solution. These referenced papers may already provide a rationale for undertaking your proposed study, and if not, you need to provide a logical one for yourself. This justification or rationale will provide information to the reader that will help them understand the purpose of the study and how the findings could develop midwifery knowledge and/or clinical practice. During process, take a look at some published papers and see how the authors have introduced their study, what the literature review looks like, and the rationale that the author(s) provide. A box is now presented for you to construct an introduction to your research proposal, your actual literature review, and rationale for carrying out your proposed research study.

STEP (5): Construct an introduction that contains a relevant literature review and rationale

Introduction:
Literature review:
Rationale:

11.2.6 STEP (6): STATE THE OBJECTIVES, AIM(S), RESEARCH QUESTION(S), SUB-QUESTION(S), HYPOTHESES, AND NULL HYPOTHESES OF THE PROPOSED RESEARCH STUDY

Chapter 4 presents a synopsis on how to capture the objectives, aim(s), research question(s), sub-question(s), hypotheses, and null hypotheses, within (STEP 5) of your research proposal. A short reminder of what these terms mean now follows:

Objectives
The research objectives should describe what you intend the research project to achieve. Objectives are designed to summarize your approach and help focus your study. An example objective is: Determine how the delivery suite environment affects midwives' happiness in the workplace.

Aim(s)
The research aim(s) refer to the overarching purpose of your research study and are usually brief and to the point. An example aim is: To explore factors within the delivery suite that affect midwives' happiness whilst at work.

Research question(s)
A research question is precisely what your study sets out to answer. This question usually addresses the issue or problem under investigation and always has a question mark at the end. An example research question is: (1) What factors within the delivery suite affect midwives' happiness in the workplace.

Sub-question(s)
Your overarching research question is often too large to answer easily, and so it may be subdivided into sub-questions that are specific, narrow, and can be directly answered by the data you collect. Example sub-question are:

1a. What factors within the delivery suite working environment make midwives *unhappy* at work?

1b. What factors within the delivery suite working environment make midwives *happy* at work?

1c. What factors would improve the delivery suite working environment for midwives?

Hypotheses and Null Hypotheses
Writing the hypotheses and null hypotheses are only relevant if you have elected to use a quantitative research method. If you are planning a qualitative study, hypotheses are *Not Applicable* (NA). If a quantitative numerical approach is to be taken, the secondary sub-questions are additionally captured in hypotheses. A hypothesis is a coherent statement that the statistical results will either support or reject. Each hypothesis is a statement that underpins a specific sub-question and ultimately the overarching research question. Each hypothesis indicates the expected difference between two variables and may be stated in a directional or non-directional form. A directional hypothesis indicates the expected orientation of the results, while a non-directional hypothesis indicates no association (relationship) between the variables. The stated hypotheses should be:

1. A tentative answer to the stated problem

2. Testable

3. Be specific, logical, and not vague

4. Supported or rejected post statistical analysis

For example:

> ### Hypothesis 1
> Maternal activity shortens length of first stage of labour.
>
> ### Null Hypothesis 1
> Maternal activity makes no difference to length of first stage of labour.

A box is now presented for you to construct your objectives, aim(s), research question(s), sub-question(s), hypotheses, and null hypotheses (if applicable) of the proposed research study. Chapter 4 elaborates on this process in far greater detail.

STEP (6): State the objectives, aim(s), research question(s), sub-question(s), hypotheses, and null hypotheses of the proposed research study

Objectives:
Aim(s):
Research question(s):
Sub-question(s):
Hypotheses:
Null hypotheses:

11.2.7   STEP (7): OUTLINE THE RESEARCH METHOD

A well-designed research proposal should be written in such a way that an unfamiliar person could pick it up and repeat the study. Each research method (recipe) follows a recognizable schedule of steps, with examples of research methods we have discussed in Chapter 5 including *randomized controlled trial (RCT), grounded theory, phenomenology, ethnography*, or *survey* (to name but a few). The selected research method is declared immediately under the subheading 'method' of the research proposal. The researcher then proceeds to outline the steps prescribed for their selected research method. It is not enough to follow the sequenced steps without understanding that the stated method directs the whole endeavour. The entire process is a unified effort, as well as an appreciation of its component parts. When published research papers are read, similar methods follow the same sequenced steps. That is, the steps involved in an RCT reported in one paper, will be similar to the steps reported in an RCT in another paper. This makes it a good idea for the devisor of the research proposal to look at published papers that have used the same research method they intend to use and mimic the steps. A recap of some research methods introduced in this book include:

Quantitative methods (recipes)

- Descriptive
- Randomized controlled trial (RCT)
- Quasi-experimental
- Quantitative survey
- Action research
- Clinical audit

Qualitative methods (recipes)

- Grounded theory
- Phenomenology
- Ethnography
- Qualitative Surveys
- Case study

It is now time to select an appropriate method to answer your research question and provide justification for this choice. To help you write the rationale, an example of how to justify why you have selected a specific research method (see Chapter 5, Table 5.14).

STEP (7): Outline the research method
Method:

Rationale for choice of method:

11.2.8 STEP (8): SELECT SETTING, PARTICIPANTS, SAMPLING METHOD, INCLUSION, AND EXCLUSION CRITERIA AND METHOD OF RECRUITMENT

Chapter 6 of this book addresses each aspect of (STEP 8) in depth and detail, with the following just a recap. What follows is a brief reminder. In relation to (STEP 8), first describe the setting (e.g. *named maternity unit(s), antenatal clinic(s), or community base(s)*). State who your participants' will be (e.g. *primiparous women, multigravida women, or women with a multiple pregnancy*), and exactly how many participants you want to present fully completed data from for analysis (e.g. $n = 40$). If a quantitative research method has been selected, a power analysis may be appropriate to justify the chosen number of participants needed to yield an acceptable significant difference between groups. In addition, you require to specify the sampling method intended to select potential participants (e.g. *convenience sampling, purposive sampling, or simple random sampling*), along with participant inclusion and exclusion criteria (see Chapter 6, Tables 6.2 and 6.3 for examples) (e.g. *age range and native English speaker*). The recruitment method should be detailed and how informed consent will be obtained, with the *participant information sheet* (PIS) and consent form presented as appendices that are referred to in text (e.g. see Appendix 1). A box is now presented for you to enter the details of (STEP 8).

STEP (8): Select setting, participants, sampling method, inclusion, and exclusion criteria and method of recruitment

Setting:
Participants:
Sampling method:
Inclusion criteria:
Exclusion criteria:
Method of recruitment:

11.2.9 STEP (9): DESCRIBE DATA COLLECTION INSTRUMENTS

Chapter 7 of this book addresses STEP 9 in detail, and so it would be of value to revisit it. Also, look at a peer-reviewed published research paper that has used the same method as you intend to, and view how the authors have described their data collection processes. It is now time to detail the data collection instruments you intend to use in your study (e.g. *survey questionnaire(s), semi-structured interview schedule(s), or weighing scales*). Justification for your choice of data collection instruments should be provided, along with referenced reports of reliability and validity if these tools were not designed specifically for your study. Describe in detail how your data will be collected, and remember to appendix your protocol for data collection, the data collection instruments, and the data collection sheets, and refer to them in text. A box is now presented for you to enter these details.

STEP (9): Describe data collection instruments

11.2.10 STEP (10): DETAIL INTENDED DATA PROCESSING AND ANALYSIS

Chapters 8 and 9 of these book address procedures involved in processing and analyzing data intended for collection. Chapter 8 advises on qualitative data analysis, and Chapter 9 on quantitative data analysis. Perhaps consider revisiting these chapters for a recap before writing up your proposed data processing and analysis plan. For a qualitative example, see Table 11.2.

It is now time to outline your intended data processing and analysis. For instance, if you have selected a qualitative method, outline the processes involved (see Table 11.2 and Chapter 8), and if you have selected a quantitative method, outline the intended descriptive and inferential statistics and how you intend to report them (see Chapter 9). Again, look at a peer-reviewed published research paper that has used the same method as you have selected, and view how the authors have described their forthcoming data processing and analysis. A box is now presented for you to enter details of your intended data processing and analysis.

Table 11.2 Example plan for proposed analysis of qualitative data.

The qualitative comments will be analysed using Braun and Clarke's (2006) method, with thematic analysis a system for identifying, analyzing, and reporting themes within the data. This method has been selected because the data-analysis trail can be audited. Appropriate software (e.g. NVivo will be used to store and analyse the transcripts).

(1) *Familiarizing self with data.*
The written comments will be transcribed and read and reread to identify patterns.

(2) *Generate initial codes.*
Numerical codes will be applied to quotes to afford participant anonymity.

(3) *Search for themes.*
Statements interpreted as representing similar ideas will be brought together to build themes and subthemes.

(4) *Review themes*
The chosen themes that have emerged from the data will be reviewed by an independent researcher for validation.

(5) *Define and name themes.*
The identified themes will be labelled using statements documented by the participants themselves.

(6) *Producing the report.*
The identified themes and their significance in relation to the research questions will be discussed.

STEP (10): Detail intended data processing and analysis

11.2.11 STEP (11): DECLARE ANY ETHICAL CONSIDERATIONS AND OUTLINE DATA PROTECTION PROCEDURES

Chapter 10 of this book has addressed (STEP 11), and so a revisit may be valuable. Detail in your research proposal any ethical considerations and how these will be dealt with. Discuss how confidentiality for participants will be managed, and what approval(s) from specified research ethics committees will be sought. Also, declare any conflicts of interest that you may have and explain these. Remember to refer to any relevant appendixes in text (e.g. PIS, consent forms, and data protection plan). A box is now presented for you to enter these details.

STEP (11): Declare any ethical considerations and outline data protection procedures
Ethics committee(s):
Ethical considerations:
Informed consent:
Confidentiality:
Data protection:
Conflicts of interest:
Proposed publications:

11.2.12 STEP (12): PRODUCE A TIMETABLE AND CONSIDER POTENTIAL PROBLEMS THAT MAY OCCUR

Chapter 1 of this book provides a detailed timetable under (STEP 10) of the exampled research proposal, and a revisit could be useful. Within any research proposal, it is important to outline to the examiner or funding body the steps embedded within an achievable timeframe. This may be presented in a variety of way (e.g. *bar chart, Gantt chart*, or *table*). Reflect upon the 16-STEP model and consider at what point you intend to complete each task (e.g. *complete the literature review, recruitment, data collection,* and *data analysis*). An example empty box is now presented into which you can enter these details.

STEP (12): Produce a timetable and consider potential problems that may occur

The duration of the proposed project will be (e.g. 36-months) and in accordance with the following timetable. Tweak this timetable to match your own research proposal, and place X's in the boxes for the months each activity will take place in (see STEP 12, Chapter 1).

*Q = quarter of a year (3-month period) Place the marker in the time point for expected delivery, e.g.

Gantt Chart Project PAL	Project Year 1 1/1/24 – 31/12/25 1–12 months					Project Year 2 1/1/25 – 31/12/26 13–24 months				Project Year 3 1/1/26 – 33/12/27 25–36 months		
Preparation (P) for Named Project	Q1	Q2	Q3	Q4	Q5	Q6	Q7	Q8	Q9	Q10	Q11	Q12
P.1: Research Fellow-advertising and recruitment												
P2: Ethics submission/approval												
P3: Meet with partner institutions												
P4: Set up steering group (SG)												
P6: Develop optimal recruitment strategy												
Study (S) process	Q1	Q2	Q3	Q4	Q5	Q6	Q7	Q8	Q9	Q10	Q11	Q12
S.1: Full research team meeting (incl co-applicants, collaborators and research fellow)												
S.2: Steering group (SG) meetings												
S.3: Literature review-update												
S.4: Develop study protocol												
S.5: Data collection –qualitative												
S.6: Data entry and transcription												
S.7: Data analyses												
S.8: Write up report/paper(s)												
S.9: Annual report to funder												
Final acts	Q1	Q2	Q3	Q4	Q5	Q6	Q7	Q8	Q9	Q10	Q11	Q12
F.1: Dissemination to stakeholders – Conferences												
F.2: Finished report to funders												

11.2.13 STEP (13): ESTIMATE RESOURCES THAT MAY BE REQUIRED

Chapter 1 of this book provides a detailed costing sheet under (STEP 13) of the exampled research proposal, with a revisit possibly of value. Within any research proposal, it is important to outline with accuracy what the expected costs of your study will be. These costings may be presented in a variety of way (e.g. Gantt chart or table). An example box is now presented for you to enter costing details.

STEP (13): Estimate resources that may be required

	Year 1	Year 2	Year 3	*TOTAL*
Personal Support of Applicants				
Named person (e.g. 1 day a week)	State amount (330 hours)	State amount (330 hours)	State amount (330 hours)	State amount (990 hours)
Named person (e.g. 1 hour a week)	State amount (52 hours)	State amount (52 hours)	State amount (52 hours)	State amount (156 hours)
Named person (e.g. 1 hour a week)	State amount (52 hours)	State amount (52 hours)	State amount (52 hours)	State amount (52 hours)
NB: Add increments on salaries per year				
Research Assistance Grade: 7 (e.g. Full time (FT)	State amount (FT)	State amount (FT)	State amount (FT)	State amount (FT)
NB: add increments on salaries per year				
Consumables • Print costs x e.g. 800 etc.	State amount	0	0	Stated amount
Patient public involvement (PPI) e.g. (*n*=?) service users e.g. 2 steering groups a year • Venue • Refreshments and lunch • Thank you voucher • Travel costs • Stationary	State amount(s)	State amount(s)	State amount(s)	State amount(s)
Travel and subsistence home University–maternity unit– participants home	State amount	State amount	State amount	State amount
Travel and subsistence To international conferences			State amount	State amount
Payment to partner university e.g. named statistician)	State amount	State amount	State amount	State amount
Contribution to maternity unit • Lighting • Toilets • Water • Heat	State amount(s)	State amount(s)	State amount(s)	State amount(s)
Equipment e.g. Monitors X 6	State amount	0	0	State amount
Estates charge	State amount	State amount	State amount	State amount
Indirect costs	State amount	State amount	State amount	State amount
TOTAL COSTS ESIMATED RECOVERY (80%)				State amount State amount

11.2.14 STEP (14): DETAIL A PUBLIC ENGAGEMENT PLAN

Public engagement is the practice of asking members of the public to review the research proposal to secure their ongoing comment throughout development and delivery of a research study. Engaging members of the public serves to improve quality, value, and impact of the proposed project. Ordinarily, a report should be submitted as part of the research proposal. The process involves, gathering 3–6 relevant members of the public and asking them: (i) If the study is worthwhile undertaking, (ii) What they think of the proposed participant activities, and (iii) If they themselves would in fact want to participate in such a study. You should also indicate ways in which the public will be actively involved throughout delivery of the proposed study. An example box is now presented for you to enter your public engagement plan.

STEP (14): Detail a public engagement plan

(1) Public perceptions of the importance of the proposed study:

(2) Public acceptance of activities involved in taking part in the study:

(3) Personal motivation to participate in study and what would prevent interest:

(4) Members of the public will be involved in:
- Design of the study. YES / NO
- Management of the research (e.g. steering group (SG). YES / NO
- Developing Participant Information Sheets (PIS). YES / NO
- Undertaking the project and/or analyzing the data. YES / NO
- Contributing to reporting or writing of the study report. YES / NO
- Dissemination of research findings. YES / NO

(5) Details of user group(s):

(Group 1) User group (e.g. will consist of 3 women from . . . etc.):
(1) Name, place of work, and email
(2) Name, place of work, and email
(3) Name, place of work, and email

(Group 2) Expert group (e.g. will *consist* of 2 midwives, 1 physiotherapist from . . . etc.):
(4) Name, place of work, and email
(5) Name, place of work, and email
(6) Name, place of work, and email

The above e.g. 6 people have agreed to be part of the *steering group* (SG).

11.2.15 STEP (15): APPEND A REFERENCE LIST

A reference list is an inventory of the studies and reports that have been cited in the research proposal. This list will inform the reader of the location and source of cited works, along with everything paraphrased or quoted within the research proposal. The recommended referencing system should be used (e.g. Harvard). The reference list should be presented in alphabetical order and be consistent and accurate, all of which will improve face validity of the research proposal. An example box is now presented for you to enter the references that underpin your research proposal.

STEP (15): Append a reference list
References:

Author(s) Surname, Initials. (Publication Year). Article title, Journal name. Volume (issue), Pages. Doi or Available at and date accessed.

11.2.16 STEP (16): APPEND RELEVANT ADDITIONAL MATERIAL

Appendix CV's, questionnaires, interview schedules, diagrams of equipment and/or any relevant information that will aid readers' understanding of the intended project. Remember to reference each appendix in text (e.g. see Appendix 1), and provide a contents list at the front of collated appendixes, which should be sequenced in order at the back of the research proposal.

Please note, at the end of a well-designed research proposal there will be a statement of intention to evaluate the success and impact of the research study post implementation. You will also be asked to sign, name, and date the final version that you submit.

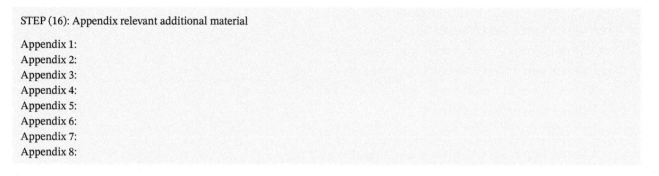

STEP (16): Appendix relevant additional material

Appendix 1:
Appendix 2:
Appendix 3:
Appendix 4:
Appendix 5:
Appendix 6:
Appendix 7:
Appendix 8:

11.3 BOOK CONCLUSION

Research Recipes for Midwives has endeavoured to walk the up-and-coming midwifery researcher through the 16-STEPS involved in writing a *research proposal*. From a well-written research proposal, the researcher(s), supervisor(s), and clinical midwifery staff can claim common understanding of what is required to make the study run smoothly within the projected timeframe. Per se, the final research proposal becomes the recipe from which responsibilities are discussed and tasks allocated. Once the 16-STEPS of your research proposal have been populated, the agreed and polished version should be submitted to the ethics committee, grant funding body, or as the prescribed modular assessment. I do hope that you have found this book a helpful chef when writing your recipe. I also wish you the best of luck with all your research endeavours.

References

Ahbel-Rappe, S. (2011). *Socrates: A Guide for the Perplexed*. London (UK): Bloomsbury Publishing.

Akyıldız, D., Çoban, A., Gör Uslu, F., and Taşpınar, A. (2021). Effects of obstetric interventions during labor on birth process and newborn health. *Florence Nightingale Journal of Nursing* 29 (1): 9–21. https://doi.org/10.5152/FNJN.2021.19093.

Aldiabat, K. and Navenec, C.L. (2011). Philosophical roots of classical grounded theory: its foundations in symbolic interactionism. *The Qualitative Report* 16: 1063–1080.

Allen, D.S. (2012). *Why Plato Wrote Blackwell-Bristol Lectures on Greece, Rome and the Classical Tradition*. New Jersey (US): Wiley-Blackwell.

Aluwihare-Samaranayake, D. (2012). Ethics in qualitative research: a view of the participants' and researchers' world from a critical standpoint. *International Journal of Qualitative Methods* 64–81. https://doi.org/10.1177/160940691201100208.

American College of Obstetricians and Gynaecologists (ACOG) (2021). The APGAR score. https://www.acog.org/en/clinical/clinical-guidance/committee-opinion/articles/2015/10/the-apgar-score

Apgar, V. (1953). A proposal for a new method of evaluation of the newborn infant. *Current Researches in Anesthesia & Analgesia* 32 (4): 260–267.

Aravind, M. and Chung, K.C. (2010). Evidence-based medicine and hospital reform: tracing origins back to Florence Nightingale. *Plastic and Reconstructive Surgery* 125 (1): 403–409. https://doi.org/10.1097/PRS.0b13e3181c2bb89.

Arksey, H. and O'Malley, L. (2005). Scoping studies: towards a methodological framework. *International Journal of Social Research Methodology* 8 (1): 19–32. https://doi.org/10.1080/1364557032000119616.

Ayala, R.A. and Koch, T.F. (2019). The image of ethnography – making sense of the social through images: a structured method. *International Journal of Qualitative Methods* 18: https://doi.org/10.1177/1609406919843014.

Baranowska, B., Pawlicka, P., Kiersnowska, I. et al. (2021). Woman's needs and satisfaction regarding the communication with doctors and midwives during labour, delivery and early postpartum. *Healthcare 9*: 382. https://doi.org/10.3390/healthcare9040382.

Bargaje, C. (2011). Good documentation practice in clinical research. *Perspectives in Clinical Research* 2 (2): 59–63. https://doi.org/10.4103/2229-3485.80368.

Bartl, M., Kannan, V.K., and Stockinger, H. (2016). A review and analysis of literature on netnography research. *International Journal of Technology Marketing* 11 (2): 165–196.

Bauchner, H. and Vinci, R. (2001). What have we learnt from the Alder Hey affair? That monitoring physicians' performance is necessary to ensure good practice. *British Medical Journal* 322 (7282): 309–310. https://doi.org/10.1136/bmj.322.7282.309.

Bedwell, C., Levin, K., Pett, C., and Lavender, T. (2017). A realist review of the partograph: when and how does it work for labour monitoring? *BMC Pregnancy and Childbirth* 17: 31. https://doi.org/10.1186/s12884-016-1213-4.

Bee, P., Brooks, H., and Callaghan, P. (2018). *A Research Handbook for Patient and Public Involvement Researchers*. UK: Manchester University Press.

Berndt, A.E. (2020). Sampling methods. *Journal of Human Lactation* 36 (2): 224–226. https://doi.org/10.1177/0890334420906850.

Birks, M. and Mills, J. (2023). *Grounded Theory: A Practical Guide*, 3e. Thousand Oaks, California (US): SAGE Publications Ltd.

Braun, V. and Clarke, V. (2006). Using thematic analysis in psychology. *Qualitative Research in Psychology* 3 (2): 77–101. https://doi.org/10.1191/1478088706qp063oa.

Briggs, D.J.S., Gololoboy, I., and Aimar, V. (2015). Ethnographic research among drinking youth cultures: reflections from observing participants. *Journal of Folklore* 61: 157–176. https://doi.org/10.7592/FEJF2015.61.youth_culture.

Buran, G. and Aksu, H. (2022). Effect of hypnobirthing training on fear, pain, satisfaction related to birth, and birth outcomes: a Randomized Controlled Trial. *Clinical Nursing Research* 31 (5): 918–930. https://doi.org/10.1177/10547738211073394.

Burns, N. and Grove, S.K. (2001). *The Practice of Nursing Research: Conduct, Critique and Utilization*, 4e. WB Saunders: Philadelphia.

Burns, E., Fenwick, J., Schmied, V., and Sheehan, A. (2012). Reflexivity in midwifery research: the insider/outsider debate. *Midwifery* 28 (1): 52–60. https://doi.org/10.1016/j.midw.2010.10.018.

Burrows, T. (2019). *The Nuremberg Trials: Volume 1: Bringing the leaders of nazi Germany to justice*. London (UK): Arcturus, Bermondsey.

Charmaz, K. (2014). *Constructing Grounded Theory*, 2e. London (UK): Sage publications.

Charmaz, K. (2017). The power of constructivist grounded theory for critical inquiry. *Qualitative Inquiry* 23 (1): 34–45. https://doi.org/10.1177/1077800416657105.

Clark, L.A. and Watson, D. (1995). Constructing validity: basic issues in objective scale development. *Psychological Assessment* 7 (3): 309–319.

Clarke, E. (2015). *Law and Ethics Midwifery*. London (UK): Routledge https://doi.org/10.4324/9781315691053.

Cloitre, M., Shevlin, M., Brewin, C.R. et al. (2018). The International Trauma Questionnaire: development of a self-report measure of ICD-11 PTSD and Complex PTSD. *Acta Psychiatrica Scandinavica* https://doi.org/10.1111/acps.12956.

Cox, J.L., Holden, J.M., and Sagovsky, R. (1987). Detection of postnatal depression: development of the 10-item Edinburgh Postnatal Depression Scale. *British Journal of Psychiatry* 150: 782–786.

Creswell, J.W. (2013). *Qualitative Inquiry and Research Design choosing among five approaches*, 3e. Thousand Oaks, California (US): Sage Publications.

Critical Appraisal Skills Programme (CASP) (2018). CASP qualitative checklist. https://casp-uk.net/casp-tools-checklists/

Cronbach, L.J. (1951). Coefficient alpha and the internal structure of tests. *Psychometrika* 16 (3): 297–334.

Crown. https://assets.publishing.service.gov.uk/government/uploads/system/uploads/attachment_data/file/1064302/Final-Ockenden-Report-web-accessible.pdf

Cunen, N.B., Jomeen, J., Poat, A., and Xuereb, R.B. (2022). 'A small person that we made'- Parental conceptualisation of the unborn child: a constructivist grounded theory. *Midwifery* 104: 103198. https://doi.org/10.1016/j.midw.2021.103198.

Czech, H., Druml, C., and Weindling, P. (2018). Medical ethics in the 70 years after the Nuremberg Code, 1947 to the present. *Wiener Klinische Wochenschrift* 130 (Suppl 3): 159–253. https://doi.org/10.1007/s00508-018-1343-y.

Daniels, E., Arden-Close, E., and Mayers, A. (2020). Be quiet and man up: a qualitative questionnaire study into fathers who witnessed their artner's birth trauma. *BMC Pregnancy and Childbirth* 20: 236. https://doi.org/10.1186/s12884-020-02902-2.

Data Protection Act (DPA) (2018). Legislation.gov.uk. https://www.legislation.gov.uk/ukpga/2018/12/contents/enacted

Denzin, N.K. (2012). Triangulation 2.0. *Journal of Mixed Methods Research* 6 (2): 80–88. https://doi.org/10.1177/1558689812437186.

Descartes, R., (author), Moriarty, M (translator) (2008). *Meditations on First Philosophy with Selections from the Objections and Replies*. (UK): Oxford World Classics (Oxford University Press).

Dewan, M. (2018). Understanding ethnography: an 'exotic' ethnographer's perspective. In: *Asian Qualitative Research in Tourism. Perspectives on Asian Tourism* (ed. P. Mura and C. Khoo-Lattimore). Singapore: Springer https://doi.org/10.1007/978-981-10-7491-2_10.

Divall, B. and Spiby, H. (2019). Online forums for data collection: ethical challenges from a study exploring women's views of birth plans. *Nurse Researcher* 27: 26–30. https://doi.org/10.7748/nr.2019.e1632.

Doran, G.T. (1981). There's a S.M.A.R.T. way to write management's goals and objectives. *Management Review* 70 (11): 35–36.

Dykes, F. and Flacking, R. (ed.) (2016). *Ethnographic Research in Maternal and Child Health*. Milton Park, Abingdon, Oxon (UK): Routledge.

Ellis, P. (2016). *Understanding Research for Nursing Students*, 3e. London (UK): Sage Publications.

English, W., Gott, M., and Robinson, J. (2022). Being reflexive in research and clinical practice: a practical example. *Nurse Researcher* 30 (2): 30–35. https://doi.org/10.7748/nr.2022.e1833.

European University Institute (EUI) (2022). Guide on good data protection practice in research. https://www.eui.eu/documents/servicesadmin/deanofstudies/researchethics/guide-data-protection-research.pdf

Flacking, R. and Dykes, F. (2013). 'Being in a womb' or 'playing musical chairs': the impact of place and space on infant feeding in NICUs. *BMC Pregnancy and Childbirth* 23 (13): 179. https://doi.org/10.1186/1471-2393-13-179.

Garra, G., Singer, A.J., Taira, B.R. et al. (2010). Validation of the Wong-Baker FACES pain rating scale in pediatric emergency department patients. *Academic Emergency Medicine* 17 (1): 50–54. https://doi.org/10.1111/j.1553-2712.2009.00620.x.

Gizzo, S., Di Gangi, S., Noventa, M. et al. (2014). Women's choice of positions during labour: return to the past or a modern way to give birth? A cohort study in Italy. *Biomed Research International* 2014: 638093. https://doi.org/10.1155/2014/638093.

Glaser, S. (1967). *The Discovery of Grounded Theory Strategies for Qualitative Research*. Chicago (US): Aldine Publishing Company.

Glaser, B. (1992). *Basics of Grounded Theory Analysis*. Mill Valley, California (US): Sociology Press.

Glaser, B.G. (2002). Conceptualization: on theory and theorizing using grounded theory. *International Journal of Qualitative Methods* 1 (2): 23–38. https://doi.org/10.1177/160940690200100203.

Gov.UK (2022). Data protection. https://www.gov.uk/data-protection

Gov.UK Service Manual (2022). Getting informed consent for user research. https://www.gov.uk/service-manual/user-research/getting-users-consent-for-research

Groves, R.M., Fowler, F.J., Couper, M.P. et al. (2009). *Survey methodology*, 2e. New Jersey (US): Wiley.

Hall, P.M. (2016). Symbolic interaction. In: *Blackwell Encyclopedia of Sociology. EncyclopediaSociology*. https://doi.org/10.1002/9781405165518.wbeoss310.pub2.

Heidegger, M. (2005). *Introduction to Phenomenological Research*. Bloomington, Indiana (US): Indiana University Press.

Heidegger, M. (2010). *Basic Writings: Martin Heidegger*. Abingdon (UK): Routledge Classics.

Hewitt, L., Dadich, A., Hartz, D.L. et al. (2022). Midwife-centred management: a qualitative study of midwifery group practice management and leadership in Australia. *BMC Health Services Research* 22: 1203. https://doi.org/10.1186/s12913-022-08532-y.

Hollins Martin, C.J. and Fleming, V. (2010). A 15-step model for writing a research proposal. *British Journal of Midwifery* 18 (12): 791–798.

Hollins Martin, C.J. and Reid, K. (2022). A scoping review of therapies used to treat psychological trauma post perinatal bereavement. *Journal of Reproductive and Infant Psychology* 6: 1–17. https://doi.org/10.1080/02646838.2021.2021477.

Hollins Martin, C.J., Kenney, L., Pratt, T., and Granat, M.H. (2015). The development and validation of an activity monitoring system for use in measurement of posture of childbearing women during first stage of labour. *Journal of Midwifery and Women's Health* 60 (2): 182–186. https://doi.org/10.1111/jmwh.12230.

Hollins Martin, C.J., Anderson, L., and Martin, C. (2019). A scoping review to determine themes that represent perceptions of self as mother ('ideal mother' vs 'real mother'). *Journal of Reproductive and Infant Psychology* 37 (3): 224–241. https://doi.org/10.1080/02646838.2018.1556786.

Hollins Martin, C.J., Patterson, J., Paterson, C. et al. (2021). ICD-11 Complex Post Traumatic Stress Disorder (CPTSD) in parents with perinatal bereavement: implications for treatment and care. *Midwifery* 96 (2021): 102947. https://doi.org/10.1016/j.midw.2021.102947.

Hollins-Martin, C.J. and Martin, C. (2014). Development and psychometric properties of the Birth Satisfaction Scale-Revised (BSS-R). *Midwifery* 30: 610–619. https://doi.org/10.1016/j.midw.2013.10.006.

Husserl, E. (1997). *Psychological and Transcendental Phenomenology and the Confrontation with Heidegger (1927–1931)*. Dordrecht, Netherlands: Kluwer.

IBM Corp. (2020). IBM SPSS Statistics for Windows (Version 27.0) [Computer software]. IBM Corp.

Independent Maternity Review (2022). *Ockenden report: final: findings, conclusions, and essential actions from the independent review of maternity services at the Shrewsbury and Telford Hospital NHS Trust* (HC 1219).

Inskip, H., Crozier, S., Baird, J. et al. (2021). Measured weight in early pregnancy is a valid method for estimating pre-pregnancy weight. *Journal of Developmental Origins of Health and Disease* 12: 561–569. https://doi.org/10.1017/S2040174420000926.

Irwing, P., Booth, T., and Hughes, D.J. (ed.) (2018). *The Wiley Handbook of Psychometric Testing: A Multidisciplinary Reference on Survey, Scale and Test Development*. Wiley Blackwell https://doi.org/10.1002/9781118489772.

Ismaila, Y., Bayes, S., and Geraghty, S. (2021). Midwives' strategies for coping with barriers to providing quality maternal and neonatal care: a Glaserian grounded theory study. *BMC Health Services Research* 21: 1190. https://doi.org/10.1186/s12913-021-07049-0.

de Jong, M., Kamsteeg, F., and Ybema, S. (2013). Ethnographic strategies for making the familiar strange: struggling with 'distance' and 'immersion' among Moroccan-Dutch students. *Journal of Business Anthropology* 2 (2): https://doi.org/10.22439/jba.v2i2.4157.

Kadam, P. and Bhalerao, S. (2010). Sample size calculation. *International Journal of Ayurveda Research* 1 (1): 55–57. https://doi.org/10.4103/0974-7788.59946.

Keck, J., Gerkensmeyer, J., Joyce, B., and Schade, J. (1996). Reliability and validity of the FACES and Word Descriptor scales to measure procedural pain. *Journal of Pediatric Nursing* 11 (6): 368–374. https://doi.org/10.1016/S0882-5963(96)80081-9.

Kingdon, C. (2013). Reflexivity: not just a qualitative methodological research tool. *British Journal of Midwifery* 13 (10): 622–627. https://doi.org/10.12968/bjom.2005.13.10.19835.

Kiserud, T., Piaggio, G., Carroli, G. et al. (2017). The World Health Organisation Fetal Growth Charts: a multinational longitudinal study of ultrasound biometric measurements and estimated fetal weight. *PLoS Medicine* e1003526. https://doi.org/10.1371/journal.pmed.1002220.

Kline, P. (2000). *A Psychometrics Primer*. London (UK): Free Association Books.

Kongsved, S.M., Basnov, M., Holm-Christensen, K., and Hjollund, N.H. (2007). Response rate and completeness of questionnaires: a randomized study of Internet versus paper-and-pencil versions. *Journal of Medical Internet Research* 9, 3: e25. https://doi.org/10.2196/jmir.9.3.e25.

Kozinets, R.V. (2019). *Netnography: The Essential Guide to Qualitative Social Media Research*. North Tyneside (UK): Sage.

Krejcie, R.V. and Morgan, D.W. (1970). Determining sample size for research activities. *Educational and Psychological Measurement* 30: 607–610.

Larkin, M., Watts, S., and Clifton, E. (2006). Giving voice and making sense in Interpretative Phenomenological Analysis. *Qualitative Research in Psychology* 3 (2): 102–120. https://doi.org/10.1191/1478088706qp062oa.

Lawrence, A., Lewis, L., Hofmeyr, G.J. et al. (2009). Maternal positions and mobility during first stage labour. *Cochrane Database of Systematic Reviews* (2) Issue 2. Art. No. CD003934. https://doi.org/10.1002/14651858.CD003934.pub2.

Liu, S.Y., Lu, Y.Y., Gau, M.L. et al. (2020). Psychometric testing of the support and control in birth scale. *BMC Pregnancy and Childbirth* 20: 293. https://doi.org/10.1186/s12884-020-02888-x. https://cpb-eu-w2.wpmucdn.com/blogs.city.ac.uk/dist/b/1267/files/2015/06/SCIB-English-version-1rdhrcv.pdf.

LoBiondo-Wood, H. and Haber, J. (2016). *Nursing Research: Methods and Critical Appraisal for Evidence-Based Practice*, 9e. Amsterdam, Netherlands: Elsevier.

Lupton, D. (ed.) (1999). *Risk and Sociocultural Theory: New Directions and Perspectives*. Cambridge University Press https://doi.org/10.1017/CBO9780511520778.

Martin, C.R. and Savage-McGlynn, E. (2013). A 'good practice' guide for the reporting of design and analysis for psychometric evaluation. *Journal of Reproductive and Infant Psychology* 31: 449–455.

Mehretie Adinew, Y., Kelly, J., Marshall, A., and Hall, H. (2021). "I would have stayed home if I could manage it alone": a case study of Ethiopian mother abandoned by care providers during facility-based childbirth. *International Journal of Women's Health* 24 (13): 501–507. https://doi.org/10.2147/IJWH.S302208.

Milgram, S. (1963). Behavioral study of obedience. *Journal of Abnormal and Social Psychology* 67: 371–378.

Milgram, S. (1974). *Obedience to Authority*. London (UK): Tavistock Publications.

Minooee, S., Simbar, M., Sheikhan, Z., and Alavi Majd, H. (2018). Audit of intrapartum care based on the national guideline for midwifery and birth services. *Evaluation & the Health Professions* 41 (3): 415–429. https://doi.org/10.1177/0163278718778095.

Mirzaee, F. and Dehghan, M. (2020). A model of trust within the mother-midwife relationship: a grounded theory. *Obstetrics and Gynecology International* 2020: Article ID 9185313 https://doi.org/10.1155/2020/9185313.

Moher, D., Liberati, A., Tetzlaff, J., and Altman, D.G. (2009). Preferred reporting items for systematic reviews and meta-analyses: the PRISMA statement (Reprinted from Annals of Internal Medicine). *Physical Therapy* 89 (9): 873–880. https://doi.org/10.1093/ptj/89.9.873.

Monaghan, T.F., Agudelo, C.W., Rahman, S.N. et al. (2021). Blinding in clinical trials: seeing the big picture. *Medicina (Kaunas, Lithuania)* 57 (7): 647. https://doi.org/10.3390/medicina57070647.

Nagael, J. (2014). *Knowledge: A Very Short Introduction (Very Short Introductions)*. (UK): Oxford University Press.

Nakić Radoš, S., Martinić, L., Matijaš, M. et al. (2021). The relationship between birth satisfaction, posttraumatic stress disorder and post-natal depression symptoms in Croatian women. *Stress and Health* 2021: 1–9. https://doi.org/10.1002/smi.3112.

National Institute for Health and Care Research (NIHR) (2022). Involve patients. https://www.nihr.ac.uk/health-and-care-professionals/engagement-and-participation-in-research/involve-patients.htm

Nishimwe, A., Conco, D.N., Nyssen, M. et al. (2022). A mixed-method study exploring experiences, perceptions, and acceptability of using a safe delivery mHealth application in two district hospitals in Rwanda. *BMC Nursing* 21: 176. https://doi.org/10.1186/s12912-022-00951-w.

NMPA Project Team. National Maternity and Perinatal Audit: Clinical Report (2022). *Based on Births in NHS Maternity Services in England and Wales Between 1 April 2018 and 31 March 2019*. London (UK): RCOG.

Norris, G., Hollins Martin, C.J., and Dickson, A. (2020). An exploratory Interpretative Phenomenological Analysis (IPA) of childbearing women's perceptions of risk associated with having a high Body Mass Index (BMI). *Midwifery* 89 (2020): 102789. https://doi.org/10.1016/j.midw.2020.102789.

Nursing and Midwifery Council (NMC) (2015). The Code: professional standards of practice and behaviour for nurses, midwives, and nursing associates: prioritise people, practise effectively, preserve safety, promote professionalism and trust. https://www.nmc.org.uk/standards/code/read-the-code-online/#fifth

NVivo 1.0 (2020). Windows & Mac. https://www.qsrinternational.com/nvivo-qualitative-data-analysis-software/try-nvivo

O'Reilly, K. (2012). *Ethnographic Methods*, 2e. Abingdon (UK): Routledge.

O'Brien, D., Butler, M.M., and Casey, M. (2021). The importance of nurturing trusting relationships to embed shared decision-making during pregnancy and childbirth. *Midwifery* 98: 102987. https://doi.org/10.1016/j.midw.2021.102987.

Paltridge, B. (2021). *Discourse Analysis: An Introduction*. University of Easy Anglia (UK): Bloomsbury Discourse.

Patterson, J., Hollins Martin, C.J., and Karatzias, T. (2019). PTSD post-childbirth: a systematic review of women's and midwives' subjective experiences of care provider interaction. *Journal of Reproductive and Infant Psychology* 37 (1): 56–83. https://doi.org/10.1080/02646838.2018.15042.

Petrova, E., Dewing, J., and Camilleri, M. (2016). Confidentiality in participatory research: challenges from one study. *Nursing Ethics* 23 (4): 442–454. https://doi.org/10.1177/0969733014564909.

Pieper, I.J. and Thomson, C.J. (2014). The value of respect in human research ethics: a conceptual analysis and a practical guide. *Monash Bioethics Review* 32 (3-4): 232–253. https://doi.org/10.1007/s40592-014-0016-5.

PRISMA (2020). Creating a PRISMA flow diagram. https://guides.lib.unc.edu/prisma

Ralph, N., Birks, M., and Chapman, Y. (2015). The methodological dynamism of grounded theory. *International Journal of Qualitative Methods* 14 (4): https://doi.org/10.1177/1609406915611576.

Rees, C. (2011). *Introduction to Research for Midwives*, 3e. London (UK): Churchill Livingston.

Reid, K., Flowers, P., and Larkin, M. (2005). Exploring lived experience: an introduction to Interpretative Phenomenological Analysis. *The Psychologist* 18 (1): 20–23.

Richardson, L. (2000). Evaluating ethnography. *Qualitative Inquiry* 6 (2): 253–255. https://doi.org/10.1177/107780040000600207.

Rishard, M., Fahmy, F.F., Senanayake, H. et al. (2021). Correlation among experience of person-centered maternity care, provision of care and women's satisfaction: cross sectional study in Colombo, Sri Lanka. *PLoS One* 16 (4): e0249265. https://doi.org/10.1371/journal.pone.0249265.

Romain, P.L. (2015). Conflicts of interest in research: looking out for number one means keeping the primary interest front and center. *Current Reviews in Musculoskeletal Medicine* 8 (2): 122–127. https://doi.org/10.1007/s12178-015-9270-2.

Romero-Gonzalez, B., Peralta-Ramirez, M.I., Caparros-Gonzalez, R.A. et al. (2019). Spanish validation and factor structure of the Birth Satisfaction Scale-Revised (BSS-R). *Midwifery* 70: 31–37. https://doi.org/10.1016/j.midw.2018.12.009.

Rosenberg, M. (1965). *Society and the Adolescent Self-Image*. Princeton, NJ (US): Princeton University Press https://fetzer.org/sites/default/files/images/stories/pdf/selfmeasures/Self_Measures_for_Self-Esteem_ROSENBERG_SELF-ESTEEM.pdf.

Rymer, R. (1994). *Genie A Scientific Tragedy*. New York (US): Harper Paperbacks.

Schreier, M. (2012). *Qualitative Content Analysis in Practice (Jacobs University Bremen)*. Thousand Oaks, California (US): SAGE Publications Ltd.

Scott, I. and Mazhindu, D. (2014). *Statistics for Healthcare Professionals: An Introduction*, 2e. Sage Publications.

Sharmer, L. and Navar, K. (2020). *Dictionary of Terms in Research Methodology*. New Deli, India: The Readers Paradise.

Shih, W.J. and Aisner, J. (2021). *Statistical design, monitoring, and analysis of clinical trials: principles and methods*, Chapman and Hall/CRC Biostatistics Series. Abingdon (UK): Routledge Taylor and Francis Group.

Skvirsky, V., Taubman-Ben-Ari, O., Hollins Martin, C.J., and Martin, C.R. (2019). Validation of the Hebrew Birth Satisfaction Scale - Revised (BSS-R) and its relationship to perceived traumatic labour. *Journal of Reproductive and Infant Psychology* 1–7: https://doi.org/10.1080/02646838.2019.1600666.

Smith, J., Flowers, P., and Larkin, M. (2009). *Interpretative Phoneomological Analysis: Theory, Method and Research*. London (UK): SAGE Publications.

Souček, I. and Karásek, M. (2022). The wedding with a stolen goddess: the ethnography of a cult in rural Tamil Nadu. *Journal of Religion and Health* 61 (3): 2500–2513. https://doi.org/10.1007/s10943-020-01010-x.

Speziale, H.S., Streubert, H.J., and Carpenter, D.R. (2011). *Qualitative Research in Nursing: Advancing the Humanistic Imperative*. Philadelphia (US): Lippincott Williams & Wilkins.

Spielberger, C.D. (1983). *Manual for the State-Trait Inventory STAI (Form Y)*. Palo Alto, California (US): Mind Garden.

Stålberg, V., Krevers, B., Lingetun, L. et al. (2022). Study protocol for a modified antenatal care program for pregnant women with a low risk for adverse outcomes: a stepped wedge cluster non-inferiority randomized trial. *BMC Pregnancy and Childbirth* 22: 299. https://doi.org/10.1186/s12884-022-04406-7.

Strauss, A. and Corbin, J.M. (1997). *Grounded Theory in Practice*. London (UK): Sage.

Tassone, B. (2017). The relevance of Husserl's phenomenological exploration of interiority to contemporary epistemology. *Palgrave Communications* 3: 17066. https://doi.org/10.1057/palcomms.2017.66.

Tawfik, G.M., Dila, K.A.S., Mohamed, M.Y.F. et al. (2019). A step by step guide for conducting a systematic review and meta-analysis with simulation data. *Tropical Medicine and Health* 47: 46. https://doi.org/10.1186/s41182-019-0165-6.

Temple University Libraries (2022). https://guides.temple.edu/c.php?g=78618&p=4178713

Vignato, J., Inman, M., Patsais, M., and Conley, V. (2022). Computer-assisted qualitative data analysis software, phenomenology, and Colaizzi's method. *Western Journal of Nursing Research* 44 (12): 1117–1123. https://doi.org/10.1177/01939459211030335.

Wager, E. and Kleinert, S. (2014). Responsible research publication: international standards for authors. *Pril (Makedon Akad Nauk Umet Odd Med Nauki)* 35 (3): 29–33.

Wanamaker, A.M. (2018). Tuskegee and the health of black men. *The Quarterly Journal of Economics* 133 (1): 407–455. https://doi.org/10.1093/qje/qjx029.

Wong-Baker FACES Foundation (2021). Wong-Baker FACES Pain rating scale. https://wongbakerfaces.org/

World Health Organisation (WHO) (1994). *Preventing Prolonged Labour: A Practical Guide: The Partograph. Part 1. Principles and Strategy*. Geneva: WHO.

World Health Organisation (WHO) (2011). Standards and operational guidance for ethics review of health-related research with human participants. https://www.who.int/publications/i/item/9789241502948

World Health Organisation (WHO) (2021). Maternal and perinatal health. www.who.int.

World Health Organization (WHO) (2018). The ICD-11 for mortality and morbidity statistics. https://icd.who.int/browse11/l-m/e.

World Medical Association (2013). World Medical Association Declaration of Helsinki: ethical principles for medical research involving human subjects. *JAMA* 310 (20): 2191–2194. https://doi.org/10.1001/jama.2013.281053.

Ybema, S.B. and Kamsteeg, F.H. (2009). Making the familiar strange: a case for disengaged ethnography. In: *Organizational Ethnography: Studying the Complexities of Everyday Life* (ed. S. Ybema, D. Yanow, H. Wels, and F. Kamsteeg). London (UK): Sage.

Zahavi, D. (2003). *Husserl's Phenomenology*. Stanford (US): Stanford University Press.

Zahavi, D. (2019). *Phenomenology: The Basics*, 1e. Routledge.

Zigmond, A.S. and Snaith, R.P. (1983). The hospital anxiety and depression scale. *Acta Psychiatrica Scandinavia* 67 (6): 361–370. https://doi.org/10.1111/j.1600-0447.1983.tb09716.x.

Index